Patient Education:

Issues, Principles, and Guidelines

Sally H. Rankin, R.N., M.S.N.
Assistant Professor
University of Southern California
Los Angeles, California

Karen L. Duffy, R.N., B.S.N.
Program Coordinator
Staff Education and Development
Durham County General Hospital
Durham, North Carolina

With a contribution from
Diane Shea Pravikoff, R.N., B.S.N.
Cardiac Rehabilitation Coordinator
Glendale Adventist Medical Center
Glendale, California

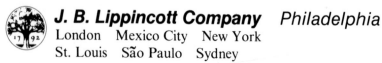
J. B. Lippincott Company   *Philadelphia*
London   Mexico City   New York
St. Louis   São Paulo   Sydney

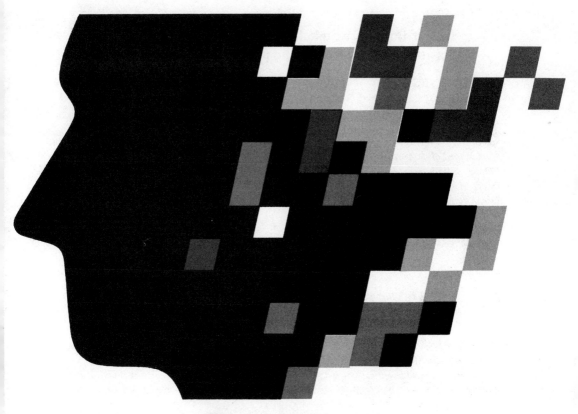

Patient
Education:
Issues,
Principles,
and Guidelines

To our families who helped us grow
sensitive to the needs of the people around us.

Sponsoring Editor: David T. Miller
Manuscript Editor: Barbara Farabaugh
Indexer: Julia B. Schwager
Designer: William Boehm with Earl Gerhart
Production Supervisor: J. Corey Gray
Production Coordinator: Edward Scirrotto
Compositor: McFarland Graphics and Design
Printer/Binder: R.R. Donnelley & Sons Company

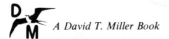 *A David T. Miller Book*

6   5   4

Library of Congress Cataloging in Publication Data

Rankin, Sally H.
  Patient education.

  Bibliography: p.
  Includes index.
  1. Patient education. 2. Nursing. I. Duffy, Karen L. II. Pravikoff,
Diane Shea. III. Title. [DNLM: 1. Patient education—Nursing texts.
WY 105 R211p]
RT90.R35 1983   610.73   82-22929
ISBN 0-397-54398-0

Foreword

The importance of health education in nursing practice is no longer debatable. The research of Lindeman and Van Aernam (Lindeman C: Symposium: Education of patients. Influencing recovery through preoperative teaching. Heart Lung 2:515–521, 1973; Lindeman C, Van Aernam AB: Research program for nurses. Hospitals 44:89+, 1970) has established the effectiveness of structured preoperative teaching in care of the surgical patient. Hall's work with the Duke University Distributive Nursing Project (Hall JE: Nursing as process. In Hall JE, Weaver BR (eds): Distributive Nursing Practice: A Systems Approach to Community Health, p. 173–191. Philadelphia, JB Lippincott, 1977) identified health teaching as an essential component of the nursing process and as one of the several nursing strategies that compose the power armamentarium used by the nursing practitioner to create change in clients and in the health-care system. Reynolds and Bingle, as a part of the Conduct and Utilization of Research in Nursing Project, under the direction of Horsley and Crane (Horsley JA, Crane J: Conduct and Utilization of Research in Nursing (CURN) Project. Project of the Michigan Nurses Association. New York, Grune and Stratton, 1982) at the University of Michigan, developed a nursing protocol that synthesizes the findings of relevant and meritorious research in preoperative teaching into a guide for nursing intervention in acute-care practice settings. These events, and many others, have established health education as a major intervention strategy in nursing practice.

The use of health education in nursing practice is widespread. Its applicability is easily seen in all clinical settings, with all patients and their families, by all practitioners of nursing representing all clinical specialties. What is less obvious is the necessity of providing for the acquisition of knowledge, the mastery of skills, the development of roles, and the recognition of values related to health teaching in nursing-education programs.

Educators teaching the nursing process have focused primarily on nursing assessment at the expense of other, equally essential, phases of the process. Courses in physical assessment, health assessment, and nursing assessment are highly visible in undergraduate and graduate nursing curricula and in continuing-education programs. Less often do nursing educators frame courses around what practitioners do to help patients and their families to change their lifeways in the direction of health. The time has come to focus on the strategies and tactics of nursing intervention with the same vigor that so successfully raised nurses' awareness of the importance of assessment in providing effective health care.

Patient Education: Issues, Principles, and Guidelines is a valuable resource for nursing practitioners and students. It focuses on health education as a major strategy of nursing intervention and presents a vast array of specific tactics for assisting patients and their families to live healthier, more functional lives. The authors draw from their own professional practices and the strengths of their personal experience in assisting their clients to acquire a sense of mastery over their environments and health problems. At the time this book was written, the senior author, Sally Rankin, was involved as a nursing educator in the development of a curriculum for undergraduate students based on Orem's self-care approach to nursing practice, in which health teaching is a major intervention strategy. Thus, the authors speak from knowledge and experience that have influenced their beliefs in the centrality of health education in nursing practice.

The underlying theme of the book is that therapeutic change through the creation of healthy lifeways helps people to enjoy life more abundantly, regardless of their health status or circumstances. By helping people to live functional lives, the authors and the practitioners who employ their approaches contribute to their clients' sense of competency, which is so essential to health. The nursing interventions presented are aimed toward preventing disease and disability, supporting lifeways that maintain health, and interrupting and replacing nontherapeutic patterns of living with more adaptive health behaviors.

The authors are realistic in the practical approaches they offer as solutions to problems encountered in practice settings. They have applied the nursing process to patient education through a pragmatic approach that will be helpful for nursing students and practitioners alike. The text maintains a strong family focus that recognizes that patients do not exist in isolation, but rather are members of family systems, which also require nursing assessment, intervention, and evaluation. The reader is given guidance in patient-care situations that cover the life span and cross the spectrum of human dysfunction, from chronic physical illness to psychiatric disorders and from the acute-care inpatient situation to health promotion in the community.

Although the authors are nurses and draw their examples from their own discipline, health-care providers from other disciplines also will find assistance for their health-education activities within this volume. Thus I commend this book to readers of all health professions in the belief that it will prove helpful as they endeavor to assist clients and their families to live healthier, more functional lives.

Joanne E. Hall, R.N., Ph.D.
Professor and Chairperson
Department of Family Nursing
Oregon Health Sciences University
Portland, Oregon

November 3, 1982

Preface

Threading his way through the tangled web of prescriptions and proscriptions for health and illness, the frustrated patient frequently turns to nurses for guidance and support. One of the more concrete means of providing this guidance has been patient education. Because we believe that this is one of the most important aspects of nursing, we have attempted to integrate sound principles into our own practice and into our teaching and supervision as nurse educators. Noting the concerns expressed by our colleagues in their attempts to implement patient education and the confusion of perplexed students who frequently do not know where to begin the process of patient education, we decided to compile *Patient Education: Issues, Principles, and Guidelines* to meet these different needs.

The *issues* chapters (2–5) evolved from our frustrations in attempting to provide innovative approaches to patient education. As we became more involved as providers of patient education, we found that we were confronted by major issues. We recognized these issues as decision-making, philosophical, political and power, economic, implementation, evaluation, and legal and ethical aspects. These issues can become major obstacles to both students and practitioners of nursing. It is hoped that these chapters will enlighten providers of patient education so that the needs of the patient may be better met. We believe that, by sensitizing the student nurse to issues she will confront in her own practice, we will enable her to be better prepared to manage the vagaries and vicissitudes of nursing in the difficult practice contexts in which she will find herself.

The *principles* chapters (6–9) combine the nursing process with patient education. This approach helps the student nurse to structure her work with patients and to plan her patient care. Throughout the four chapters in this section we use a case study and derive a nursing-care plan for a patient and her family. Our readers will notice throughout the book a strong propensity to consider the patient's entire family, not just the patient, as the client. We believe that the family should be assessed from a systems perspective and, therefore, that goals, interventions, and evaluations should include the entire family.

The *guidelines* chapters (10–12) answer questions that arise in many different patient-education contexts—inpatient, home, community, pediatric, psychiatric, geriatric, and terminally ill patient settings, to name a few. We offer some practical guidelines for developing new programs. Because there is an abundance of how-to-educate books aimed toward specific patient populations, we have avoided such an approach. The use of case studies and examples of our own successes is meant to help our readers to apply basic principles to their own practice settings and to evaluate their own situations.

In order to provide our student readers with a better understanding of their place on the health-care team, we have included an initial *overview* chapter (Chap. 1), which describes the participation of other health-care professionals in patient education. Although we believe that the nurse and physician are central to the management of patient education, we do not want our profession to become insular or lack cognizance of the contributions of other health-care workers.

We wish to extend our sincere thanks to the nurses, physicians, pharmacists, dietitians, social workers, and physical therapists who shared their thoughts on patient education with us. Although our interviews did not include dentists, we also want to acknowledge their active involvement in teaching patients and their contributions to preventive health education.

The evolution of this book has been a growth-producing experience for us. We have had to examine more deeply our own feelings about ourselves as nurses and educators and about how we relate to others, especially patients. Our belief is that patient education enhances the lives of people in health and illness by better empowering them to express themselves cognitively and emotionally and that it returns to them a greater measure of control over their own lives. The powerlessness of patienthood is perhaps the most devastating aspect of illness. Patient education can reduce the feelings of helplessness and enhance the patient's ability to be the chief decision maker in the management of his health and illness problems.

Without the enthusiasm and creativity of the students we have taught, or the probing questions, problems, and perseverance of our patients, this book would not have been possible. We would like to express our appreciation to the faculty, residents, staff, and patients at the Duke–Watts Family Medicine Center, where we were encouraged to attempt innovative programs. We wish also to thank our colleagues Cecily Betz, Mary McRee, Tom Gambill, Tom Wooters, Terry Monahan, and Godfrey Hochbaum for their ideas and suggestions. To Lois Heller and Sarah Haskell for their help in editing, and to Lois Marski, Betty Hilliard, and Vi Woorster, we gratefully acknowledge assistance in preparation of the manuscript.

Sally H. Rankin, R.N., B.S.N.
Karen L. Duffy, R.N., B.S.N.

Contents

Chapter 1
Overview of Patient Education

How Does Patient Education Begin?

It was a rainy Saturday. In an upstairs bedroom, four sisters opened a doll hospital. Dolls of various sizes were placed carefully in shoe boxes, and the end of each box was labeled with the patient's name. The patients were all sick; it didn't much matter with what. The four little nurses scurried busily about the patients, giving baths, administering shots with straight pins from their mother's sewing basket, and applying scarf bandages, Band-Aids, and plasters of baking soda with water or toothpaste. While doing so, they reassured their patients that they would be better soon, and that the nurses would take care of everything. Eventually, their mother's voice at the bottom of the stairs called the sisters down to lunch. This reaffirmed that the recovery of all the patients was complete. The sisters dressed the dolls, put them back in their usual places, and cleaned up the messy bandages so that their magic treatments would not be discovered.

Years later, the sisters went off to college. One went into nursing. The first day of clinical was, in many ways, as full of adventure as those rainy Saturdays.

As nursing students, we walked onto the floors of the hospital with excitement, fear, and a certain reverence. We watched the floor nurses rush about, answering bells and caring for sick patients. Each of us was assigned a patient and we reached anxiously for his chart. We hoped for a patient who needed dressing changes, injections, or treatments we had never performed. We hoped we would be able to decipher the doctor's handwriting and understand the medical jargon. Would we have to make an occupied bed? Was there an intravenous or central venous pressure line?

Many of us were attracted to the profession of nursing during our childhoods. We were prompted by the desire to help people become healthier and happier and to take away their pain. The fields of medicine and nursing seemed to be enveloped in mystery, and we hoped to be able to evoke cures. We discovered during nursing school, or early in our first jobs, that we could not fix everything or take away all the pain. There was no easy cure, panacea, or magic remedy. We came to terms with our own strengths and limitations. Our effectiveness was determined more by our ability to influence people than by our ability to control them. We found out that the control we exercised in the hospital did not necessarily help patients, or their families, to survive at home after they were discharged. In spite of our well-meaning and knowledgeable advice, patients did not always follow our directions.

Finally, we learned that nurses do not interact with patients in a vacuum. Rather, nurses are members of a larger team, which is composed of a variety of health-care professionals. The patient and family are at the head of the team. Each team member has a special expertise or contribution that should not be ignored.

Learning to work in harmony with other team members is much more difficult than learning technical skills. It is often hard to change from focusing on merely doing things to the patient to viewing him as the head of the health-care team. We begin by recognizing the patient's right to choose his future and by being willing to share our knowledge with him. This is known as *patient education*, a practice based on influence, not control. We must also learn to appreciate the roles of the other team members and find a way to articulate our respective contributions in helping the patient and his family.

This chapter is intended as an overview of the contributions of all health-care professionals in the delivery of patient education. Experiences between nurses and other team members are varied. It seems to be human nature to remember problems more clearly than successes. This chapter begins by recounting the progress nurses have made in defining their roles as patient educators, and then considers how they interact with the team.

The Role of Nurses

It was always easy to distinguish nurses from doctors in storybooks. Nurses were girls. Doctors were boys. Furthermore, nurses wore caps and white uniforms. The nurse's job was to help the doctor, usually by giving the patient an injection.

As we grew older, most of us became aware, by becoming either nurses or patients, that nursing was more than giving injections. We learned that boys could be nurses and girls could be doctors. Some nurses did not wear uniforms, and most did not wear caps. We heard parents, patients, and physicians comment that they did not recognize nurses without their caps and that nurses just did not seem like nurses if they were not wearing white. Professionals and consumers detected that the nursing profession was changing. They worried that nurses were trying to do the doctor's job.

Yes, nursing has changed and is changing. It is not competing with medicine, but rather trying to establish its own professional identity. Nurses are more clearly defining what it is they do, in which settings they practice, and with which patient populations they intervene. Nursing subscribes to the holistic model rather than to a traditional, disease-oriented, medical model.

The word *nurse* is derived from the Latin word *nutricius*, meaning nourishing. Our aim is to nourish patients and families, helping them to grow and achieve their fullest potential. We intervene not only when disease stands in the way of growth but also at times of family crisis. We are involved in health promotion— the prevention of disease. It is natural that nurses are found not only in hospitals, but also in the community, in schools, in outpatient clinics, and in occupational-health settings.

Nurses foster growth through the application of the nursing process, a professional model designed to meet client needs in a systematic way. The nursing process is discussed in Chapter 6. Through this approach, the nurse gathers information with which she assesses client needs, defines goals, intervenes, and evaluates the outcome of care. She recognizes significant others, especially the family, who have a direct influence on the client. She must be prepared to perform technical skills and to counsel clients regarding behaviors that promote health. Through patient education, the nurse assists the patient and family to perform self-care activities to the extent they are able. She works closely with physicians and other health professionals contributing to the patient's care.

It is crucial to prepare nurses not only as technicians, but also as teachers. Although teaching has always been an integral part of nursing practice, nursing education has not always prepared nurses for the teaching role. In the early part of this century, the National League for Nursing voiced concern that nursing education dealt only with disease and not with preparation for teaching.[1] The League has continued to speak out on the importance of educating nurses to teach.

In 1975, the American Nurses' Association (ANA) published a document entitled *The Professional Nurse and Health Education*. It stated that the professional nurse's responsibility includes "teaching the patient and family relevant facts about specific health care needs and supporting appropriate modification of behavior."[2] The ANA's *Model Nurse Practice Act* defines patient education as a component of the registered nurse's practice.[3] Licensed practical nurses are responsible for reinforcing what is taught. In many health-care institutions, the job descriptions of nurses include patient education. This function has become a professional expectation of nurses.

Nursing schools have responded by including teaching/learning skills in their curricula. We have observed that recent graduates display new willingness and confidence in teaching patients. Many patients and health professionals recognize the effectiveness of nurses as teachers. Others, unaccustomed to this nursing role, may be suspicious of its intent. Nurses, in addition to teaching patients about health problems, often find themselves having to inform the public about their capabilities.

We stated that it is important for nurses to articulate their contributions with other professionals involved in patient care. This involves an understanding of how other health professionals see their roles, particularly as they relate to patient education. It necessitates effective communication during the patient-education process. Many professional groups have published official statements describing patient-education responsibilities.

The Roles of Other Health Professionals

We have found that more recently educated members of other health professions tend to be as involved as nurses in patient teaching. Nurses often assume that, because they have received opposition or lack of cooperation in the past, no physicians, for example, are supportive of patient education. These assumptions thwart collaboration and the delivery of patient education.

Rather than drawing our own conclusions or focusing on negative experiences, we have been able to grow in our patient-teaching roles by getting to know people in other health professions who practice patient education. We asked them how they see their patient-teaching roles and how they perceive ours. We asked each to consider how his role is connected with the nurse's role in patient teaching and to suggest ways to increase collaboration. The responses from attending physicians, resident physicians, dietitians, physical therapists, pharmacists, and social workers follow.

Physicians

In 1975, the American Medical Association's House of Delegates adopted a statement on the physician's role in patient education. It addressed the physician's responsibility to provide the patient and his family with patient-education services designed to help them effectively manage individual health.[4] Many specialty groups have also adopted statements related to patient-education responsibilities.

Attending Physicians

What is your involvement in patient education?

"I teach patients one to one. I try to tell them what they want and need to know in language they understand. I want them to understand and agree with the plan, to know what the goals are, and to participate in decision making."

"I try to help the patients to tell me in their own words what's wrong and the costs, benefits, and risks of treatment."

"Ten percent of the time I teach the patient and his family together."

How do you see the nurse's role in patient education?

"I see it as necessary and important. Nurses have a different perspective from mine. Patients tend to confide different information to nurses. For example, patients are more open about fear of cancer with the nurse, and talk with me about stomach pain. Nurses can teach about diets and urine testing much better than I can. Nurses clarify and reinforce a lot of what I teach."

"Nurses teach patients and families, especially in dealing with chronic diseases."

How do you see your role in patient education interfacing with the nurse's role ideally?

"The two roles are complementary. The doctor teaches about diagnosis and prognosis. The nurse teaches daily management. There is combined strength."

"Doctors and nurses teach in different ways but there is significant overlap, so crucial information gets reinforced."

How do your roles interface presently?
"I don't know what the nurses teach."

"We get rushed and don't communicate well. Sometimes, when we have planning meetings about a patient's care, we work out our roles very well."

"I usually don't have time to track the nurse down. Nurses' notes are crucial to communication. Sometimes they're helpful and sometimes not."

What increases your collaboration with the team in patient education?
"Knowing what different people can do and like to do. Personal knowledge and trust."

"Having time to get to know other members of the team."

"Reading nurses' notes. I read them daily. Checking in with the day-shift nurse. If I can't find her I write a note on the nurses' notes to let her know I read them."

"I ask the patient who is teaching him. The patient is really the center of the team and can help me work with the team."

"Recognizing my own limitations. This makes me want to work with other people. Some physicians are scared. They're afraid to admit they don't know something, like diet teaching. The nurse or dietitian can unobtrusively make suggestions on the chart to help them out. This increases trust and team development. The physician can still save face. People on a team need to recognize their own limitations."

"We should start by trying to model the team approach in patient management."

Resident Physicians

What is your involvement in patient education?
"I think it's important that what my role is and what my role should be are different. Many residents lack both the skill and desire to do patient education. The role of educating the patient doesn't always seem to fall to you. I've chosen to be actively involved in it. I think patient education is essential, not just important."

"The role of the family-medicine specialist is prevention. It doesn't exist without patient education."

"I try to incorporate patient education into my interaction with the patient, but I don't feel I have the skills to do that right now. I think you need to be consciously aware of patient education, and you have to have a good feeling that your patients are understanding and doing what you, together, agree is appropriate. I think we assume that more than we should."

"I think it's clear that if patient education is to be a valid concern for the future, to get third-party payment we have to be able to show it's valid and necessary. I don't think most physicians are convinced that it's valid or necessary."

How do you see the nurse's role in patient education?
"Patient education is often left to the nurse."
"Nurses do the majority of patient education as it stands. The role is often assumed by females. It's an interesting thing. If you look around, most of those who are interested in patient education seem to be female residents or nurses. I don't think it's been considered the masculine thing to do. It seems nursing-like by tradition."
"Nurses often lack confidence in their ability to teach."

How do you see your role in patient education interfacing with the nurse's role ideally?
"The nurse's role complements mine."
"In a busy practice, the physician usually doesn't have the time it takes to teach. Ideally you want to work with a nurse who knows enough about the problem to teach it, and who knows how to do it so the patient will understand."
"I don't think it has to be a very formal approach. It's a physician-nursing role. The physician recognizes and uses patient education, as does the nurse. The nurse reinforces what the physician begins. That's the meat of what's going on in the patient interaction—not just the pamphlets and the materials and tricks of patient education."
"We work side by side on the same team."
"The roles of physician and nurse are broken down. You need to take a health-team approach. The nurses have to accept this approach. If they don't interact well, it's counter to patient education. Often, now, the nurses don't have a good idea of what to teach the patient because they don't have a good idea of what the physician is thinking. So they teach routine things. And physicians, because they don't have a good feeling for what the nurses are doing, don't have a good feeling for what the patient wants to know. That's usually conveyed to the nurses. The key is to merge into a health-team approach—have good communication between the physician and nurse, with both contributing the different skills they bring to patient management."

How do your roles interface presently?
"A lot of nurses aren't interested in patient education."
"One instance sticks in my mind—it really bothered me. It was the night I had a patient die of lung cancer. It was a difficult family to work with. I couldn't, in good conscience, resuscitate the patient but the family expected that. There was a lot of denial and a lot of anger. That night I thought there was no question—he was going to die. I had a conference with the family. I made an effort to find the nurse who had been involved in his care and said, 'I'm having a conference with the family; would you like to be there?' I just got a negative response. That particular nurse never did show up. It was probably the most crucial thing in the management of that patient for the entire hospitalization. The nurse did not care to be part of it. That's not typical of every nurse. Primary

nurses in particular are very concerned. But this situation has arisen over and over. I think that's too bad. When you're working long hours, any extra effort seems like ten times as much as it really is. You don't have to make that effort too many times before you discover it's wasted. I get discouraged. And I believe in it enough to make the attempt, fairly persistently, to involve the nurses. I'm sure if I got discouraged, and I think it's important, anyone who doesn't feel that strongly about it isn't doing it anymore."

What increases your collaboration with the team in patient education?

"The most important thing is discussion. There has to be desire on all parts. People can find the time to do it. Take a half hour to discuss a difficult patient, and bring in everyone who's involved in the care. It's difficult to do with team nursing (as opposed to primary nursing). You formulate an approach and cross-educate one another. It optimizes patient care for that particular patient, but it also teaches people how to deal with difficult patients."

"It helps if we have similar interests."

"I don't know what the nurses want. I've tried to make rounds with nurses who feel as if they're just tagging along as handmaidens of the doctor. It's a prevalent attitude. I don't know if other doctors would want to do this. I do know it has worked in university settings. I find it enjoyable and educational."

"You have to teach nurses in school to develop a positive attitude about patient education. I think nurses could be happier to find this other dimension in patient care. I think nurses are generally better trained in patient education than physicians are. They have to use it."

"There has to be desire and awareness. There have to be people with the desire to get it rolling."

"*SOAP* notes and assessment should clarify what the nurse thinks. The same is true of physician notes. If you use the *SOAP*-note system as Larry Weed set it up, the last part of that note, as part of the plan, should say what you told the patient. Spelled out in the beginning of that system is that one of the most crucial things you do for the patient is document how you educated him."

Dietitians

Professional dietitians are registered by the American Dietetic Association (ADA). The ADA supports the role of dietitians in patient education, specifically with regard to counseling individuals and families in nutrition and dietary planning, documenting nutritional care data, and developing nutrition-education materials.[5]

What is your involvement in patient education?

"We educate patients about the diets they need to follow at home. We try to find out what the patient usually eats and how we need to modify this."

"Sometimes we have to discuss the diet with the doctor because what he orders is inappropriate. We make the necessary changes and teach the patient."

How do you see the nurse's role in patient education?

"Nurses reinforce what the dietitian tells the patient. That involves a fair amount of knowledge about dietetics. Many nurses aren't comfortable doing this, though."

"Nurses let us know what's going on with the patient and this helps us to evaluate whether the patient understands his diet plan."

"Nurses teach patients about medications and treatments."

"Nurses teach patients basic survival skills."

"They explain what the doctor has said to the patient after the doctor leaves."

How do you see your role in patient education interfacing with the nurse's role ideally?

"It would be nice if the nurses also knew the information we gave to the patient about diet so they could reinforce our teaching."

"The nurse could emphasize to the patient the importance of following his diet plan."

"It would help if the nurse could give us an idea as to when the patient would be discharged. I got a call today to teach a patient fifteen minutes before he was to go home. That's just not enough time."

How do your roles interface presently?

"Nurses don't really know what the patient has been taught by the dietitian, so they are unable to reinforce it."

"Sometimes the patient has questions about his diet that the nurse can't answer. It's great if she calls us and we can either answer the question or come to see the patient. But sometimes we never get called, and the patient doesn't get an answer to his question."

What increases your collaboration with the team in patient education?

"We need team-planning meetings. We need to know what other people are teaching the patient. The patient should not have to hear things over and over again. We could each contribute in the area of our expertise."

"Protocols for teaching help. You know what other people are teaching, although you don't always know at what level the patient is understanding."

"It would really be a team if people would go out of their way to communicate with one another."

"It's really individual, depending on the nurse and the dietitian. Some nurses are more alert to dietary problems patients are having and will call the dietitian to work things out. Others don't do this. Some dietitians are more outgoing than others. The more open the communication is, the better—even if it's a quick note in the chart."

"Nursing notes—as much information as possible. The nurse's assessment of the patient's readiness to learn is especially helpful. Some physicians write thorough notes. Others never do. Good written communication always helps. Documentation of patient teaching is highly variable, depending on the person. Dietitians are trying to be very conscientious about writing notes in the chart. We resort to extraordinary measures to see that physicians read our notes. Sometimes we take them out of our section and slip them on top of the physician's notes to be sure he sees them."

"Nurses and shifts change frequently. Good communication between shifts, and especially with third shift, is very important if the team is going to work."

Physical Therapists

What is your involvement in patient education?

"We inform patients about their disease, about what to expect, and about any procedures that are done."

"We teach them about ambulation, functional activities, and safety, especially postsurgically. Physical therapists have a large role in educating patients about rheumatic diseases and how to deal with and prevent flare-ups."

"Physical therapists give daily instruction in exercise programs, including pre- and postoperative teaching. We discuss prostheses and help patients with them."

How do you see the nurse's role in patient education?

"I see the nurse's role as one of educating and orienting the patient to his disease and reinforcing the teaching of other health-care personnel."

"Nurses give patients emotional support, teach them about activities of daily living, and give general instructions about medications."

"The nurse's role is very important in teaching about medications, exercise, and rest and reinforcing what physical therapists teach."

"Nurses reinforce precautions in transfer and positioning. This is extremely important. They can help to motivate the patient and coordinate pain medications with the treatments."

How do you see your role in patient education interfacing with the nurse's role ideally?

"We are working toward the same goal—getting the patient ready to handle discharge."

"We should plan teaching together for all patients."

"We should construct a postoperative teaching program."

"Ideally, we would have a team approach in which nursing, physical therapy, occupational therapy, social services, and the doctor would reinforce teaching and give emotional support from admission to discharge."

How do your roles interface presently?

"There is little carry-over of patient teaching. We function independently of each other."

"Due to staffing problems there is not much time for interaction between physical therapists and nurses."

"Nurses change so frequently that there is little consistency. We don't know enough about one another's roles to reinforce one another."

What increases your collaboration with the team in patient education?

"Frequent team meetings, especially with primary nursing."

"Mutual respect among the disciplines, cooperation, and knowing to use the other's expertise in different cases."

"Good written and verbal communication."

Pharmacists

In 1975, the American Society of Hospital Pharmacists (ASHP) approved a statement that defined the specific functions of the pharmacist that relate to patient education. It stated that the pharmacist should "inform, educate, and counsel patients about each medication in the patient drug regimen." Included are the name of the drug, the reason it has been prescribed, how it is to be prepared and taken, precautions, side-effects, contraindications, and storage.[6]

What is your involvement in patient education?

"The pharmacist is often the first person to see patients when they have problems. When patients ask for advice, the pharmacist must know if a referral to other health-care providers is needed."

"We tell patients how to take drugs and about side-effects. We have to understand the patients to know how much to tell them."

"The main job of the hospital pharmacist is to dispense medications. He is involved in administration and may not see patients very often. The pharmacist can be a resource person."

"The pharmacist has to teach about how the drug works in the body. If the patient knows the reason for taking the drug, he's more likely to take it as he should. A lot of patients know nothing about their medication. They don't know what it is or how to store it. Sometimes they don't even take it, depending on how they feel. This is especially true of hypertensive patients."

"The pharmacist has to sense how the patient is feeling and whether he's ready to learn. A lot of pharmacists toss out information but have no idea whether the patient is comprehending. The patient may be asking leading questions because he has high anxiety. Sometimes we unintentionally brush off those questions."

"On the retail basis, there is a minimum amount of information the pharmacist is required to communicate: how to take the medicine, what to avoid, precautions, and so forth."

How do you see the nurse's role in patient education?

"They do a good job teaching what they know about. I don't really know how much nurses know about diseases or if they can handle teaching that. I don't know how much nurses know about drugs."

"Nurses see the patient more than others do. They coordinate the teaching in the hospital. Especially with primary-care nursing, they teach the family. I think patients relate better to nurses than to other health professionals."

How do you see your role in patient education interfacing with the nurse's role ideally?

"If nurses question drugs that are prescribed or need information, they should call us. There are so many new drugs. If nurses are going to teach patients about these drugs, we need to collaborate."

"All patients have the right to know what medications they're taking, how much, and why. Nurses can teach this when they administer medications."

"The pharmacist and nurse would work together. The pharmacist would take a drug history, the nurse would coordinate teaching, and the pharmacist would talk with the patient at discharge."

"Traditionally, the relationship between pharmacist and nurse is poor because we're so departmentalized and because nurses are caught in between when the doctors and pharmacists disagree. We need a better mutual understanding of what our jobs are, how we're trained, and in what areas we have expertise."

"It's important for nurses to appreciate that pharmacists are interested in patient education. Nurses have a big job to do and the patients expect a lot of them. If a patient doesn't understand something about his medication, teaching usually falls to the nurses. Pharmacists in the hospital really don't go up to the floors and teach patients. This is something I would like to see happen. The role of the clinical pharmacist should be developed."

"The nurse can reinforce the teaching done by the team and communicate with other team members to meet the patient's learning needs."

"We need to work together with an orientation toward prevention, not just disease."

How do your roles interface presently?
"There is little interaction. Occasionally nurses call the pharmacy with questions about a drug."

"We often confuse patients because we don't have our story together. We explain things in different ways or give contradictory information."

What increases your collaboration with the team in patient education?
"Satellite pharmacies on the patient units would increase communication."

"Pharmacists could review charts and look for compliance problems related to medications. This could happen if the pharmacists had more time to get involved."

"Pharmacists could be more open to nurses' questions and encourage their calls."

"There should be organized continuing education for nurses, with the person who has expertise sharing it. Pharmacists could teach nurses as new drugs come out, making nurses better able to teach the patients."

"Nurses make valuable assessments about the patient and family and what their supports are like. Nurses can often predict compliance or noncompliance. Nurses can offer the pharmacist guidance in how much to tell the patient or how to present the information. The nursing assessment could be shared more, especially in the nurses' notes."

Hospital Social Workers

What is your involvement in patient education?
"Our biggest role is as a hospital/staff and staff/community liaison. If the patient, for instance, has a question about what will happen when he leaves the hospital, and if he cannot take care of himself, we review organizations that

can help. We talk with patients, doctors, and staff about these resources. We coordinate with agencies."

"We do counseling in the broadest meaning of the term. We teach the patient about nursing homes and what they can offer. We prepare them, and help them understand that it does not have to be a bad experience. We teach families about the same things. Families come in with so much guilt and in such crisis about what they are going to do, they may be at the end of their limits. We try to help the family understand what a nursing home can offer. We teach them who is appropriate for home health care and how they might try it. We help them consider whether it will work."

"Many families have problems before they even come into the hospital. They need help with these, too."

"We counsel patients, especially poor patients, about how to use health-care services."

"I answer preoperative questions—the things patients are really afraid of. Patients worry about exposing themselves, about the anesthesia wearing off. Patients have told me how unprepared they were to wait down in the holding area before surgery, how they were cold, yet afraid to ask for a blanket, with people joking all around them. Patients tend to tell things to social workers that they're embarrassed to tell nurses or doctors."

"Nurses do a lot of the medical teaching. But it so often helps to have someone not in a white coat who comes in and sits down and doesn't have to run off to the next room or get the medicine cart out. The patient says, 'Gee, I'm worried about my bandage,' or, 'I'm scared about surgery tomorrow.' We can reinforce what the nurse has taught. We must know our own limits and help get the doctor or nurse in to answer questions. Somehow patients don't worry about bothering social workers. They feel that we always have time."

"We give emotional support. We teach a lot of families about dealing with the aged patient. We do a lot of the 'what-can-I-expect' kind of teaching, especially with surgical patients."

"We try to get patients hooked up with support groups and information agencies."

How do you see the nurse's role in patient education?

"The nurses I know do a tremendous amount of patient teaching, especially with surgical patients. They're there 24 hours a day, always answering questions for patients and families."

"They tell patients what they need to know. They answer questions patients never ask their doctors. The nurses keep themselves up to date in their fields."

"In the surgery area, I see their teaching as strongest with postoperative care. I think the two weakest points are preoperative care and discharge."

"Some nurses are very aware of the situations the patients are going home to. Others are not."

How do you see your role in patient education interfacing with the nurse's role presently?

"Sometimes nurses don't know enough about what we do to make referrals, but we need to work together."

"I get my best referrals from nurses. There's something about hanging an IV bag, giving a shot, washing hair, giving a bath—patients tell things to nurses while the nurse is doing these things. Nurses do involve us when we are better able to handle certain kinds of crises."

How do you see your roles interfacing ideally?

"Nurses need to know where their limits are. The patient needs follow-up after discharge to learn and to reinforce learning. I can help with this by making referrals that go beyond hospitalization but we have to work together, to focus less narrowly on rescuing."

"We all need to realize that patients do want to know what's going on. Being in the hospital is a dehumanizing situation. People lose control and identity. If we can do anything to give them a little element of control to hang on, it's valuable. Even if they only remember one thing about what we teach (they never retain it all), it's something. We all feel the same way if we're patients in the hospital; even doctors, when they are patients, feel the same way. When we go down for that barium enema, or put on that hospital gown slit up the back, we're all the same, rich or poor. Everyone needs his identity and to have a little bit of control."

What increases your collaboration with the team in patient education?

"Grand rounds with the physicians and nurses are a good opportunity to communicate. Communication with other team members is very fragmented. It just depends on who you're working with. We generally have better contact with dietitians than with pharmacists. What we could tell pharmacy is incredible. We see patients harboring medicines. We have the family bring in every pill bottle so that we can go through them and throw out what medication has passed its expiration date. Many patients go to several doctors for the same thing and then to a psychiatrist who also prescribes medicine. We tell the nurses about this, but the lines of communication are not very good."

"Good notes in the chart are very important. I read all the notes. The nursing assessment often tells me in a nutshell what I need to know. Some doctors' notes are good. Others are not. Sometimes I have to help the family fight to keep the patient in the hospital. Noting things like the patient's response to the nurses is very helpful. Details also help me assist the family in planning for discharge. I need to know things such as whether the patient is incontinent or nonambulatory. Notes from the health team validate what I see."

Promoting the Team Approach

While those health-care team members we interviewed stressed the importance of protocols and organization, they frequently stated that the attitudes and skills of individuals directly influenced the success of teamwork in patient education. They emphasized the following criteria for successful teamwork:

1. Communication (verbal and written), facilitated by planning meetings, care conferences, telephone consultation, good documentation, and "the willingness to go out of our way to communicate with one another"
2. Mutual respect among disciplines, recognizing respective areas of expertise, knowing our limitations
3. The desire to work as a team
4. Recognition of our common goal

By meeting the challenges mentioned above, members of all disciplines on the health-care team can continue to build a base of support for patient education within their settings. The question remains: how do we change the attitudes of people who pose opposition to patient education?

Building a Base of Support for Patient Education

First, we as nurses must determine where our strength is found. Second, we must look for support from influential administrators, health-care professionals, and consumers.

One of our nursing colleagues has had experience in nursing practice, education, and administration, and is now the patient-education coordinator in a county hospital. She has been able to bring together representatives from different disciplines, to facilitate their dialogue about patient education, and to help them formulate interdisciplinary teaching programs. We looked to her for her thoughts on building support for patient education.

What makes the nurse's contribution to patient education unique, setting her apart from the rest of the team and making her role different?

"I think the uniqueness in nursing, as opposed to the other health professions is the continuous, intimate contact with the patient. The one-to-one presence, the laying on of hands, the advocacy . . . I see the patient and nurse as a team. The nurse does direct teaching and coordinates the teaching of others. That's where we get into facilitating other people's knowledge, including the physician's."

A lot of us look for a system that would make coordinating patient education easier. How important do you think it is to have institutional support to do this?

"If the top corporate administration does not support it, and if the total mission statement does not contain some commitment to a patient-education system, I'd scrap the whole idea. You must have a philosophical commitment institutionally or the system will not be accepted."

So, without support, a system could not work. But could nurses continue patient-education efforts on an individual level?

"The teaching will go on, but it will be catch-as-catch-can. I believe so strongly in a systematic approach—one that will feed into other systems. For example, take a system of nursing administration and services: nurses come into that system believing that one of their primary responsibilities is to help the patient learn from his encounter with the health-care system; the system of patient education, then, has to be a support to bring that responsibility to the forefront."

One of the points that came out in our interviews with health professionals was that the success of patient education is highly dependent on individuals and how they perceive their roles. It seems that patient education is dependent on personalities: specifically, those who like to teach and are confident doing it. If we say that patients have a right to know and should be taught by nurses, what can we do to get those nurses who don't like to teach to join the patient-education team?

"Why not capitalize on personalities and look at why certain personalities not only get teaching done but also encourage others? Tap that as your core leadership group. Identify what they believe their skill and knowledge deficits are. Help them to learn the skills they are lacking, and then to use and market those skills confidently. By marketing I mean growing more and more confident, saying to the physician: 'This is happening. This is what I'm doing. What are you doing? Let's get together.' I would say the same thing about the dietitians, physical therapists, and whatever health professionals are coming into the picture in terms of patient teaching. There's got to be some way to communicate through both documentation in the medical record and a verbal face-to-face contact."

"We toss around these terms *interdisciplinary* and *multidisciplinary*. I prefer *interdisciplinary*. You bring in people with different knowledge and skills but they have a common goal. They plan and do things together and at some points they articulate. *Multidisciplinary* means to me that they have different resources; they sit and plan together, but then each goes his own separate way in implementation."

You mentioned building a broad base of support with enthusiastic nurses rather than going right after those who present obstacles. Can the same be true for physicians? Pharmacists? Dietitians? Other professionals? Should we look to those in each group who enthusiastically try to model patient education? Is that more worthwhile than going after, for example, the obstinate physician?

"Yes, I certainly think it is. One strategy that seems to work effectively is to say to those people who are supportive: 'OK, what are you willing to do? What do you see as your role to help stimulate this interest? In what way are you going to find opportunities to influence others?' We waste time trying to drag people along. Let's start with that core group."

So you recommend that individuals look at their own commitment to teach patients and at how much they're willing to do to influence others.

"Yes. I see it with other things in nursing besides patient teaching—like assessment. Registered nurses have a very strong responsibility to do this—to make their own observations and care plans, and to communicate with the physician to make both plans work together. But nurses must have the commitment and the skills to do this. I would love to see the time in nursing when employers find a way to assess these competencies and select the people we need. We've seen this happen with pharmacists. Some like to teach and some are very happy filling pill bottles. Both are fine, but the latter may not be clinically oriented. We have to bring in clinical pharmacists and nurses who want to teach patients. The employer needs to examine philosophy and preparation."

How can we better prepare nurses for the teaching role?
   "I wonder if there may be a need to help nurses change a bit of their commitment, so that they are devoted not only to caring for the patient but also to helping the patient control his situation. Some nurses get frustrated because patients may not do what the nurse has told them."

One of the issues we will examine in Chapter 4 is that in the past, patient education has been undertaken by some with the hope that it would make the patient do what he was told. Maybe one goal should be to teach the patient, so he can make an informed choice. But this is not for the purpose of control. It is for the purpose of a relationship, among the health-care provider, patient, and family, in which people are given guidance and allowed to make choices.
   "You really said something when you said *relationship.* That is the opportunity that nurses have, to make the difference between patient–nurse interaction and patient–nurse relationship. I think we get a little sidetracked. I don't think enough time is really given to this in basic nursing programs or in nursing practice."

We talked about the need for nurses to take a unified stand on issues such as patient education. Do you think that we might gain more freedom to use teaching programs without having a formal doctor's order if we worked together?
   "Yes. Use a unified approach. You can't just sneak up on them [doctors]. I think we should have a little more feeling for physicians. The medical community has gone through some pretty traumatic experiences in the past ten years. They've never before become so exposed to the public. The public's knowledge has increased; the public is saying, 'Hey, I don't have to put up with this. I have a right to second opinions.' They read about it in *Reader's Digest.* It's the consumerism movement."

What aspects of the consumer movement do you think have really had an impact on health care—particularly on patient education?
   "Increasing costs. Historically, up until right after World War II, there had been very little increase in costs. Then some hospital managements (boards of trustees) started including businessmen who said, 'This is a losing game.' And over a period of five to ten years, costs went way up. It was the feeling among a lot of people that it was not right to charge for hospital services. The public rose up. The increase in costs affected industries that insured their employees. They organized alternative health-care services. The rural health-care movement spread. Physician's assistants, nurse-practitioners, and lay workers joined in. The competition scares physicians. The public is going after what it wants."

What about the Patient's Bill of Rights?
   "A lot of people organized, began to address consumer health-care issues, and pressured their legislators. Consumers came to the forefront. People

began looking not only at hospitals but also at doctors. They're not gods. The public has stopped looking at them as gods."

Do you think people began to realize how much collective power they had? The Civil Rights Movement and the Women's Movement showed us this. Did the same thing happen with the Health-Care Movement?

"Yes, and consumers learned to use the channels for change. The media had a lot to do with consumer success. The portrayal was not always accurate, but it raised the public consciousness."

We talked about influence. Nurses can influence other nurses. Health-care teams can influence other health-care teams. What about consumers? Do you see them as being able to contribute to this broad base of support for patient education? If so, how can we tap their strength to get patient-education systems off the ground?

"Yes, we can use their strength. I think the best way for nurses to start is with assessment. Ask them: 'What do you want? This is your hospital.' Ask about satisfaction. Ask them who they know. Sometimes families who have a positive experience will know someone on the board of trustees and can use their influence."

Do you think most patients want to be educated?

"Yes, I do. Some may not think they do."

A social worker commented to us that sometimes what we think *people want to know and what they really* do *want to know are two different things. Sometimes they are afraid to tell the nurse or the doctor what they really want to know—whether they'll be exposed during surgery, or what will happen if the anesthesia wears off. They may not be concerned about the generic name of their drug or other things we think they want to know.*

"They want to know what that drug is going to do: 'What kind of trouble am I going to have?' I still think everyone has a right to his beliefs and values."

Most health professionals believe they have the patient's best interests in mind when they try to take care of him totally. We don't think beyond discharge. We don't help him go through that problem-solving process. He gets home and doesn't know what to do.

"Yes, he goes home from that structured, protected environment. He has to develop new skills. When the patient has surgery, for example, patient education should be more than getting him up and helping him understand why he has pain. You can take advantage of having him walk, sit, and get out of bed to teach him body mechanics. All students of nursing should appreciate that the patient's hospital stay ought to be a learning experience for him. Nursing and medicine need to have a new perspective on what hospitalization is all about."

Summary

The nurse's involvement in patient education is mandated by the *Nurse Practice Act* in most states, by professional statements of the American Nurses'

Association, by the American Hospital Association's well-known *A Patient's Bill of Rights,* and by the Joint Commission on the Accreditation of Hospitals' *Standards for the Accreditation of Hospitals.*[7,8] These standards and legal guidelines formalize the nurse's responsibility to teach. Every nurse is called upon to provide patients and families with an opportunity to learn in their health-care encounters. Patient education is built on nurse–patient relationships that foster growth through respecting one another, caring, and working together.

References

1. National League for Nursing Education: Standard Curriculum for Schools of Nursing. Baltimore, Waverly Press, 1918
2. American Nurses' Association: The Professional Nurse and Health Education. Kansas City, American Nurses' Association, 1975
3. American Nurses' Association: Model Nurse Practice Act. Kansas City, American Nurses' Association, Pub. Code: NP-52M5/76, 1979
4. American Medical Association: Statement on Patient Education. Chicago, American Medical Association, 1975
5. American Dietetic Association: Position Paper on Recommended Salaries and Employment Practices for Members of the American Dietetic Association. Chicago, American Dietetic Association, 1976
6. American Society of Hospital Pharmacists: Statement on Pharmacist Conducted Patient Counseling. Bethesda, American Society of Hospital Pharmacists, 1976
7. American Hospital Association: A Patient's Bill of Rights. Chicago, American Hospital Association, 1972
8. Joint Commission on the Accreditation of Hospitals: Accreditation Manual for Hospitals. Chicago, American Hospital Association, 1982

Bibliography

Books

Brill NI: Working With People: The Helping Process. Philadelphia, J B Lippincott, 1973
Brill NI: Teamwork: Working Together in the Human Services. Philadelphia, J B Lippincott, 1976
Bower, FL, Bevis EO: Fundamentals of Nursing Practice: Concepts, Roles and Functions. St Louis, C V Mosby, 1979
Dorroh T: Between Patient and Health Worker. New York, McGraw-Hill, 1974
Orem DE: Nursing: Concepts of Practice. New York, McGraw-Hill, 1974
Redman BK: The Process of Patient Teaching in Nursing. St Louis, C V Mosby, 1980
Rogers ME: An Introduction to the Theoretical Basis of Nursing. Philadelphia, F A Davis, 1976

Journals

Barrett M, Schwartz MD: What patients really want to know. Am J Nurs 81, No. 9:1642, 1981
Fuhroz LM, Bernstein R: Making patient education a part of patient care. Am J Nurs 76, No. 11, 1798–1799, 1976
Lespare M: The patient as a health student. Hospitals 44, No. 6:75–80, 1970
Levine ME: Holistic nursing. Nurs Clin North Am 6:253–263, 1971
Linn LS: A survey of care–cure attitudes of physicians, nurses and students. Nurs Forum 64, No. 2:245–259, 1975

Miller M: Patient education: A growing concern for many. Patient Education, NLN Pub. No. 20-1633:19–28, 1977

Partridge KB: Nursing values in a changing society. Nurs Outlook 26:356–360, 1978

Pender NJ: Patient identification of health information received during hospitalization. Nurs Res 23:262–267, 1974

Ramsden EL: The patient's right to know: Implications for interpersonal communication processes. Phys Ther 55:133–138, 1975

Reader GG: The physician as a teacher. Health Educ Monogr 2:34–38, 1974

Richards RF: Patients are learning. Health Educ Monogr 2:30–33, 1974

Ulrich MR, Kelly KM: Patient care includes teaching. Hospitals 46:59–65, 1972

Chapter 2

Philosophical and Political Issues

When nurses are interviewed about their experiences with patient education, they invariably mention issues that can be categorized as philosophical, political, and power issues. *Philosophical* issues concern one's approach to patients and basic beliefs about how patient education should be put into operation. Philosophical issues tend to vary with educational background: the nurse tends to practice patient education in a manner consistent with her own nursing education.

Power and *political* issues usually concern control—who teaches what, to whom, and when. Power and political issues produce more tension than any other patient-education issues. Most practicing nurses are poorly prepared to deal with power and political issues. This chapter presents skills that will enhance the effectiveness of the practicing nurse, who confronts philosophical, power, and political issues daily, and that will help prepare the student nurse to become an agent for change.

Other areas explored in this chapter are differences in professional roles and institutions in relation to their impacts on the delivery of patient education, criteria that can help a practicing nurse to determine who has power in a given setting and to gain power herself to improve patient education, methods used to bring about planned change and the use of change-agentry skills, and, finally, practical suggestions for managing philosophical and political issues.

Differences Between Traditional and Progressive Health Professionals

We have found, during our years of nursing practice, that we generally interact with two different types of health-care professionals. We have classified them as the traditional health-care professional and the progressive health-care professional. When we refer to health-care professionals we include the entire health-care team: physicians, registered nurses, dietitians, pharmacists, social workers, and occupational, physical, and respiratory therapists. The following discussion will focus primarily on the physician and the nurse.

Our image of the traditional health-care professional is that of an older man or woman accustomed to a hierarchical approach to medical care, in which the physician is the dominant decision maker and the focus of patient-care activities. Nurses, physicians, and other health-care professionals who subscribe to this model view the physician as totally responsible for all aspects of the patient's care and tend to regard the patient as "belonging" to the physician. The physician operates from a position of centralized power. Such traditional models assume that the physician always knows what is best for the patient and that the patient concurs with this attitude. The patient exhibits this concurrence by responding without question to the medical regimen.

We note that physicians who represent this approach generally practice in the areas of surgery and internal medicine, and are less frequently found in obstetrics, pediatrics, psychiatry, or family medicine. This impression is supported by a recent study that examined physicians' opinions of clinical pharmacy. Physicians were found not to favor the expanding role of clinical pharmacy, and those least in favor were older physicians, those in high-malpractice-risk specialties, and those who write a large number of prescriptions. Interestingly, physicians with a high risk of malpractice suit tend to be unfavorable toward *any* extraprofessional involvement in physician–patient relationships.[1] Physicians practicing in some of the medical and surgery specialty areas are among those with a high risk of medical malpractice suit. This may account for this group's less-than-enthusiastic acceptance of nurse-sponsored patient education. Implications for nursing are that this group of physicians must be persuaded that patient education can actually reduce litigation. Accurate and concise documentation will establish a channel of communication, keeping the physician aware of all information given to his patients.

Nurses who fall into the category of traditional health-care professionals tend to be educated below the baccalaureate level (*i.e.,* either associate-degree or diploma graduates). Their orientation is most likely related to their educational preparation as a bedside nurse. The bedside nurse who is trained to fit into the traditional model will have fewer problems with role inconsistency and role insufficiency than will the nurse educated in the progressive model. We have seen more traditional nurses in hospitals than in community, public school, college and university nursing, or other outpatient settings.

In contrast to the traditional health-care professional, the progressive health-care professional may be younger, more accustomed to a team approach with the patient as the focus, and less likely to view the physician as the dominant or only decision maker. The progressive health-care professional eschews centralized power in favor of decentralization, so that all members of the team have authority in their specialty areas.

As our readers can probably tell, our bias is in favor of the progressive health-care professional. We have worked successfully with traditional nurses and physicians, but we feel that the progressive professionals offer better patient-education services and greater job satisfaction for all. Table 2-1 uses broad generalizations to illustrate many of the differences between the traditional and progressive approaches to patient-education issues.

Examination of the Issues

Philosophical Issues

Self-care

A term coined by Dorothea Orem, *self-care* connotes a conceptual basis for nursing practice. Self-care behavior " . . . is the practice of activities that individuals personally initiate and perform in their own behalf in maintaining life, health, and well-being."[2] The function of the nurse is to assist the client in achieving a level of wellness consistent with the client's own life-style and value system, but not necessarily with the value system maintained by the health-care purveyors. *Self-care* means that the client has control over his medical regimen and makes choices regarding his medical management. The traditional health-care system in the United States, with its emphasis on acute management, leaves the physician very little opportunity to assist the client in accomplishing self-care activities.

Patient education is an integral part of self-care practice because most patients lack the requisite knowledge to promote health or to manage problems

Table 2-1. **Approaches to Issues in Patient Education**

Issue	Traditional Approach	Progressive Approach
Philosophical		
Self-care	Not subscribed to; health-care providers make most decisions with belief they are acting in best interest of client; engenders paternalistic attitude and client dependency	Subscribed to; original impetus from nursing; promotes client's active participation as member of health-care team
Patient-education model	Medical model: diagnosis, treatment, prognosis	Educational: teaching/learning principles
Sharing information	Less willing to share information; sometimes withholds information	More willing to share information; relates to patient on appropriate level for patient function

(continued)

Table 2-1. **Approaches to Issues in Patient Education** *(continued)*

Issue	Traditional Approach	Progressive Approach
Philosophical *(continued)*		
Holism	Not subscribed to	Subscribed to; avoids mind–body–spirit trichotomy
Teaching the chronically ill	Teaches in terms of medical regimen	Is oriented toward assisting client to obtain highest level of wellness possible in a manner consistent with his life-style.
Preoperative teaching	Believes that preoperative teaching promotes compliance; gives information to obtain consent for diagnostic and operative procedures	Includes more than informed consent; promotes self-assertive behavior and decreases patient's feeling of powerlessness in preoperative context
Power and Political		
Compliance	Bases patient education on desired compliance	Is not directly compliance oriented; promotes patient decision making; encourages positive and cooperative health behaviors
Responsibility for teaching	Believes physician or clinical teaching specialist should do all the teaching	All members of health-care team actively involved in patient education; team concept ensures coordination of health professionals; maintains planned, coherent approach
Patient-education referrals	Is unwilling, based on some paternalistic attitudes; unaware of other patient-education resources	Is very willing to refer; makes referrals based on patient's autonomy and desire for extramural help
Knowledge and use of community resources	Is unknowledgeable, often unwilling to refer	Is usually knowledgeable, willing to refer; has increasing appreciation for contribution of individuals and groups that promote wellness
Attitudes toward self-help groups	Views with skepticism, is frequently unwilling to refer; occasionally co-opts self-help groups	Is interested in concept and willing to refer; avoids co-optation of self-help enterprises

related to disease. Ideally, patient education is offered to a client in order to reduce his dependency on the health-care system, not to increase his need for services. Self-care activities promoted by the nurse attempt to make the system conform to the client's needs. Patient-education activities encourage self-care and greater independence from the traditional health-care system.

We believe that the traditional health-care professional is changing his attitude toward the self-care approach. This is partly a result of consumer desires and pressure and partly because of a changing philosophy in many nursing and medical schools. The self-care approach is related to the growth of the self-help movement, and this issue will be examined later in the chapter.

Patient-Education Model

Progressive and traditional health-care professionals differ over the model used in patient education. It has been our experience that traditional health-care professionals tend to approach patient education from the perspective of the medical model: diagnosis, prognosis, and therapy. Teaching is oriented toward imparting knowledge about these three entities. Unlike medical students, nursing students (especially recent graduates) receive instruction in teaching/learning theory. Nursing students are also required to put the theory into practice, and almost all recent nursing graduates can remember being evaluated on a patient-education project. Nursing students learn that merely imparting information does not guarantee that learning will take place. Although this theoretical background has been presented, all nurses do not necessarily use the precepts of teaching/learning theory as comprehensively as they should. A recently evaluated baccalaureate student in a patient-education setting said to the patient, "Since you've had a heart attack before, I know you understand what it's all about. I'll show you a filmstrip that will give you more information." The student made no effort to assess the patient's level of understanding or his possible misconceptions about the previous myocardial infarction (MI). This student was essentially a product of the medical-model approach. (For more information on assessment in patient-education settings, see Chap. 6.)

The progressive health-care professional views patient education as part of a process with discrete steps, while the traditionalist frequently views patient education as the imparting of information. The documented lack of medical-school training in communication skills is partly to blame for this attitude.[3,4] As physician-nurse relationships become more complementary, physicians will undoubtedly become more skilled in communication techniques and nurses will gain more knowledge of medical therapeutics, so that both physicians and nurses will become better prepared to educate patients.

Sharing Information

Another philosophical issue, which also has overtones of issues relating to power and control, is that of sharing information. As noted in Table 2-1, progressive health-care providers generally tend to be more willing than traditional providers to share information with patients. One nurse related an incident that occurred in a hospital where she worked, in which a number of physicians did not want their patients told about the potential dependency effects of diazepam (Valium). In another instance, a nursing student was forbidden to make home visits to an oncology patient because the physician did not want the student to tell the patient the possible side-effects of chemotherapeutic agents. When a physician forbids a nurse to give information to a patient there are definitely issues of power and control at stake.

Obviously, there have been instances when nurses have imparted incorrect information or chosen the wrong time to attempt patient teaching. Many nurses so completely overwhelm their patients with teaching before coronary-artery bypass-graft surgery that the patients approach surgery with high, unhealthy levels of anxiety. It is the nurse's responsibility to make certain that what she teaches is correct and that she properly assesses the patient's ability to learn. It is the physician's responsibility, in keeping with the patient's "right to know," to impart all *pertinent* information to the patient in such a manner that the patient can understand the information.

Holism

The *holistic concept of man* impacts on patient education. This concept implies that we view the individual as a total, nonfragmented human being, who is a sum of all his parts.[5] When we assume the holistic approach we are interested in the total individual, not just the diseased or dysfunctional part. In the past, nursing focused on the mind–body–spirit separation, as did medicine. The medical model presumes a nonholistic approach—one looks at the child's broken leg, diagnoses it through the use of x-ray films, casts it, and prescribes an analgesic. According to the medical model, the fractured femur is the dysfunctional part and is what is treated. A holistic approach would expand the focus on the child with the broken bone to include assessing the parents' need to be taught childhood safety.

When the holistic approach to man is applied to patient education it becomes evident that patient education should include more than just teaching about a single dysfunction or problem. Another example of holism and its effect on patient teaching involves a 44-year-old man with gastric carcinoma. A nursing student who had cared for the patient in the hospital made a home visit to evaluate his status and do any necessary teaching. She found that the patient's family had learned the necessary skills of gastric lavage and jejunostomy-tube feedings and that they were doing much better with the physical care than had been expected. However, she noted that the teenage son was exhibiting inappropriate behavior by ignoring his father. During discussions with the mother and son she learned that the son feared a very bloody, gruesome death scene. The nursing student was able to clarify the misconceptions and alleviate a great deal of the adolescent's anxiety. Her holistic approach also included a referral to a local hospice group.

In the past, most nursing education paralleled medical education, and nurses were instructed according to the medical model. Some nurses still subscribe to the medical model but, as nursing education has progressed, many nurses have abandoned the old model in favor of a view of man as a unified whole. It should be added here that many young physicians are also ascribing to a holistic concept of man, and it is not unrealistic to hope for a unified nursing–medical approach in the future.

Teaching the Chronically Ill

There are differing viewpoints between traditional and progressive health-care professionals toward educating chronically ill patients. Most progressive professionals believe that patients with chronic illnesses need more in-depth teaching than is ordinarily offered by the medical regimen. Teaching patients with chronic illness involves more than indicating on a chart when medications should be taken. Nurses and other progressive health-care professionals undertake teaching about chronic illness in an effort to assist the client in attaining the highest level of wellness possible.

Ruth Wu stated in her book *Behavior and Illness* that the chronically ill person maintains a secondary role, the chronic illness role, on a permanent basis or until he becomes acutely ill, at which point he reverts back to the sick role.[6] The chronic illness role requires greater patient adaptation in most situations than does the more acute sick role. Social expectations are vague for the patient in the chronic illness role. He learns that the condition, unlike acute illness (the sick role), is not reversible, and this has great implications for the information that the patient will need to adapt. An example will clarify the need for comprehensive patient education. A nurse spent four hours with a 12-year-old juvenile-onset diabetic and her parents, attempting to educate them about the intricacies of diabetes management. This preadolescent girl and her family not only had to learn about the injection of insulin, diet, exercise, and the signs and symptoms of hypo- and hyperglycemia, but they also had to learn how to work this regimen into the life-style of a 12-year-old. At one point they realized that they had to weigh the advantages of less strict control against the possible dangers of later complications and even premature death. It is especially important to impart *all* information to the patient and his family when patient education involves a chronic illness. Long-term plans must be made and long-term goals defined by the family and nurse, working together.

The nurse educating a patient and his family about chronic illness is responsible for covering the details of the medical regimen. If, however, she does not discuss the regimen in the context of the patient's life-style (including his educational background, socioeconomic status, marital and family status, and occupation) then the teaching is virtually useless.

Preoperative teaching

An area of patient education that has recently gained attention is preoperative teaching. Physicians and nurses generally agree that preoperative teaching is helpful, but sometimes the progressive and traditional professionals have different goals for the teaching. It has been our experience that many traditionalists view preoperative teaching as a means of acquiring compliance, whereas progressive providers, although also interested in compliance, view preoperative teaching as a means of adding to the patient's psychological comfort and as one aspect of the patient's right to know.

The compliance approach to preoperative teaching is illustrated by the advertisement of one commercial patient-education company, which offered a program that would leave the patient " . . . less frightened, more cooperative . . . less likely to sue."[7] Preoperative teaching is a basic patient right, as is all patient education. The fact that preoperative teaching has been documented as a method of reducing anxiety is another important reason to program it into hospital and outpatient education.[8]

Power and Political Issues

Compliance

An important topic in any discussion of patient education is compliance. *Compliance* is defined as "the act or process of complying to a desire, demand, or proposal or to coercion" or "a disposition to yield to others."* Many traditional health-care professionals claim that the goal of patient education is compliance and that patient education is worthless if we cannot prove that it increases compliance.

Our belief is that compliance with a medical regimen is an important goal of patient education, but it is not the only goal. There is a significant process that takes place between education and compliance, in which the client internalizes the teaching and then makes informed choices about applying the teaching to his life. We would like to introduce the terms *concurrence* and *cooperation* as alternatives to *compliance.* Both suggest choice, mutuality of goals, and a patient–provider relationship based on respect and trust. Chapter 4 discusses the decision-making process and the variables that impinge upon it. As nurses we should focus on the quality and quantity of behavioral changes that result from patient education and use these data as the basis for further teaching.

It is the coercive aspect of compliance that relates this issue to power and control. Who does have power in a patient-education situation—the health-care provider or the patient? Obviously, the patient should have the control, but too often we try to control the situation for the patient, subtly threatening removal of our support or services if he does not follow our instructions. For too long, health-care providers, especially physicians, have been viewed as authority figures whose will must be obeyed. As the consumer has begun to require greater accountability of health-care professionals, many providers have responded by dropping traditional, paternalistic roles. It is our hope that all health-care professionals will eventually put aside their cloaks of authority and view compliance as one small part of the provider–client relationship, instead of as an end in itself.

Responsibility for Teaching

A second power and political issue on which progressive and traditional providers frequently disagree is that of who should teach. Nurses have a legal responsibility to provide health teaching for their patients (see Chap. 5). We have, however, found many physicians who believe that nurses should not perform health teaching. We know of cardiologists in a large medical center who refuse to let nurses teach patients who have had myocardial infarctions about management of heart disease. There are also community hospitals whose physicians require nurses to wait for an

---

*By permission. From Webster's New Collegiate Dictionary © 1979 by G. & C. Merriam Company, publishers of the Merriam-Webster® Dictionaries.

order before their patients may be shown hospital-approved filmstrips or literature. Although in some instances a physician's order is required to facilitate third-party payment for patient-teaching activities, in many situations the requirement of a physician's order for patient education is an issue of power and control.

Physicians' reluctance to allow nurses to perform this as an independent function may be related to incidents they have seen involving nurses who were clinically unprepared to teach. Licensed vocational or practical nurses (LVN, LPN) are not prepared in their educational programs to assess and plan for patient education. This is not to say that there are not many LVN/LPN patient educators who carry out effective patient teaching, but it is unrealistic to expect all of them to be as well prepared as the registered, professional nurse. Granted, there are some professional nurses who are ineffective as patient teachers because of either personality factors or lack of preparation. A few experiences with these nurses tend to dampen the enthusiasm of even the most strongly patient-education-oriented physician. On the other hand, nurses who have been rebuffed in their patient-education efforts by physicians are inclined to lose some of their enthusiasm. Patient education must be a team effort and, in our discussion of change-agentry skills, we will further discuss the positive effects of collaboration for patient education.

Most nurses are not interested in appropriating the physician's role in discussing the diagnosis, prognosis, and therapy with the patient. Instead, they interpret their role in patient education as that of making themselves available for clarification and discussion of daily management of the problem. Such a role seems appropriate for the nurse if we accept the goal of nursing as the promotion and maintenance of health in individuals, families, groups, and the community.[9,10] Again, collaboration is a key to effective patient education.

Patient-Education Referrals

The third and last political issue is the willingness to refer patients to other patient-education resources, especially self-help groups. Frequently, it seems appropriate to refer patients to extramural patient-education resources because of various factors (*e.g.,* the need for ongoing support from like-affected individuals, and the need for ongoing teaching, as in the case of the education, specialized teaching, and support found only in certain programs such as ostomy clubs and Alcoholics Anonymous).

Too often nurses and physicians are unaware of the existence of groups and resources to which patients could be referred. Ignorance of such resources is undoubtedly partly a result of the proliferation of literature with which health professionals must be familiar, but it is also representative of a lack of concern regarding the development of patients' coping and adaptive resources.

A more disturbing attitude, however, is the paternalism found among traditional health-care professionals who refuse to suggest community resources unless they can vouch for their value. The idea of "ownership" of patients by physicians, and occasionally by nurses, is not a viewpoint congruent with the prevailing belief that adults are responsible, autonomous human beings who make their own choices about health care. Thus, when a physician or nurse refuses or neglects to give a patient information about self-help groups, he has single-handedly decided that the patient is unable to judge for himself whether such a self-help group might be useful. We heard one physician who taught in a large medical center affirm his belief that it was unwise to refer patients to community self-help agencies unless the physician could personally verify the integrity of the group. Such an attitude denies the adulthood of patients and effectively places the power for decision making in the physician's hands instead of in the patient's, where it rightfully belongs.

Considering our mutual interest in patients and their welfare, it behooves all physicians and nurses to acquaint themselves with self-help groups and support groups that may aid the patient in his acquisition of an optimal level of health. The health-care consumer has already recognized the need for self-help groups, along with his growing awareness that the traditional social and medical institutions are not able to provide complete support for the handicapped, the needy, the deviant, or the socially isolated. With our recognition that we cannot be all things to all people it is imperative that, as health professionals, we hand over some of our power to self-care and self-help support groups if the client desires it.

How Differences Among Roles and Settings Affect Patient Education

In our discussion of philosophical and political issues we outlined some of the major differences between physicians and nurses in their approach to patient education. We have also discovered some areas needing change. These are discussed later in the chapter. We will now consider some of the differences in roles and settings that influence different approaches to patient education.

Differences among physicians and their approaches to patient education parallel the differences among nurses and their diverse strategies. Roles of nurses vary among institutions and even inside institutions. Some institutions employ specially prepared nurses who do all the patient teaching in one area, such as diabetes management or ostomy teaching. These nurses may be referred to as *nurse clinicians* or *clinical specialists*. Staff nurses in these institutions conduct either no patient teaching or only minimal instructing in these areas. Other institutions employ a patient-education coordinator, who may or may not be a nurse, and she is responsible for making certain that staff nurses are prepared to teach all aspects of management with which they come in contact.

Many outpatient settings are placing greater importance on the teaching role of the nurse than are most acute-care institutions. Thus, community-health nurses, school and occupational-health nurses, and nurses employed in outpatient clinics are generally spending a greater proportion of their time in patient-teaching functions than are nurses working in acute-care settings. We believe that this is changing in acute-care settings since the Joint Commission on Accreditation of Hospitals (JCAH) mandated in 1979 that patient education be documented in many clinical areas. Also, a greater emphasis recently on patient education in nursing schools has produced a young cadre of professional nurses who are aware of the benefits of, and the need for, patient education. Because most of these younger nurses are employed in acute-care settings, this has also brought about a change in the emphasis placed on patient education in secondary and tertiary care.

Our experience with physicians indicates that younger, less specialty-oriented, and less traditional physicians tend to stress the importance of patient education. They are more encouraging toward nursing efforts in patient education, and are more willing to try various innovative teaching modalities. A group of family-medicine residents with whom we worked was very enthusiastic about patient education, forming a patient-education committee with nursing personnel to enhance and promote patient-teaching efforts in the outpatient setting. On the other hand, we have had experiences with pulmonary-medicine specialists who refused to let nurses who were working on a respiratory unit initiate teaching of new asthmatics without specific orders. Other unfortunate experiences, such as with internists who have prevented our colleagues from informing patients of the side-effects of antihypertensive medications and with obstetricians who refused to let nurses prepare patients psychologically for postpartum depressions, have made us believe that the more "medicalized" a physician is, the less likely he is to respond favorably to the prospect of patient education.*

We suspect that one of the reasons patient education is so frequently a battleground for physicians and nurses is the lack of definition between roles. The nurse–physician relationship was formerly a narrowly prescribed role in which both the nurse and the physician knew what was expected of them. A role transition has taken place in nursing, engendered by nursing education and by new, expanded roles for nurses. However, many physicians have been unaware of, or unwilling to respond to, the role transition.[5] This has produced role conflict and a lack of definition of physician–nurse boundaries. Patient education is not the only arena of practice that has been affected by role conflict. A few of the other areas of conflict are diagnosis, prescription of medications, and midwifery.

Experience with such health professionals as dietitians and pharmacists supports our contention that the more clearly the role boundaries are drawn, the less likely issues of territoriality and ownership of patients are to arise. Dietitians have a long history of involvement in patient education, and nurses and physicians have characteristically called upon their expertise in therapeutic dietary teaching. Dietary teaching is a discrete area of patient education and the need for such teaching can be readily recognized. Likewise, pharmacists occupy a specific role whose boundaries with nursing are easily defined. The pharmacist–nurse relationship is complementary, as is the dietitian–nurse relationship, in that the role functions of each are very clear. Pharmacists historically have not been as involved in inpatient teaching as have dietitians and nurses, although this is changing.[11] In outpatient situations, however, pharmacists have been involved in patient education for many years in drugstores and, more recently, in outpatient

---

* Medicalization is a term coined by Ivan Illich in *Medical Nemesis* to describe the abrogation by the medical structure of functions that previously were performed societally. A medicalized physician or nurse, then, would buy into this value system and attempt to perpetuate the supremacy of medicine. (Illich I: Medical Nemesis: The Expropriation of Health. New York, Pantheon, 1976)

clinics. We have observed effective medication teaching with lower-income patients in outpatient settings where clinical pharmacists were hired for the express purpose of teaching.

In summary, we note that patient education practices vary among institution, as well as in conception and implementation of roles. We believe that patient education is undertaken with greater ease and effectiveness when roles are discrete and when respect for the various roles and for personnel on a human level is manifest.

Power in the Patient-Education Setting: Who Has It and How to Get It

We have been referring to power throughout this chapter, assuming that our readers are familiar with our use of the term. Perhaps it is appropriate now to review a few definitions. Stephen Robbins defines power as the influence an individual or group has upon the decision-making process.[12] John Wax's definition supplements Robbins's: it is "the control of resources essential to the functioning or survival of individuals and the organization."[13] Traditionally, nurses have been afraid of power and have viewed it as a magical tool possessed by physicians or as "unladylike." More recently, nurses have begun to recognize power as a legitimate function in nursing, and nurse educators have promoted its use. In this section we outline how one recognizes who has power, what the sources of power are, and how to obtain power in order to implement patient education.

Power is frequently believed to originate from some legendary, mystical source. Many of us believe it is a quality that some of us are fortunate enough to acquire at birth, rather than recognize what it truly is—a quality that is developed, over time, with a great deal of hard work. The clues to recognizing power and influence in others are subtle. In implementing patient education, ask the following questions:

- Who decides if this patient is to receive teaching?
- Who assesses the value of my teaching program and mandates its operation in the hospital?
- Whom do I approach for obtaining necessary funding for audiovisual equipment to enhance patient education?
- Who has the "word" on what is really going on in this institution?
- Who seems to be "in control" at meetings on patient education?

Since power includes decision making and control of resources, learn to answer the above questions correctly and approach the power source or sources.

Power emanates from various sources, which in turn strengthen or lessen the power. The following typology of power outlines power sources, starting with the most influential and ending with the least effective type of power:

1. Expert power
2. Positional power
3. Personality or charismatic power
4. Social power[14]

Expert power is the most effective type of power. The person with expert power knows what she is talking about and people respect what she has to say. This person may or may not possess positional power. The person who is attempting to coordinate or initiate a patient-education program must have expert power if she is to be successful in patient-education efforts. Expert power may be a type of formal power, such as that invested in a nurse–clinical specialist, or it may be informal power, as exhibited by the staff nurse to whom everyone turns when a diabetic patient needs teaching. Expert power can be developed by formal education or on-the-job training, but expert knowledge must be present to make this person credible.

Positional power is always formal power, because it is invested by the institution or organization in the individual. Persons with positional power have the ability to hire and fire, to authorize pay increases, and to set limits of acceptable behavior. Positional power is an obvious asset to the nurse who is trying to initiate a patient-education program in her institution. In the chapter on implementation of patient education we further discuss the advantages of positional and expert power.

A third type of power, which is less effective than expert or positional power, is *charismatic power* or *power by personality*. All of us have known individuals with tremendous power because of a dynamism that set them apart from others. We can readily think of political and religious leaders with charismatic power. There are also people in institutions with power based on their personalities. We know a physician who began a very successful in-house patient-education program that was quickly adopted by the medical and nursing staff because of the power of his personality. Power by personality is more efficacious if it is combined with either expert or positional power. The support of an individual with charismatic power can be a tremendous asset in beginning a patient-education program.

The fourth, and least effective, type of power is *social power*. Social power is the power that one has through social relationships and friendships. It is power given by a group to its informal leader. The aspects of social power that make it least useful are its dependence on relationships, its lack of substantiveness, and the underlying premise that something is owed in return for the granting of social power.

Social power, like expert power and personality power, can be a type of either formal or informal power. Head nurses frequently use social power in an attempt to get a staff to accept changes. It is not unusual for the director of nursing in a large hospital to employ charismatic power or expert power; in fact, she is probably a more productive director if she is able to use these types of power as well as the more formal kinds. A combination of power types is usually very effective, but expert power is a necessity for anyone who wants to be recognized as an able patient educator.

Once the questions about who has the power have been answered and the type of power has been identified, a number of directions can be taken. An obvious response is to develop expert power. Since this usually takes some time to develop, it may be desirable to gain knowledge from the one with expert power by spending time observing her *modus operandi*. This is also the time to gather as much formal training and education as possible, through reading books and journal articles and attending seminars and classes. For instance, one nurse who was hired to develop and assume a job as coordinator for patient education in a community hospital spent the first six months in her new position identifying powerful figures among physicians, nurses, and other hospital personnel. She also improved her already formidable knowledge about patient education by attending conferences on patient education, by reading extensively, and by working closely with graduate students in health education to develop a needs assessment for the hospital. After six months she solidified her power, which was previously positional, by displaying her knowledge of patient-education needs in the hospital and being recognized as an expert in her field. Positional power continued to undergird her authority, and expert power enhanced and strengthened her power in the hospital.

After assessment of the institutional power structure and establishment of a power base, change may be necessary. The following section addresses the planned change process, and appropriate change-agentry skills are introduced and elaborated.

Planned Change and Change-Agentry Skills

The nature and process of change is still not well understood, although many social scientists and some nursing leaders have recently developed theories and models that attempt to explain it.[15,16,17,18] Planned change entails organizing for change or applying scientific-method/problem-solving skills: assessment, planning, implementation, and evaluation.[19] Examples of situations in which change-agentry skills have been applied to patient education illustrate the usefulness of these skills.

The Duke University School of Nursing, during a series of nine conferences, developed three levels of process skills for nurses. These skills were designated as Level I, Basic Process Skills for Nursing; Level II, The Components of Nursing Practice; and Level III, Change Process Skills.[19] The Level III skills are those we are interested in introducing here. As Joanne Hall states, these " . . . skills are those which can be employed to facilitate change in client systems and constitute the power armamentarium of the nursing practitioner as a change agent."[19] These change-agentry tools are (1) inquiring, (2) helping, (3) teaching, (4) supervising, (5) coordinating, (6) collaborating, (7) consulting, (8) bargaining, (9) confronting, and (10) lobbying. To increase her power in the patient-education arena, the nurse–change agent must become proficient in skills 5–9. The other five skills should also be employed, but we chose to concentrate on the five named above. This is partly because these skills greatly enhance the professional image of the nurse, and it is also because many nurses are somewhat afraid to develop proficiencies in such powerladen areas. We are introducing two other change-agentry skills we have found useful in diverse patient-education settings. We are referring to the first of these as *reframing*, realizing that this term is frequently used in psychotherapy but also appreciating that it is useful in our context. The second skill we are introducing is *coercion*.

Coordinating

Change agentry in patient education involves organizing and bringing together various approaches and health-care professionals in such a way that high-quality patient education is delivered. The nurse who uses this type of coordination as a change-agentry skill recognizes the contributions and capabilities of others involved in patient education and arranges patient-education programs to meet the needs of varied client groups.

In a community hospital that had recently hired a master's-prepared nurse to establish a hospitalwide patient-education program, the change-agentry skill of coordination was used in the following manner. In committee decision-making situations the patient educator repressed her tendency to want to control and, instead, facilitated the decision making by *not* asserting her power or authority. She openly recognized the nurses and physicians on the patient-education task force as the experts, and she assisted them in designing teaching protocols.

Coordination skills were also used to assist the patient-education task force in setting goals. The goal was to create a product that would be strongly desired and then to make that product very visible. By developing a product, the members of task force enjoyed an enhanced image and the entire task force was given increased credibility.

Collaborating

The process of working in a creative and egalitarian manner can be used to further promote the welfare of the client in the patient-education setting. The nurse who integrates such collaboration as a change-agentry skill is respected by physicians, pharmacists, dietitians, and other health professionals because she is willing to share her expertise with others. Collaboration precludes the negative approaches of territoriality and ownership of patients.

In the community hospital discussed above, collaboration was used creatively by the patient educator to set a tone of cooperation. She employed *validation* as a strategy to prevent members of the task force from becoming entangled in the decision-making process. Validation consisted of documentation and carefully written minutes that were circulated before every meeting. By validating the process that was taking place, she was able to establish a spirit of mutual cooperation and appreciation of others' contributions.

Another way in which she used collaboration was through her obvious ability to work within the environment of the community hospital and to deal with the constraints imposed by the institution. The fact that she was able to work creatively with administrators, physicians, and the director of nursing immeasurably improved her chances of successfully implementing a hospitalwide patient-education program.

Consulting

There is a reciprocal relationship between the nurse with proficiency in patient education and the consultee seeking her skills. The nurse shares her expert knowledge in order to further the practice of sound patient-education concepts. The nurse as consultant has effective communication skills and uses them to assist the consultee in developing patient-education resources and programs. In using consultation as a change-agentry skill, the introduction of the consultant into the consultee's work setting is avoided.

In our example, the patient-education coordinator assumed her role as consultant by first clarifying her own understanding of her role. She realized that she occupied a staff position and not a line position; thus, there were limits on her authority and ability to discipline, hire and fire, or set policy. Instead, she had been employed for her considerable managerial and organizational skills and to provide the impetus for the establishment of a patient-education program.

She avoided a common consultant mistake by refusing to actually practice patient education. She thus did not interject herself into the nurses' work setting. When a patient-education coordinator uses consultation to effect change it is inappropriate for her to assume the actual task of educating patients. Instead, she should teach the nursing staff the principles of teaching/learning theory and other relevant information.

Furthermore, this coordinator herself took on the role of consultee when she sought help from other departments. In addition to increasing her visibility in the hospital, she also managed to secure some valuable contacts for later use. For example, the coordinator consulted the medical-records department to determine the most frequent diagnoses on admission. Her ability to move from the consultee to the consultant role provided beneficial role modeling for the nursing staff.

Bargaining

The nurse–patient educator and another person (or persons) often must negotiate agreements. The agreements usually involve the procurement or delivery of patient education to a needy client group. Bargaining is a positive process through which both parties derive satisfaction. In the patient-education setting, bargaining may also occur between a nurse and a client, with both bargaining for mutually satisfactory and achievable goals.

Bargaining is a splendid change-agentry skill that many of us rarely use. Like all such skills, it must be accomplished in a setting where rationality and calmness prevail. Emotional debates were avoided by the patient-education coordinator, and if someone exhibited obnoxious, strident behavior during meetings it was ignored and not held against him in future meetings.

The coordinator bargained effectively when the goals of certain patient-education programs were questioned. Instead of compromising goals, however, she agreed to changes in content and strategy. When bargaining is used as a change-agentry skill, the nurse must remember that negotiating a bargain is a give-and-take proposition and that some important ideas may have to be traded away.

Confronting

The various perceptions held by different people in a patient-education setting must be clarified and compared. Confrontation involves face-to-face communicative encounter between the nurse and another health professional or the patient. Reserve the powerful change-agentry tool of confrontation for situations involving a lack of direct, open communication. Use confrontation only after other change-agentry skills have been exhausted.

When using confrontation as a change-agentry skill, be aware of the two levels of response it usually evokes: emotional and intellectual. Recognize and identify the emotional response, but do not respond to it. The intellectual response allows room for reasoning. Do not use confrontation in an attempt to impose beliefs on another, but to establish an environment that will encourage a new approach to the problem. For example, when the patient-education coordinator realized that territoriality was becoming an issue, she turned the decision-making focus toward patient care and patients' rights.

When involved with confrontation, consider the amount of authority and support held by the person being confronted. If he is not powerful, the optimal method of confrontation may be to override him. If he does possess support and authority, summon the committee members to attempt to change his mind. These group members must have equal influence and power for this method of confrontation to work. The term *confrontation* often has negative overtones. Attempt to remove the emotional, "battle-lines" aspect of the term.

Reframing

When a situation is viewed in an entirely new light, old ideas and methods can be replaced with new approaches.[20] This reframing is different from confronting in that the nurse reworks or restates the situation for the patient or client group. This frequently involves introducing an entirely different perspective into patient education. When old problems are broached in a different light, new avenues can be taken.

This different perspective in patient education may be brought by the patient or the institution, or it may be the perspective of a particular committee member. An example of reframing occurred when we spoke to the medical staff of an outpatient center, presenting patient education as more than an attempt to gain compliance and as a basic feature of the patient's right to know. One physician who had obviously been pondering this idea said, "I see what you are saying; it's like informed consent."

Coercing

Legal authority can be used to gain an end that is not attainable in any other, less forceful, fashion. Coercion avoids emotional overtones, focusing instead on institutional and federal regulations. Coercion is better applied to recalcitrant groups of health professionals who are unwilling to institute patient education than it is to individual clients. Coercion is usually a last-resort change-agentry tool; apply it only when all else has failed.

When a patient-education coordinator was stymied by one "blocker" physician, she used coercion by having an administrator exert power from above, after showing him that the blocker was obstructing the goals of the organization. This change-agentry skill makes many of us feel uncomfortable; it is not a skill we are taught as nursing students, and women in general are not encouraged or taught to use coercion. At times, however, it is the only effective way of achieving the desired goal.

The use of critical incidents, such as a high rate of diabetic readmissions or JCAH probationary accreditation, can coerce reluctant people or institutions to effect change. When the staff of a community hospital was informed that they did not meet JCAH criteria for acceptable patient education, they ceased arguing the merits of patient education and began planning better programs.

Other Strategies

Using open-ended questions to probe the attitudes of recalcitrant patient-education task-force members has led to greater understanding of some unspoken, underlying issues. When opposition to the matter at hand becomes very strong, another good tactic can be to retreat and compromise rather than continue waging war. When using this strategy, however, it is unwise to go back to the beginning of the process, as all gains would thus be nullified. A third strategy is to reinforce the base of support and make it stronger. A change agent needs all the help she can get, and she should constantly reinforce her position through the help of others. It is also important to look inward if things are not going well. Perhaps an undesirable response has been provoked by the nurse–change agent. Increasing credibility is another strategy to effect change. Showing is better than talking, and it is imperative that other health professionals believe the change agent is an expert in her area. High visibility in an institution does not guarantee credibility.

Nursing Suggestions

In other chapters we suggest specific implementations for patient-education plans and programs. We wish, however, to caution nurses that expectations must remain realistic in all patient-education contexts. Nursing's battle for professionalism and respect is still being waged and, while the struggle continues, philosophical and political issues will remain intense. Even with our armamentarium of change-agentry skills, we will not be able to change some of the entrenched, traditional attitudes that prevail. While planning for the future, we also need to concentrate on the moment at hand, and that includes accomplishing necessary patient-education tasks and persevering as strong advocates for the patient.

Deal with the issues of territoriality and ownership of patients in all institutional settings in an open, honest manner. It is true that physicians have a legal responsibility for the care of the patient, and they are probably the most vulnerable in terms of lawsuits. It is also true, however, that nurses have a responsibility, mandated by many states' nurse-practice acts, to educate clients in health practices. When ownership of the patient becomes the battleground, no one wins, least of all the patient. An adult patient is an autonomous, free human being and, as such, is not owned by either physician or nurse. Once we all accept this point, many philosophical and political issues will wane.

Another suggestion is to look at the situation in a positive light. Instead of assuming that a physician who wants to write orders for patient teaching is against nursing's efforts to promote patient education, consider him as contributing to the team effort. We frequently draw battle lines too sharply, creating polarization over a relatively minor issue. We need to save our energies for the important debates, not dissipate them over trivial matters.

We suggest that nurses strengthen their natural alliance with other allied-health professionals in order to increase their power base. Many other allied-health professionals are also contending for more autonomous, independent roles. It behooves nurses to offer support when pharmacists attempt in-house patient teaching about discharge medications, or dietitians attempt to get third-party reimbursement for community classes on obesity and weight control. Group patient-education classes that have been co-taught by nurses and other health professionals have experienced success and are a positive initial means of forging the alliance.

References

1. Ritchey R, Raney M: Medical role-task boundary maintenance: Physicians' opinions on clinical pharmacy. Med Care 19, No. 1:90–93, 1981
2. Orem D: Nursing: Concepts of Practice, p 13. New York, McGraw-Hill, 1971.
3. Perrin E, Goodman H: Telephone management of acute pediatric illnesses. N Engl J Med 298, No. 3:130–135, 1978
4. Farsad P, Galliguez P et al: Teaching interviewing skills to pediatric house officers. Pediatrics 61, No. 3:384–388, 1978
5. Menke EM: Conceptual basis for nursing intervention with human systems: Individuals. In Hall JE, Weaver BR (eds): Distributive Nursing Practice: A Systems Approach to Community Health, p 82. Philadelphia, JB Lippincott, 1977
6. Wu R: Behavior and Illness. Englewood Cliffs, Prentice-Hall, 1973
7. Levin L: Patient education and self care, how do they differ? Nurs Outlook 26, No. 3:174, 1978
8. Lindeman CA, Stetzer SL: Effect of preoperative visits by operating room nurses. Nurs Res 22, No. 1:4–16, 1973
9. Hall JE: Distributive health care and nursing practice. In Hall JE, Weaver BR (eds): Distributive Nursing Practice: A Systems Approach to Community Health, p 5. Philadelphia, JB Lippincott, 1977
10. Roy C: Introduction to Nursing: An Adaptation Model, p 18. Englewood Cliffs, NJ, Prentice-Hall, 1976
11. Witte K, Gurwich EL, Anzalone R, Campagna MA: Audit of an oral anticoagulant teaching program. Am J Hosp Pharm 37:89–91, 1980
12. Robbins SP: The Administrative Process. Englewood Cliffs, NJ, Prentice-Hall, 1976
13. Wax J: Power theory and institution change. Social Service Rev 45, No. 3:284, 1971
14. EC Murphy Associates: Managerial Power. In-house consultant series. Buffalo, Communications in Learning
15. Bennis WG, Benne KD, Chin R: The Planning of Change. New York, Holt, Rinehart, & Winston, 1969
16. Watzlawick P, Weakland J, Fisch R: Change: Problem Formation and Problem Resolution. New York, WW Norton, 1974
17. Lewin K: Field theory and social science: Selected theoretical papers. In Cartwright D (ed): New York, Harper & Row, 1951
18. Brooten DA, Hayman L, Naylor M: Leadership for Change: A Guide for the Frustrated Nurse. Philadelphia, JB Lippincott, 1978
19. Hall JE: Nursing as process. In Hall JE, Weaver BR (eds): Distributive Nursing Practice: A Systems Approach to Community Health, pp 173–191. Philadelphia, JB Lippincott, 1977
20. Clark CC: Reframing. Am J Nurs 77:840–841, 1977

Bibliography

Books

Aiken LH (ed): Health Policy and Nursing Practice. New York, McGraw-Hill, 1981

Berger MS (ed): Management for Nurses: A Multidisciplinary Approach. St Louis, CV Mosby, 1980

Beyers M, Phillips C: Nursing Management for Patient Care. Boston, Little, Brown & Co, 1979

Caplan RD: Adhering to Medical Regimens: Pilot Experiments in Patient Education and Social Support. Ann Arbor, Research Center for Group Dynamics, Institute for Social Research, University of Michigan Press, 1976

Clark CC: The Nurse as Group Leader. New York, Springer-Verlag, 1977

Claus KE, Bailey JJ: Power and Influence in Health Care: A New Approach to Leadership. St Louis, CV Mosby, 1977

Cohen SJ (ed): New Directions in Patient Compliance. Lexington, MA, Lexington Books, 1979

Douglass LM, Bevis EO: Review of Leadership in Nursing. St Louis, CV Mosby, 1977

Douglass LM: The Effective Nurse: Leader and Manager. St Louis, CV Mosby, 1980

Epstein C: Effective Interaction in Contemporary Nursing. Englewood Cliffs, NJ. Prentice-Hall, 1974

Loomis ME: Group Process for Nurses. St Louis, CV Mosby, 1979

Mauksch IG, Miller MH: Implementing Change in Nursing. St Louis, CV Mosby, 1981

Moloney MM: Leadership in Nursing: Theory, Strategies, Action. St Louis, CV Mosby, 1979

Redman BK: Issues and Concepts in Patient Education. New York, Appleton-Century-Crofts, 1981

Squyres WD: Patient Education: An Inquiry into the State of the Art. New York, Springer-Verlag, 1980

Stevens WF: Management and Leadership in Nursing. New York, McGraw-Hill, 1978

Yura H, Ozimek D: Nursing Leadership: Theory and Process. New York, Appleton-Century-Crofts, 1981

Journals

Becker MH, Maiman LA: Strategies for enhancing patient compliance. J Community Health 6, No. 2:113–135, 1980

Bernstein R, Andrews E, Weaver L: Physician attitudes toward patients' requests to read their hospital records. Med Care 19, No. 1:118–121, 1981

Borman LD: Self-help and the professional. Soc Policy 7:46–47, 1976

Glanz K, Kirscht JP, Rosenstock IM: Linking research and practice in patient education for hypertension. Med Care 19, No. 2:141–152, 1981

Green LW: Research and demonstration issues in self-care: Measuring the decline of mediocentrism. Health Educ Monogr 4:161–189, 1977

Robbins JA: Patient compliance. Primary Care 7, No. 4:703–711, 1980

Schain WS: Patients' rights in decision making: The case for personalism versus paternalism in health care. Cancer 46, No. 4:1035–1041, 1980

Tax S: Self-help groups: Thoughts on public policy. J App Behav Science 12:448–454, 1976

Chapter 3

Economic, Implementation, and Evaluation Issues

Patient education is an appealing concept. Our visceral reaction is that the instructed patient fares better than the uninstructed one. It is, however, very difficult to evaluate concretely the positive outcomes of patient education. Because of this difficulty, problems arise in financing, implementing, and evaluating patient education. This chapter explores these problems.

The section on financial issues discusses funding sources for programs in both the inpatient setting and the community. Third-party payments, hospital-assessed fees, and other funding agencies such as private foundations are considered as possible long- and short-term revenue sources. The reciprocal relationship of power and political issues and funding issues is noted.

The section on implementation views the issues, taking into account their interrelations with financial and evaluation issues. Specifically, acquisition of the support and advisory aid of administrators, physicians, and other health professionals is addressed, as are the later steps that must be taken to activate a patient-education program. Examples involving hospital-based and community-based patient-education programs are shared to help the reader gain some knowledge of the many issues and problems involved in implementation.

The evaluation issues confronting the nurse and other health professionals are discussed in the third section of the chapter. A model for evaluating patient-education outcomes is presented to aid the practitioner in developing an evaluation model. The problems involved in evaluating the outcomes in individual or small-group patient-education programs as opposed to those in the mass-education approach are defined. (See also Chap. 9.)

Finally, we offer suggestions for enhancing the implementation process, as well as for sharing and alleviating the burdens of funding and evaluation.

Financial Issues

When a group of nurses was interviewed about patient education, all expressed a need for patient-education services in their institutions; however, all raised the issue of payment. As one stated, "Everyone's bill will increase and this is unacceptable to the consumer." She also voiced her observation that many hospital administrators consider patient education a "frill." Although evidence exists that some consumers are willing to pay for education, many are unable or unwilling to foot the bill for patient education programs.

Not surprisingly, hospital administrators also tend to be reluctant to approve spending of increasingly tight money for patient education. As some hospital administrators have said, "If patient education really works, then eventually our census will go down and we'll be unable to keep the hospital afloat." Others ask, "If we cannot prove that patient education works, then why attempt it?"

Because of inflationary times, coupled with governmental attempts to seriously curtail federal spending for all health care, many must ask, "Where on the priority list is patient education placed in my institution?" Many of us have heard administrators give lip service to patient education, only to find that there is no money to implement plans, or that nurses are expected to conduct patient education on either their own time or an overtime basis. We know of one outpatient clinic that established very successful prenatal classes for its own patients and other interested patients from the community. Nurses developed, taught, and evaluated the five-part series. Patients were charged for the classes through a "prenatal package," but when the nurses requested compensatory time for the hours they spent teaching, the clinic was frequently unable to guarantee it. These same nurses were unable to channel income from the classes toward buying a badly needed labor-and-delivery film. It is difficult to believe that an institution highly values patient education when it is unwilling to allocate resources for implementation.

Nursing-Staff Time: How Much Is There and Who Pays for It?

Nursing-staff time is one of the thorniest problems involved in financial issues. Nursing administrations, prompted by patient-education enthusiasts or prodding by the Joint Commission on the Accreditation of Hospitals (JCAH), frequently mandate patient teaching by staff nurses. In addition to the motivational, organizational, and training aspects of beginning a new patient-education program, the question of time allocation arises. The three questions of time allocation are the following:

1. How do we find enough time in a busy 8-hour shift to implement patient education?

2. If extensive patient education is going to be planned and implemented, what *type* of staffing hours will be required (*i.e.,* how many RN and LVN/LPN hours must be allocated)?

3. If extra hours beyond regular nursing-staff hours are allocated for patient education, who pays for them?

The first question is the one most frequently raised by nursing-staff members when approached about patient education. Frequently we hear, "I'd love to do patient education but I don't have the time with all the paperwork and other demands placed on me." We feel that many golden opportunities for patient education are lost during the typical day. For instance, bath time can be used for teaching the diabetic about good skin and foot care, the surgical patient about dressing or cast care, the chronic-respiratory-disease patient about breathing exercises, and so on. Medication time can be used to teach the congestive-heart-failure patient how to take his pulse before self-administering digitalis or to teach the rheumatoid-arthritis patient how he can safely taper off steroids. Any time we enter a patient's room can be a golden opportunity to do some patient teaching. The astute nurse who does make use of these moments must also remember to document her teaching in the patient's chart.

The second question, involving types of staffing for patient education, must be faced straightforwardly. It does require more RN hours to accomplish high-quality patient education. There are very few LVN/LPNs in any setting who have been taught to design, execute, and evaluate patient-teaching activities. Such sophistication requires RN staffing. As many hospitals increasingly move toward primary nursing and all-RN staffing, this problem will be alleviated. The small community hospital that is heavily dependent on LVN/LPNs and aides, however, will not be able to deliver as much high-quality patient education as will the larger or more professionally staffed institution. We found LVNs involved in prenatal education in an outpatient setting to be willing and enthusiastic about attending classes but unprepared and unable to lead patient discussions or teach didactic or lecture components of the class.

The question of who pays for patient-education time must be faced realistically. Although we do believe that many golden moments are lost during the course of a working day, there is no doubt that extensive and comprehensive patient education requires time above and beyond the work requirements of a normal nursing shift. The only way to obtain extra hours for patient education is to document carefully the amount of time required to complete each patient-education activity. One hospital that was already involved in extensive patient education for myocardial-infarction (MI) patients examined medical records retrospectively and realized that only 14% of all patient teaching was completed during the highest census month, while 80% was achieved during the lowest census month. The staff then began to keep careful records of patient-teaching needs and managed to document that an extra two hours each week would be sufficient time to organize necessary patient-teaching activities.[1]

Figure 3-1 provides a simple method of calculating the costs of current patient-education programs. The data obtained from this chart can be used to justify current costs as well as to plan for future needs. The data also indicate the extent of various departments' involvement. If the cost is going to be distributed throughout the hospital or agency, each department will know the extent of its share.

Staff time needed for patient education will vary with the number of disease processes covered, the sophistication and experience of the nurses involved, the usefulness of the patient-teaching protocols, and the amount of preparation the

PATIENT EDUCATION PROGRAM/ACTIVITY

Activity	Personnel involved	Hours spent	Cost/ hour	Resources used (materials, equipment, other)	Costs
		Total	Total		Total

Fig. 3-1. *Patient Education Program Chart. (Reprinted, with permission, from* Implementing Patient Education In the Hospital, *published by the American Hospital Association, copyright 1979.)*

staff has had in teaching/learning theory. Documenting the number of hours required for patient education can be combined with documenting the patients' responses to education; this eventually helps in evaluating the overall effects of the patient-education program.

The third question, that of who pays for nurse–patient instructional hours, leads to our discussion on sources of funding.

Funding Sources

Anne Somers estimated in 1976 that it takes approximately $25,000 to $50,000 for a medium-sized community hospital to initiate a patient-education program.[2] Included in this estimate are the salary for a patient-education coordinator and secretarial, office, and promotional expenses. Somers further estimates that this budget would be equal to about 5% or 6% of the hospital's budget. Patient-education costs are considerable, but they are small compared with many other hospital expenses. Part of the funding dilemma in patient education can be blamed on the relative lack of knowledge among nurses about budgetary and financial matters.

Most staff nurses do not have to worry about the financial exigencies of their institutions. This tends to be true whether the institution is a hospital, doctor's office, group practice, Visiting Nurse association, or public-health department. Thus, when administrators ask nurses how they would obtain reimbursement for patient education, the nurses are usually unprepared to produce a plan. Nurses, beginning with nursing students, need to be taught the financial bases for operating large institutions. Ignorance among nurses in such areas serves only to exalt administrators and keep nurses in a subservient role.

Financial preparation could help a nurse understand which patient-education expenses would constitute legitimate, reimbursable costs. In addition, she would have increased understanding of what types of costs must be limited to handling by specific departments and which can be "floated," or carried by other departments.

Many of us complete nursing school with the belief that it is unethical to charge patients for nursing services. Therefore, when we first encounter the financial aspects of patient education we are inclined to offer patient education as *part of basic nursing care.* Admirable as this idea may be, it does not work well as the funding basis for patient education. In effect, it means that patient education is free and that it will be one more service added in the interests of good patient care. The most common product of this approach is the frustrated nurse, who quickly realizes she is unable to deliver high-quality patient education as well as attend to her myriad other duties.

Nurses' own perceptions of themselves and their profession also influence their attitudes about charging for patient education. The old image of nurses as merciful angels of charity is a difficult one to shake. We see ourselves as delivering a service—at times, indeed, a charitable service—and we frequently feel that we should not accept payment for this service. Hand in hand with this image, and related to our own feelings of worth as women, goes the question of how much our time is worth. If we view our time as relatively worthless, it is likely that the public will reflect this image back to us. A profession is defined partly by the public's perception of it, and as long as we are viewed as nonprofessional technicians we will have little luck in enhancing our own self-image. It is a vicious cycle that at times seems to spiral out of control.

Once the goodwill of nursing service as a basis for providing patient education has been exhausted, the next logical step is to approach hospital administrators. Hospital administrators are frequently envisioned as villains. Unfortunately, nursing administrators frequently use them as scapegoats in an attempt to justify their own actions to unhappy nursing-services employees. Frequently, the hospital administrator will support the idea of patient education and take the path of least resistance in funding it—*an increase in patients' room or bed costs.* In essence, every patient is assessed a fee that is added to the basic daily hospitalization fee. Since the daily costs of patient education is assumed by all, the fee per patient is generally very small—about $1 per day. Since this fee is usually "hidden" in the room rate, it appears as if patients are receiving patient education for free. Third-party payments cover this fee and, compared with the cost of a liter of intravenous fluid ($10), medication expenses, or the cost of virtually any nursing procedure, the fee seems minuscule. Such funding also supplies enough revenue to accomplish broad-spectrum patient-education efforts; a 500-bed hospital with 80% use of beds could expect to realize as much as $146,000 a year from the $1/day fee. It must be recognized that most administrators and patient-education coordinators are unable to estimate the daily cost of patient education. Because patient education is subsumed under the daily room charge, most of those questioned simply stated that patient-education costs were absorbed by the hospital.

Arguments against this type of funding include the fact that the majority of patients pays for the teaching of a few. If the only teaching program in a hospital is oriented toward teaching post-MI patients, then it would seem unfair to charge every patient for these services. A second argument against such funding is that the consumer seems to learn better, and more, when he is taking the financial responsibility for his own patient education. In the United States, many people subscribe to the philosophy that "you get what you pay for," and their logical conclusion is that if you cannot tell what you are paying for, it cannot be worthwhile.

It is our feeling that these arguments are somewhat specious. First, as patient education becomes more important in inpatient and outpatient settings and as consumers demand more education, patient-education programming will become more comprehensive. Second, we are observing a trend toward prevention among the better-educated public. As the cost of health care skyrockets, the public's openness to patient education and preventive approaches increases correspondingly.

We have observed that most hospitals of more than 400 beds offer some sort of patient-education program. Many of these hospitals have classes and tours for expectant parents, nurses for teaching ostomy patients and diabetics, and programs for comprehensive cardiac rehabilitation, as well as plans to expand into other areas. The argument that one expects to get what one pays for does apply to the middle-class, motivated, and well-informed patient. These patients will, however, probably make the effort to become informed on their own. The patient who needs patient-education services the most (*i.e.,* the poor, unmotivated, semiliterate patient) is at a disadvantage if patient education is not paid for by all. This patient is the least likely to have health insurance and also the least likely to be able to pay out-of-pocket fees for patient education.

Another source of funding is to *charge each patient individually* for patient teaching. An example of this type of funding is teaching by a community-based dietitian who conducts group classes for diabetics for a flat fee of $5 or $10 per class. It has been our experience, however, that this type of funding is very similar to third-party reimbursement because insurance companies frequently cover such fees if classes are ordered by physicians. We know of one outpatient clinic that offers five individual one-hour sessions to diabetics, taught by nurses at the cost of $5 per session. Most third-party agencies have been willing to pay for the sessions as long as they are ordered by physicians. When a client is not covered, the cost of the classes is waived. The state of California has recently adopted a plan whereby third-party carriers are mandated to reimburse diabetic patients for education in self-management of diabetes. There is speculation that such legislation may open the door to other program reimbursement by third-party carriers. Reimbursement for diabetic self-management is not dependent upon a physician's order.

We have mentioned *third-party reimbursement* as another avenue to explore for the financing of patient education. Essentially, this involves obtaining approval from local third-party-payment agencies for specific patient-education programs. If the third-party agency agrees to pay expenses for all patients who participate in a program they have approved, then it is unnecessary to have a physician's order to gain reimbursement. However, most insurers are loath to reimburse the consumer if the teaching is not ordered by a physician. This is an unfortunate policy because it effectively deprives the individual patient of his efforts at self-care, it reduces the important role of prevention, and it denigrates the nurse's role in prescribing patient education for needy clients. Nurses are attempting to gain autonomy in this arena and, at present, the American Nurses' Association is working toward this goal.

The role of third-party payments in the financing of patient education is substantial. Presently, Blue Cross and Blue Shield carry more than half of all insured individuals participating in private health-insurance plans. Blue Cross is also the agency named by the federal government to act as "fiscal intermediary" for Medicare in most parts of the United States.[3] This means that Blue Cross approves and sets standards for Medicare claims. Thus, if Blue Cross approved a patient-education program for third-party reimbursement, then payment for such a program should also be covered by Medicare.

Other third-party-payment agencies are the private-for-profit type, such as the Paul Revere Insurance Company and Aetna Insurance. The nurse looking for patient-education revenue is advised to start her quest with her area's largest provider. If Blue Cross approves a patient-education program, the chances of the smaller, private-for-profit carriers' approval are enhanced.

One outpatient clinic with which we are familiar was able to obtain third-party reimbursement for the participation of nurses in patient education by following this plan:

Physicians referred patients to nurses for home teaching and counseling in the following areas: diet teaching, contraceptive counseling, diabetes review, prenatal nutrition, and breast-feeding problems. Nurses made home visits during the early morning or late afternoon because both were slow times at the clinic. During the home visits, the nurses were able to assess the patients' home environments and do the necessary teaching in a setting that usually allowed for greater patient comfort than the clinic could provide. After the visits were made, the nurses documented their teaching and any other pertinent information on the progress-notes section of the chart.

Billing for such teaching visits was handled in the following manner. The visits were each billed as one of four types of "professional fees" and were submitted as such to the third-party-payment agencies. For purposes of internal record keeping, however, the clinic's computer registered each encounter as a home visit by a nurse. At the end of a year it was possible to tell how many home visits were made by nurses and for what teaching purposes. The patients benefited from such a charging system because the costs of the visits were not as high as those for office visits with a physician. Benefits that accrued as the result of this approach were increased credibility of the value of nurses' contributions to patient education, increased physician appreciation of the team approach, an improved image of nursing among patients, and increased administrative appreciation of the nursing staff's concern for a balanced budget and realistic fees for service.

Besides third-party reimbursement there are other sources for funding that should be considered. An appendix at the end of Chapter 8 lists *voluntary and commercial agencies* that may be helpful in supplying media useful in patient education. We have also found some of these voluntary groups helpful in providing start-up funding.

Another source of funds that should be considered by any institution initiating a pilot patient-education program is private *grants from foundations.* Appendix A to this chapter lists the names of some foundations as well as a directory of foundations. Foundation grants are usually time-limited, but they can be very helpful when an institution needs funds to persuade recalcitrant staff, through a pilot project, of the efficacy of patient education.

An example of a successful statewide patient-education program that received its impetus from foundation grants is the system in New Jersey. The College of Medicine and Dentistry of New Jersey (CMDNJ) organized a plan in 1972 whereby CMDNJ provides patient-education information to community hospitals in a partnership created by the medical school and a network of hospitals and primary-care settings. In addition to leadership and technical assistance, start-up funding is also provided by CMDNJ in the form of grants from a private foundation controlled by CMDNJ's board of trustees. In order to receive a grant, a program must meet a number of criteria including participation of consumers, support from the medical staff and agency board of trustees, and ability to maintain the program after the grant expires.[2]

New Jersey's plan could serve as a prototype for other states eager to tackle patient education on a statewide, or smaller, level. The able leadership of Anne Somers, a physician, has strengthened this program. Many articles in medical, nursing, and hospital journals have made health professionals aware of the program's existence.

Interface of Political and Financial Issues

The connection between power and political issues and financial issues should not be overlooked. Obviously, if the people who control a budget are opposed to patient education, it will be much more difficult to implement a program. Our experience in hospitals has been that if hospital administrators and key physicians believe in the efficacy of patient education, then implementation becomes fairly straightforward and simple. On the other hand, if these people feel that patient education is a "frill" and not beneficial in terms of cost, it is extremely difficult to initiate patient-education programs.

In the latter type of situation it is sometimes possible to sell patient education to the nonsupportive administrative and medical staff as an image maker. In other words, patient education becomes more appealing when it is marketed to the community as an agency attempt to reduce the high cost of health care through prevention, as a purveyor of better patient services, and as a way of securing more consumer participation. In fact, in some communities with many medical facilities, patient education has been used as an advertising "come-on."

In this era of rising health-care costs caused by the technology explosion, decisions about the expenditure of increasingly tight funds must be made. Most hospitals will choose to spend funds on computed tomography (CT) scans and leasing of heart-assistive devices (intraaortic balloon pumps) before they will budget funds for patient education. Attempts to control the high costs of health care through what we believe are sane approaches, such as the Kaiser health plan and health-maintenance organizations (HMOs), are becoming increasingly frustrated. The public, urged on in many instances by health professionals, is demanding greater technocracy and more lifesaving assistive devices, which cause the costs of health care to skyrocket. The high costs of technological advances, therefore, demand that patient education be marketed in increasingly clever ways.

In addition to the influence of decisions made by hospital administrators and political influence on financial issues, we must also consider the power exerted by physicians in setting priorities for patient education. The power and influence of certain physicians will frequently dictate which programs are implemented first. If the chief of staff decides that diabetes education is the most important priority in his hospital, it would not be surprising if the initial output of funds were directed towards diabetes education. Ideally, an assessment of patient-education needs should be conducted first; however, this frequently does not occur. In such a situation the nurse who desires a strong patient-education program would be well advised to support the chief of staff's plan and implement a vigorous patient-education program in diabetic teaching, which then could serve to garner support for other patient-education programming.

Financial issues necessarily overlap with implementation issues. For instance, how does one set priorities for spending funds for patient education? Do we spend money first on human resources or on hardware (*e.g.*, audiovisual equipment)? This section covers implementation issues related to the actual establishment of a patient-education program.

Implementation Issues

Implementation is the act of fulfilling or accomplishing. Before the process of patient education is completed, a number of steps that we refer to as the *implementation process* must be accomplished. An outline of an orderly process for implementing patient education follows, along with a discussion of the issues confronted during implementation.

Although we have instituted individual patient-education programs to meet the needs of particular client groups, we do not recommend this single-shot approach to implementing patient education. This approach tends to be hurried and crisis-motivated, in that staff efforts are directed toward assuaging the needs of the most obviously needy group. Instead, we suggest conducting a systematic patient-education needs assessment.

Needs Assessment

A needs assessment requires about six months to complete, but it is the cornerstone for planning and implementing patient education. Such a needs assessment will allow for long-range planning and direction, so that continuity of program planning is assured, independent of changes in leadership or personnel.

Table 3-1, outlining the various steps that should be taken in assessing a particular institution's patient-education needs, has been prepared by the American Hospital Association. It can also be modified for use in assessing outpatient educational needs.

Table 3-1. **Institutional Assessment Guide**

Assessment Tasks and Questions	Possible Sources and Methods of Collection
Hospital Philosophy, Goals, and Policies	
Review the hospital's statement of philosophy and goals for patient care. Can these goals be met without patient education?	Obtain documents from administration or department heads.
Review the goals of hospital departments. Which departments have goals that relate to patient education?	Obtain documents from administration or department heads.
Review the medical staff's policy-and-procedures manual. Which statements or policies on informed consent have been developed?	Interview administrator. Also, obtain medical staff's policy-and-procedures manual.

Table 3-1. **Institutional Assessment Guide** *(continued)*

Assessment Tasks and Questions	Possible Sources and Methods of Collection
Organization of the Hospital Staff	
What nursing staffing patterns does your hospital have for each shift?	Interview or send a questionnaire to the director of nursing and head nurses.
How is nursing care organized by the unit and by the patient?	Interview or send a questionnaire to the director of nursing and head nurses.
What medical coverage is available at your hospital?	Interview or send a questionnaire to the chief of staff.
What other professional groups (*e.g.,* dietitians, social workers) have patient-care responsibilities? When are they in the hospital, and how is their time for patient education allocated?	Interview or send a questionnaire to department heads.
Patient-Care Support Staff	
Who on the nursing staff (*e.g.,* clinical specialists) has clinical responsibilities but is not assigned to patient care on a specific unit?	Interview the director of nursing.
What are the assignments of these members?	Interview the director of nursing.
Who on the staff is responsible for orientation and continuing education of the clinical staff?	Interview or send a questionnaire to department heads.
Are patient-education skills or performance included in job descriptions or performance evaluations?	Interview or send a questionnaire to department heads. Also, interview appropriate personnel-department staff.
Which students use the hospital as a clinical setting? When are they on the units? What kinds of responsibilities do they have on the units?	Interview or send a questionnaire to those responsible for different student groups or instructors.
How are volunteers being used at your hospital?	Interview the head of the volunteer department.

(continued)

Table 3-1. **Institutional Assessment Guide** (continued)

Assessment Tasks and Questions	Possible Sources and Methods of Collection

Characteristics of the Patient Population

What are the most common diagnoses of patients admitted to the hospital?	The data systems developed by hospitals vary; interview administration to find what is available, especially from the medical-records department.
What are the most common diagnoses found on each unit? What are the average lengths of stay and ages of patients with these diagnoses?	The data systems developed by hospitals vary; interview administration to find what is available, especially from the medical-records department.
What are the trends in health-care problems presented by discharge diagnoses over the past five years? What are those predicted for next five?	The data systems developed by hospitals vary; interview administration to find what is available, especially from the medical-records department.
What are the most common diagnoses of patients who use outpatient and emergency departments?	If no data are available, do a chart audit for outpatient and emergency groups.
What does your hospital use to measure patient satisfaction with services provided? What problems have patients identified?	Interview administration or specific departments, including patient representatives if applicable.
Are there any data available to describe the patient population that uses the hospital or one of its departments (*e.g.,* by age, place of residence, or social, cultural, or economic variables)?	Interview or send a questionnaire to administration, the research-committee chairperson, the public-health department, or other community agencies.

Patient Admission

What information is currently being given to patients *before* they enter the hospital's inpatient or outpatient departments? When, by whom, and in what format is this information being given?	Interview or send a questionnaire to members of the admissions department (both inpatient and outpatient), public-relations department, and emergency room, as well as to admitting physicians, patients, and community-referral agencies if applicable.

Table 3-1. **Institutional Assessment Guide** *(continued)*

Assessment Tasks and Questions	Possible Sources and Methods of Collection

Patient Admission *(continued)*

What is the admitting process? What steps would most patients follow?	Interview or send a questionnaire to members of the admissions department.
Which staff members have contact with patients during the admitting process? Do these staff members see any problems of misinformation or unrealistic expectations during this process?	Interview or send a questionnaire to members of the admissions department.
How are bed assignments made?	Interview or send a questionnaire to members of the admissions department.

Patient-Care Process

What patient-history information is collected during the patient admission? What part of this information could be helpful in determining the patient's educational needs?	Review a sample of patient records. Interview unit staff involved in patient care.
Who determines patient-care goals? How are the goals revised? Is team planning a part of determining patient-care goals?	Interview head nurses (managers for patient-care units).
How does the staff document patient-education activities and outcomes?	Interview head nurses (managers for patient-care units).
What patient-education information is included in discharge summaries?	Interview head nurses (managers for patient-care units).
If your hospital has developed standard care plans, what are their patient-education components?	Review standard care plans.
Identify staff included in your process of audit. Define their roles.	Interview members of the audit committee.
How are the populations for development of criteria for audit determined? Are patient-education criteria part of the audit? In your completed audits, were the patient-education criteria met?	Interview members of the audit committee.

(continued)

Table 3-1. **Institutional Assessment Guide** *(continued)*

Assessment Tasks and Questions	Possible Sources and Methods of Collection
Patient-Care Process *(continued)*	
Did the last visitors from the JCAH make comments about the hospital's patient-education activities?	Interview the administrator.

Staff Perceptions of Current and Needed Patient-Education Programs

What activities do the staff members on each shift define as patient-education activities currently being implemented?	Interview or send a questionnaire to department heads, supervisors, and head nurses. Have informal meetings with staff groups.
What materials or media are being used for activities?	Same as above
Would the staff like to see these activities changed? How?	Same as above
What new patient-education activities would the staff like to see implemented?	Same as above
Which staff members on each shift have been involved in patient education for specific populations? In what specific patient education were they involved?	Same as above
Which staff members who are not yet involved in patient education are interested in participating?	Same as above
Which people do staff members identify as their patient-education resources? Which medical staff are especially supportive of hospital staff conducting patient education?	Same as above

Completeness of Existing Patient-Education Programs for Specific Populations*

Have written objectives been established for the program?	Extensive interviews with the staff responsible for the program, as well as those who participate in it. Review of written materials about the program. Observation of actual implementation of teaching activities.

*Note: This assessment should be completed for each patient population for which a program has been developed. When available, written materials such as content outlines and handouts should be collected.

Table 3-1. **Institutional Assessment Guide** *(continued)*

Assessment Tasks and Questions	Possible Sources and Methods of Collection

Completeness of Existing Patient-Education Programs for Specific Populations* *(continued)*

Is patient progress or outcome of the educational experience documented?	Same as above
Does the program use a common content outline or handouts?	Same as above
Are predetermined teaching methods defined and used?	Same as above
Has there been multidisciplinary involvement in patient-education planning and implementation?	Same as above
How is the program individualized to meet specific needs of patients?	Same as above
Are the written policies and procedures adequate for smooth running of the program?	Same as above
Have specific staff members been given responsibility to implement parts of the program?	Same as above
How are new staff members trained to participate in the program?	Same as above
What percentage of the target population is reached by the program?	Same as above
Has this program benefited the patient or his family? What is the evidence?	Same as above
What are the major program needs, as defined by the involved professionals?	Same as above
Have patients provided feedback on what they think about the program?	Same as above

*Note: This assessment should be completed for each patient population for which a program has been developed. When available, written materials such as content outlines and handouts should be collected.

(continued)

Table 3-1. **Institutional Assessment Guide** *(continued)*

Assessment Tasks and Questions	Possible Sources and Methods of Collection

Patient-Education Resources Within the Hospital

What media and materials are currently being used for patient education? Where are they housed? If some of the materials are purchased, what funds are used?	Obtain examples from the media department, library, or education or in-service departments.
What media equipment does the hospital own? Could it be used for patient education? What kind of expenditures will be made in the next year for audiovisual software and hardware? Have long-range goals for using media in the hospital been determined (*e.g.,* implementing a closed-circuit TV system)?	Interview appropriate managers to determine production and distribution processes.
Are funds budgeted for patient education within staff education or public relations?	Obtain information from appropriate managers.
Does the hospital have an active auxiliary? Is the auxiliary interested in patient education?	Explore this with the auxiliary president and members.

Patient-Education Resources in the Community

Which voluntary health agencies are located near the hospital? What is their involvement or interest in patient education?	Interview (phone) representatives of major organizations.
Which patient-education activities are performed by the health department?	Interview people responsible for health education and public-health nursing.
Which community agencies (*e.g.,* Visiting Nurses' Association) are involved in follow-up patient care? What do they see as their patient-education activities? Is there a feedback system already set up between the hospital and these agencies?	Identify agencies through staff involved in discharge planning.
Which patient-education activities are being conducted by other hospitals in the city?	Interview representatives. Talk with administration or nursing to identify.
Which are the formal and informal professional groups in the area with major interests in patient health education?	Interview representatives. Contact the local American Society of Health Education and Training groups, the Society of Public Health Educators, colleges with departments of health education, and so forth.

The needs assessment does not have to be conducted in a vacuum; other patient-education activities can be taking place while the needs assessment data is being gathered.

Appointment of a Steering or Advisory Committee

It is important that a patient-education steering committee be appointed early in the implementation process. The steering committee acts in an advisory fashion and should be composed of physicians, nurses, administrators, and others having an active interest in patient education. The patient-education coordinator is usually the person responsible for initiating the committee and she should judiciously gather recommendations for committee members. Appointment of physicians should be made by the medical staff, although the patient-education coordinator can attempt to have physicians appointed who are known proponents of patient education. Likewise, nurses at the decision-making level should be appointed to the steering committee with the input of the nursing-service coordinator. The historical involvement of such health professionals as dietitians, pharmacists, and physical therapists may make their membership valued in some institutions. Efforts should be made to include other health professionals because their cooperation can enhance patient-education programs.

After the assessment guide has been completed, the patient-education coordinator will have a data base that will aid in organizing and directing her efforts. The patient-education advisory committee can use these data to plan for future patient-education efforts.

While the needs assessment is being conducted and the advisory committee is being appointed, the patient-education coordinator and those working closely with her should begin a review of the literature to discover what types of programs have worked, why they have been successful, and where they have been located. There is a great deal of information we can gather from the successes and mistakes of others, and it is limiting to ignore the ever-increasing quantity of material about diverse patient-education programs. This is also a propitious time to make contacts with patient-education coordinators in other community and inpatient settings. They will be able to share ideas about the needs of the community, as well as help to prevent a duplication of efforts.

Establishing Goals and Priorities

Once the patient-education needs assessment is completed, it is time to set goals and priorities for the development of programs. The advisory committee should be aware of the import of wisely choosing the first specific patient-education program to be implemented. If the steering committee decides that a comprehensive preoperative teaching program should be established, but the chief of surgery is opposed to preoperative teaching, the program will be doomed to failure and future programs will emerge under a pall. It is best to start with what promises to be a very successful program. There will be many unforeseen problems along the path of implementation that will test the resolution of those involved—poor program selection will only compound these problems.

Task Forces for Specific Programs

After priorities and goals have been established, a task force willing and able to establish a specific patient-education program should be appointed. If the highest priority is to establish an adult-onset-diabetes education program, then the committee should consist of health professionals involved in caring for diabetic patients. It is important that there be physician membership on this committee because approval must be gained from the medical staff to implement the diabetic-teaching program. It should be recognized, however, that including physicians on such task forces does not always guarantee wide medical-staff approval. We are aware of one community hospital that wished to implement preoperative teaching. Its task force, including physicians, approved a comprehensive preoperative teaching plan, but when the plan went to the medical staff some surgeons refused to approve the system outlined by their colleagues.

Learning from Personal Experience

We believe that nurses can learn from the successes and mistakes of others and, therefore, we will outline some of the experiences we have had in establishing an inpatient and an outpatient education program. Neither of these programs was part of the systematic process we have outlined. Both projects, however, can be viewed as successful if measured in terms of their staying power: both are still being implemented (one is in its fifth year, the other in its third). Each can be used to illustrate some of the financial and implementation issues involved in patient education.

The first program was an innovative and immensely successful, program for diabetic patients and their families. The original impetus for the program came from a health-education graduate student, who was working in the hospital's educational and staff-training department, and me (S.R.); at the time I was a nurse in-service educator in the same department.

The patient group chosen, adult diabetics, turned out to be a wise choice because diabetics are a highly visible and needy patient group, because education of diabetics tends to be standard, and because many health professionals, including physicians and nurses, find teaching diabetics time consuming and tedious and are only too happy to turn them over to someone else for instruction. If the patient population had been a group for whom treatment is not agreed upon universally (*e.g.,* the post-MI patient), we probably would have encountered more resistance, especially from physicians.

A second implementation issue was the general appeal of the program to all hospital staff. A luncheon at which diabetics and their families could learn about diet and other aspects of diabetes management had an immediate acceptance, partly because of its rather novel approach. In fact, the program was later covered by the local newspaper, garnering some favorable publicity for the hospital.

Cooperation from ancillary health-services departments, such as dietary and pharmacy, was assured from the beginning. This alleviated the problem of gaining wider support. These departments absorbed the cost of staff time in their general operating budgets.

The needs assessment was completed in a rather perfunctory fashion, by a one-week audit of pharmacy records to determine the average daily load of patients on oral hypoglycemics or insulin. The time elapsed from the initial inception of the idea until implementation was only two months.

One of the original assumptions in creating the diabetic luncheon program was that nursing-staff time would be saved by the education of patients and their families in groups. This proved to be unfounded, however, and the issue of time required for patient education arose. Staff nurses were asked to help prepare patients for the luncheon by obtaining filmstrips for them from the education department. They were also expected to identify suitable patients for the luncheon and to secure a physician's order for each patient to attend. All of these tasks definitely added to the time nurses already spent teaching patients about insulin injection and urine testing.

A power and political issue confronted in this project was that of who would select the patients to be involved in the program. Staff nurses in the institution functioned in a traditional role and were accustomed to having a physician's order for everything. Although most physicians would have been pleased to have the nurses assume the responsibility for sending a patient to the luncheon, the nursing staff would not do so without a physician's order. An unforeseen benefit of seeking physicians' orders, however, was that the physicians became aware of the program and actively encouraged their patients to attend.

A fifth implementation issue, which interfaces with philosophical issues, arose when I (S.R.) became identified as "the diabetes-teaching nurse." My role was to coordinate the teaching on the ward and cover one segment of teaching during the luncheon. Because of my visibility in the program, however, physicians began writing orders stating "patient is to be educated by diabetes-teaching nurse." Staff nurses, accustomed in the past to performing basic diabetic-teaching activities, were very willing to give up this function and depend on me. It is highly preferable that the staff nurses with whom the patient has his primary relationships should do the bulk of the teaching.

Another experience that illustrates this dilemma is one recounted by a hospital patient educator. A young, pregnant patient with newly-diagnosed diabetes was admitted to the medical intensive care unit with ketoacidosis. After she was stabilized physiologically, the staff called the patient-education coordinator with a request for her to come to the unit and teach the patient because the diabetes nurse educator was on vacation. These nurses had become so dependent on the nurse who routinely taught diabetic patients that they felt ill prepared to teach even the basics of insulin injection.

One of the financial issues that resulted from the diabetic luncheon involved the expense of staff time. The dietary, pharmacy, and education departments assumed the costs of any of their staff who participated in the teaching project. The only charge to patients and their family members was the cost of the lunch. No effort was made to obtain third-party reimbursement for the diabetes education.

Other costs included the audiovisual materials that were purchased so that patients and their family members could watch filmstrips before the luncheon. The education department assumed this expense.

The pharmacy purchased kits for diabetic patients and charged each patient a small fee for the kit and a paperback book. The costs of the entire teaching program were so minimal in relation to each department's budget that the question of financing the program never arose. However, if similar programs had been initiated for other patient populations, financial issues would have been more prominent.

Our experiences with a prenatal outpatient program are also useful in examining some financial and implementation issues. In this case, the financial issues were more prominent than implementation issues.

Implementing the prenatal classes in the outpatient-clinic setting was relatively easy. Again, the needs assessment was very simple. Physicians, residents, and nurses were polled to ascertain their perception of the most critical patient-education needs. Many areas for teaching were mentioned, but the most frequently named need was prenatal teaching. The clinic was staffed primarily by residents participating in a three-year family-medicine residency that was sponsored by a large medical center and a county hospital. The clinic served all socioeconomic groups but, because of its low fees, attracted many indigent families.

Many of the prenatal patients were unmarried adolescents and young adults. Already operative in the community were very successful Lamaze and Bradley childbirth-preparation classes, however, because the orientation of Lamaze and Bradley is to include the coach (usually the husband) and also because these classes tend to attract middle- and upper-income couples, the young, unmarried women our clinic was serving did not feel comfortable in those classes. The Red Cross also sponsored classes, but these were held on an infrequent basis and did not meet the needs of our clients. Therefore, classes for the clinic's prenatal patients seemed appropriate.

Another reason for the clinic's eagerness to sponsor its own classes was the staff's desire for the patients to learn their approach to prenatal and obstetric care. The use of analgesics and anesthetics during delivery was discouraged; breathing exercises and breast-feeding were encouraged.

The issue of territoriality never became a problem because of the implementation process of integrating the residents into the classes. Nurses coordinated and taught most of the five classes cooperatively with the residents. Input from the residents, who followed their patients through labor and delivery and observed them postpartum, was used to evaluate the program and formulate future classes. The fact that nursing students from a local university were included in the teaching also helped to diffuse the territoriality issue.

Another benefit that accrued to the clinic was a positive community image. The prenatal classes added to the clinic's desired reputation of being oriented toward preventive medicine and education.

The prenatal classes were originally developed when I (S.R.) was a graduate student, as part of my graduate curriculum and independent study. The clinic did not initially have to involve its own staff in the creation of the classes (although the actual teaching did later become a staff responsibility); therefore, the issue of use of staff time to develop classes was not a problem.

Although implementation went smoothly, financial issues arose when I ceased teaching the classes. After graduate school, I began teaching in the nursing school of the local university, using the clinic as a setting for student experiences by continuing to teach the classes, at no charge to the clinic, and incorporating my students into the classes. When I stopped teaching the classes, the head nurse (and coauthor) began teaching and coordinating the classes. The clinic administrators first proposed compensating the head nurse for her time through a compensatory-time mechanism. Because of her heavy responsibilities, for which she had to be present during the day, this was not considered realistic. During this time the head nurse tried to involve some of the other clinic nurses, who were paid on an hourly basis, in the classes. The decision to involve these nurses was based on role and job enhancement. Most of the nurses declined involvement when compensatory time was offered as the reimbursement for evening hours of teaching prenatal classes. They found the mechanism of compensatory time as opposed to monetary compensation unsatisfactory because they had family responsibilities and children, necessitating additional child-care expenditures for those evening hours.

Some nurses were willing to teach on a time-and-a-half basis, to which the administration eventually agreed. The salaried nurses (head nurse and nurse practitioner) were usually not compensated for their evening teaching responsibilities.

The issue of financing the classes was solved by charging all prenatal patients a set fee for the clinic's prenatal package. One of the items in the package was the prenatal teaching program. Since this charge was buried in the total package cost, there was no problem with getting third-party reimbursement.

Other expenses were handled in various ways. Pamphlets handed out for each class were obtained free of charge from the U.S. Government Printing Office and pharmaceutical and infant-formula companies. Films were borrowed from the state's health-firm library, free of charge. Staff brought healthy snack foods and fruit juices, for which the clinic reimbursed them.

These experiences help to illustrate some of the implementation and financial issues we have confronted in both inpatient and outpatient settings. Obviously, various settings and diverse programs will provoke other situations, completely different from those we experienced. We hope, however, that these examples will serve to illustrate the fact that, even with such issues and problems arising, it is possible to implement patient-education programs.

Evaluation Issues

Evaluation of patient-education programs presents some of the most difficult problems encountered in the entire patient-teaching venture. What, how, and when to evaluate are all questions that must be answered before the evaluation process can begin. We will attempt to answer these questions and will propose a model for evaluating patient-education programs. A sample tool used in the evaluation of the aforementioned prenatal classes is presented in Chapter 11 (Fig. 11-1). We are referring in this chapter to the evaluation of *programs,* not the evaluation of the individual learner's experience. Evaluation of the individual patient's learning is discussed in Chapter 9.

We believe that evaluation should be an integral part of program planning. A means of evaluation should be built into the original program design. The inclusion of a design for evaluation in any proposal for funding will make third-party-payment agencies and health-care administrators more likely to approve the proposed program. Evaluation frequently occurs after a program has been operational for a while. This type of evaluation procedure is not as effective as an originally planned evaluation that is suitable to the educational intervention or planned teaching program.

Outcomes to Be Evaluated

When the program is being formulated, it is important to decide which outcomes are going to be evaluated. There are many different outcomes and it is impossible, if not inappropriate, to evaluate all of them.

As discussed in Chapter 2, many of the more traditional nurses and physicians view the outcome of patient education in terms of desired *patient compliance*. Although it is true that compliance is desirable, there are many other positive outcomes that can accrue as a result of patient education. Therefore, one of the issues in evaluation becomes how to decide which outcome should be evaluated and whether this outcome indicates that the program is, indeed, beneficial.

The desired outcome must be related to the type of intervention. For example, the desired outcome of educating a group of 13-year-olds on the relationship of cigarette smoking to cardiovascular disease and lung cancer is *prevention* of smoking. The desired effect of such education with a group of the teenagers' smoking parents, however, is obviously *cessation* of smoking.

As more research is done on the relationship of *knowledge acquisition* to behavioral change, we realize that acquisition of knowledge does not always guarantee the desired change. When we apply this to our group of cigarette-smoking parents we may decide that a more realistic immediate outcome is simply knowledge about the effects of smoking. Perhaps later a behavioral change (cessation of smoking) will take place; this may or may not be related to the knowledge acquisition. In any case, an argument can be made for improving and increasing the patient's knowledge and understanding of his health status even if it does not lead to improved adherence to, and cooperation with, the medical regimen. Increasing the patient's understanding of his health can be interpreted as part of the patient's legal right to know. We believe he deserves the information even if he does not choose to act on it.

Another outcome to be considered is the *patient's satisfaction with his health-care provider*. In the literature, this is commonly referred to as *physician satisfaction* or *nurse satisfaction*. It has been demonstrated that one of the two factors most closely associated with compliance is the patient–provider relationship.[4] Presumably, the patient who is satisfied with this relationship will feel comfortable asking questions to gain more knowledge about his condition. One of the desired outcomes of the prenatal classes was improved patient–provider relationships. Our experience indicated that patients who attended the prenatal classes frequently called the nurses who taught the classes for advice during the prenatal and postpartum periods. Because they attended the prenatal classes they became better known to the nursing staff, who in turn gave more personalized care. A spiral effect thus takes place when patient satisfaction increases, so that the patient feels more comfortable in his relationship with the provider, the provider knows the patient better and individualizes his treatment more, and the patient is able to ask more questions and improve his understanding of his health status.

We may also wish to evaluate a *reduction in patient anxiety and fear.* The relationship of preoperative teaching to positive postoperative outcome was mentioned in Chapter 2. Other studies have shown that preoperative preparation can reduce the anxiety patients experience during induction of anesthesia,[5,6] in the recovery room,[7] and in the postoperative period.[8] In addition to reducing anxiety in the surgical setting, patient education can reduce anxiety and fear in diagnostic procedures such as cardiac catheterization, in health-maintenance settings such as prepared-childbirth classes and school-health programs, and in maintaining health and controlling complications in chronic-illness situations such as arthritis and chronic renal failure. The patient who is contending with a potentially fatal illness such as breast cancer also needs education to alleviate her anxiety.[9] The anxiety and fear related to hospitalization are perhaps the most devastating concomitant of illness and the one in which we can intervene most easily. As nurses we know how to reduce unhealthy anxiety to a lower level and how to deal with patients' fears of the unknown. We can use moderate levels of the patient's anxiety to his advantage by teaching him problem-solving mechanisms and stress-reduction methods.

Knowledge is power, and by sharing information with our patients we can help them to gain a means of *controlling feelings of powerlessness.* This alleviation is important for all hospitalized patients and their families because the sensation of powerlessness may be greater in the hospital than anywhere else. A college teacher recently spoke of the experience she had when her mother died five days after the initial onset of symptoms and diagnosis of pancreatic cancer. During her mother's hospitalization she repeatedly asked for information from her mother's physicians and nurses. She asked them to explain the diagnostic tests they were doing, the surgery that was contemplated, and the treatment that was planned. As she watched her mother get progressively weaker and more jaundiced, she asked more questions but received very few answers. Her inability to understand what was happening to her mother compounded her feelings of helplessness as her mother got worse. The mother died of a massive pulmonary embolus with her daughter at her side. The daughter later said that if she had been given the information she had requested she would not have felt so powerless in the situation. She was accustomed to processing information and using intellectualization as a healthy coping mechanism, but at the time of her mother's illness and death she was denied this tool and made acutely aware of her own powerlessness.

Norman Cousins's popular book, *Anatomy of an Illness,* outlines a process for adapting to a chronic illness and lessening feelings of powerlessness.[10] One component of this process is patient education. When Cousins was able to obtain information about the pathophysiology of his disease, he was able to take control of his medical regimen and make decisions that affected his recovery. Decreasing the patient's feelings of powerlessness implies a willingness of health-care professionals to share information, a philosophical issue discussed in Chapter 2.

Patient confidence levels are another outcome we can evaluate following a patient-education intervention. Experience with many different types of clients in patient-education settings indicates that they frequently do not feel confident of their skills and information as applied to management of health or illness situations. Patient confidence is especially important when learning a skill is involved or when knowledge is related to prevention or to potentially dangerous situations. For example, it is essential for the spouse or significant other of an insulin-dependent diabetic to feel confident giving insulin so that in times of sickness or emergency the other person can intervene. Prenatal patients frequently express fears about their ability to remain in control during the contractions of labor and delivery. By teaching the patient such techniques as slow, deep breathing, we can improve the patient's confidence that she can exert some control over her pain. A sample questionnaire that tested confidence levels in a pre- and post-test situation is presented in Chapter 11 (Fig. 11-1).

Another example of the importance of an outcome of increased confidence is the prevention of potentially dangerous situations, such as can be achieved with knowledge of cardiopulmonary resuscitation (CPR) for the prevention of sudden death. Spouses of myocardial-infarction patients frequently express regret that they did not know what to do before help arrived. Many hospitals are now teaching spouses of cardiac patients how to perform cardiac massage and mouth-to-mouth resuscitation. Likewise, parents of infants frequently fear that their children may choke, and fear they would be unable to respond if their child should aspirate an object or have difficulty breathing. Teaching the Heimlich maneuver to these parents is an easy intervention that can greatly enhance levels of confidence. Another area in which parents express a lack of confidence is in taking infants' rectal temperatures. It is easy for a nurse to teach a parent how to take a rectal temperature safely, and thus help increase the parent's feeling of self-confidence in management of sick children.

Another outcome that may be evaluated is the *ability of the patient to present himself at the most propitious time for early diagnosis and treatment.* With increased emphasis on self-examination of breasts, many women are coming in earlier for diagnosis and treatment than they did in the past. Although the mortality rate remains high (about 50%), the survival rate in terms of years for breast cancer seems to be increasing.[11,12] A second example of this type of outcome is the reduction in mortality from heart disease that has been documented during the 1970s and 1980s.[13] The fact that deaths caused by heart disease have decreased is related to a number of factors, one being that people are recognizing the signs and symptoms of heart attack and gaining treatment earlier. In cities like Seattle, which initiated an intensive program to train the populace about CPR and the signs and symptoms of heart attack, more heart-attack victims arrive alive at hospitals than do victims in cities with less informed populations.[14,15]

These outcomes can be assessed many different ways, and all are worthy as evaluative measurements. Many of the outcomes overlap and influence one another, but each is worthy in itself as a positive outcome of patient education. We will now discuss sources of data, also referred to as feedback, that can be examined to determine outcomes.

Feedback: Sources of Data in Evaluation

Data can be obtained from a number of sources to evaluate patient-education programs. The broad areas from which these data can be abstracted are patient behaviors and attitudes, staff behaviors and attitudes, health outcomes such as morbidity and mortality statistics, and formal medical records.

Patient behaviors as a source of feedback data can be assessed from the staff's observation of the patient or from the patient's reported behaviors. If the outcome to be evaluated is prompt presentation of patients for diagnosis and treatment, the feedback mechanism can be staff observation of patients who are reporting symptoms and requesting treatment. For example, a group of physicians who had patients enrolled in our prenatal classes reported that after the patients attended classes there were more attempts to breast-feed, more attempts to control pain nonpharmacologically during labor and delivery, more pertinent questions asked during office visits.

Patient knowledge as an evaluation outcome can be assessed through the patient's reported behaviors. An example of reported patient behaviors is diaries, such as those submitted by asthmatic patients following a teaching intervention. In a study of asthmatics conducted at the Johns Hopkins Hospital, those patients who had attended discussion groups on asthma reported fewer symptoms of breathlessness, wheezing, and chest tightness than did those in a control group.[16]

Patient attitudes measure outcomes such as increased confidence and decreased powerlessness. These attitudes can be obtained by questionnaires or through patient interviews. For an example, see our prenatal confidence-level questionnaire (Fig. 11-1). It is often desirable to obtain the attitudes of patients' families, as well as those of the patients, toward a particular program.

Staff behaviors are an important part of the feedback mechanism in evaluating outcomes, especially when outcomes such as patient compliance and patient knowledge are desired. It is possible that the reason a desired outcome has not been achieved is that the program has failed during implementation because staff did not do their part. For example, evidence shows that physicians overreport the amount of information given to patients.[4] Therefore, if the program depends on the physician's transmission of information and this is not actually accomplished, the desired outcome of increased knowledge will not be achieved. Feedback related to staff behaviors can be obtained through a review of medical records or a review of encounter forms (the forms that detail diagnosis, treatment, and the amount of time the provider spends with the client). Other methods of obtaining even more specific data include observing or videotaping client–provider interaction. Simulations of patients interacting with providers will show how the providers respond and how well the patient-education program is being implemented.

Staff attitudes are an important source of feedback about the efficiency and value of patient-education programs. This feedback is frequently the easiest to obtain because staff are the first to observe the effects of patient education. Positive feedback about new mothers' adoption of successful breast-feeding techniques indicates to the providers of patient education that their teaching methods are beneficial. Conversely, feedback from physicians that diabetic patients are exhibiting weight gains, high blood or urine glucose levels, or lack of understanding about the exchange diet plan can be an indication that the methods of teaching the exchange diet system need reexamination.

Nursing staff members working in specialty units frequently report that they can easily distinguish which patients have received patient teaching by their responses to pain and other stresses of hospitalization. For example, delivery-room nurses are heard to say, "You can tell by her panic and screaming that she hasn't had any preparation for childbirth." In a specialty unit that receives all the coronary-artery bypass-graft and valve-repair patients, it is very simple to determine which patients have received preoperative teaching by the fear and constant anxiety exhibited by those patients who have received no preparation.

Health outcomes that can be obtained from morbidity and mortality data are another important form of feedback. Morbidity and mortality data can be obtained fairly easily for large populations, cities, counties, states, and nations from sources such as county public-health departments and state and federal bureaus of vital statistics. These data are inappropriate feedback for evaluating small patient-education programs not found throughout the community. Such data are, however, essential for evaluating the effects of such programs as the community wide CPR program instituted in Seattle or a seat-belt and car-safety campaign. Also, the fact that deaths from heart disease have decreased since 1970 was determined by examining mortality statistics for the United States. Most public-health officials believe that this reduction was related to widespread health-education efforts, which concentrated on such risk factors as diet and exercise.[13] If we are interested in studying the effects of a patient-education campaign to reduce morbidity and mortality related to brown-lung disease in a community with textile mills, we can examine the data as compared with those in a similar community without health-education practices for textile-mill employees. These feedback data take longer periods of time to collect than some of the previously mentioned feedback mechanisms, but they offer an effective manner of evaluating health education aimed at great numbers of people.

Formal medical records such as patients' charts, encounter forms, and data that hospitals and other agencies have available through records and computer systems can be examined in an effort to determine the efficacy of certain patient-education programs. For example, a study that assessed the effectiveness of a "hot-line" telephone service for diabetic patients reviewed medical records to determine the number of unnecessary clinic visits and hospital admissions that were forestalled by the institution of the hot line. Hospital admissions and unnecessary clinic visits had been significantly reduced.[17]

The use of computerized record keeping has eased the collection of such data as the most frequent diagnosis on admission in a specific hospital or outpatient agency. This makes it possible to evaluate programs by need as well as outcome. In most instances there is much more available feedback than most patient-education evaluators realize.

Evaluation Model

We have considered outcomes and feedback mechanisms for the evaluation of patient-education programs. We have also discussed implementation and financing. The evaluation model that we are presenting includes all points covered in this chapter and views evaluation from a general systems-theory perspective. We believe that evaluation is a constant, ongoing process and not a separate entity from the total educational process. Therefore, systems theory, including the processes of input, throughput, output, outcome, and feedback, lends itself well to this discussion. *Input* is the information or energy that the system brings in; *output* is the product that the system creates from its inputs. For example, total input in patient education is the patients, staff, economic and material resources, and the committees for a specific patient-education program. Output is the patient-education program derived from the total input. *Throughput* is the *process* by which the input becomes output. Throughput in patient education refers to the implementation process of planning and establishing patient-education programs. *Outcome* is the result of the output. In a patient-education system, the targeted outcome is to have patients functioning at optimal health and psychosocial levels. *Feedback* is the information that the system receives about itself to aid in achieving better performance in the future. In patient education, feedback is the information we use to evaluate outcomes. We have not, by any means, presented an exhaustive explanation of systems theory; however, these definitions will suffice for our purposes.

Figure 3-2 is a general model that can be applied to any patient-education program. It can be particularized for various patient education settings by plugging in the input, throughput, output, outcome, and feedback for each particular setting. An example of its specialized use is given in Chapter 11 (Fig. 11-2).

Evaluation of Large-Scale Health-Education Programs

Evaluation of large-scale health-education programs is also accomplished in terms of outcomes. The feedback mechanism, however, usually takes a longer period of time to become operational and data can be more difficult to collect than with small-scale programs.

As mentioned previously, there have been incidents of successful health education at the national level (*e.g.,* the decrease, demonstrated in national mortality statistics, in heart-disease deaths). Public health education that began in earnest around the turn of the century has greatly improved nutrition, promoted better sanitation, increased immunization against communicable diseases, and enhanced maternal–child health. The morbidity and mortality data of the United States for the past 80 years make these health-education efforts very apparent.

Other health-education efforts, such as campaigns to promote the use of seat belts and attempts to decrease cigarette smoking, have been singularly ineffective as measured by morbidity and mortality data. If the outcome to be evaluated for these campaigns were simply knowledge acquisition, then we could safely say that the outcome has been achieved. The American public knows that

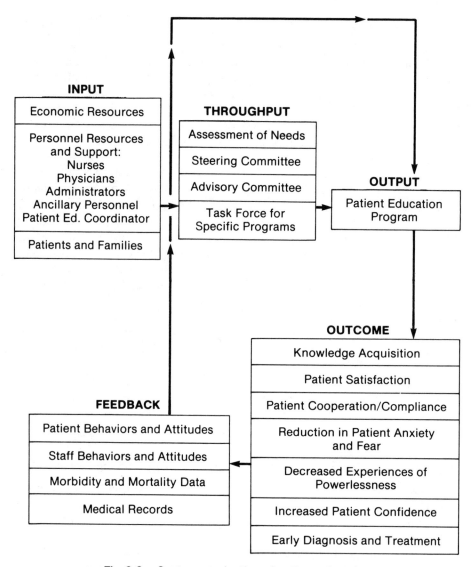

Fig. 3-2. *Systems evaluation of patient education.*

cigarette smoking is closely linked to lung cancer and vascular disease and that using seat belts reduces the number of fatalities and serious injuries from automobile accidents. Obviously, knowledge acquisition has not brought about the most desired outcome—behavioral change. Many variables affect the successful implementation of such campaigns and, until we better understand these variables, achievement of the desired outcomes will elude us.

Evaluation Research

Lawrence Green, head of the Division of Health Education at the Johns Hopkins University, has examined the dilemmas in evaluating health education and proposed a number of approaches to better evaluation techniques.[18] As he observes, the traditional research methods that attempt to reduce placebo effects, demand rigor, and increase internal and external validity also tend to dilute the strength of the intervention and alter the nature of patient education. Evaluation research is one avenue that can be used to deal with some of the dilemmas.

Evaluation research uses the scientific method to make an evaluation. Unlike basic evaluation, which is the process of making a judgment concerning the value of some activity or program regardless of the method employed, evaluation research examines a specific program using the problem-solving method. (*Research*, as distinguished from *evaluation research,* is not usually applied to a specific program but is instead intended to add to the general body of knowledge.) Therefore, evaluation research can be effectively applied to patient education programs when we need to have specific data on the basis of which we can formulate future program proposals, compete for limited resources, and analyze cost benefits. Evaluation research can contribute to improved planning, implementation, and accountability in patient-education programs.

Evaluation research focuses on *process*, *outcomes*, and *goals*. The *process* component of evaluation research, when applied to patient education, concerns the actual implementation of patient education (*i.e.,* the program or intervention and its content). It is just as important to focus on the process as on the outcomes, so that knowledge is generated about the methodologies that actually work in patient education. If only the outcomes are evaluated, it becomes impossible for others to repeat the successful program or to learn from our mistakes. In Figure 3-2, the process is the throughput component. *Outcomes* in patient-education evaluation research remain the same as those presented in the systems model. The *goal* component of evaluation research consists of the program's stated goals which are

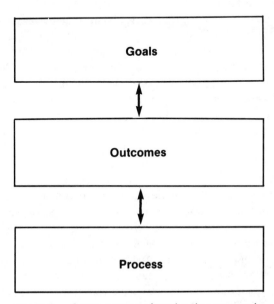

Fig. 3-3. *Components of evaluation research.*

identifiable and measurable and have been implemented. Figure 3-3 identifies the components of evaluation research.

The stated goals are at the top of the diagram; the process and outcomes support and build the program goals. Some social scientists point out that evaluation of outcomes should not be limited to stated goals because frequently positive outcomes will be derived that were unintended and not pertinent to a stated goal.[19]

For example, the stated goal of the diabetic-patient luncheon was that patients and their family members would learn about the functions of diet, medication, and exercise in the management of diabetes; this learning was measured by their correct verbal responses to questions. The desired outcome was greater patient/family knowledge about the management of diabetes at home. One of the most positive outcomes, however, was originally unplanned for; it was the confidence patients gained by relating their own experiences and successes to each other. Such an outcome would have been overlooked if evaluation research had examined only the stated goal.

Suggestions for Practice

Maintaining Nurses' Interest

Our experience has indicated that, regardless of the membership of others on task forces and advisory committees, nurses are almost wholly responsible for implementation of patient-education plans. To ensure and maintain the interest of nurses in proposed and ongoing patient-education programs, we feel that it is essential to include them in every aspect of patient education.

Nurses must be included in the initial planning phases so that their input is considered in deciding on long-term goals, in setting priorities, and in gaining widespread nursing-staff participation. It is imperative that nurses familiar with certain disease entities and the units to which patients with these diseases are assigned be included on the task force for developing patient-education protocols. If their input is neglected, failure during implementation is guaranteed. For example, if an extensive cardiac-rehabilitation program is planned to involve the coronary-care unit nurses, they need to give information about staffing time, necessary space, needed in-service training of staff members, audiovisual resources, and so forth.

In addition, it is important to involve nursing staff in the budgeting for patient education so that they understand the financial exigencies of patient education. This will ensure that plans remain realistic. Such inclusion of nursing staff is also a growth-enhancing mechanism for staff members who wish to learn more about the economic realities of health care.

Evaluation of programs is another important area in which nurses should be included. They are most able to make qualitative evaluations of the patient benefits of certain programs. The quantitative aspect of evaluation (*e.g.*, statistical analysis) should also include nurses as another means for their career enhancement and to involve them in research in the practice setting.

Nursing interest can be promoted by using involvement in patient education as part of a horizontal career ladder. Nurses are frequently heard complaining that advancement is impossible unless one moves into administration and leaves the bedside. Since patient education is a legitimate and much-needed nursing activity, it is desirable to promote those nurses who exhibit competency in patient education. Such horizontal promotions would keep the nurse who is an effective patient educator at the bedside while at the same time, through monetary and career advancement, recognize her abilities.

Consumer Participation

A second suggestion for practice is very simple and obvious, but it is one we have never observed in operation: why not include one or more patients in all phases of planning, implementing, financing, and evaluating patient education? As consumers of a service, their input is much needed. In fact, including them in the planning process would possibly make implementation much smoother and evaluation less problematic.

As funds for health-care services become more restricted, it is not unlikely that health-care professionals will have to charge fees for their patient-education services or, in some way, hold the consumer more responsible for payment than he is presently. At this time there are several completely self-supported patient-education and self-care groups in the community. For example, the American Diabetes Association has chapters throughout the country that finance all their educational activities through their members' dues and fund-raising projects. Many believe that such financial responsibility for one's own patient education guarantees better education and more adherence among patients.

Sharing Planning Efforts in a Community

Developing a consortium of patient-education coordinators in a community is a positive way to share successes and failures, to garner support for new programs, and to become more familiar with what is going on in patient education. Many of us sit in our own agencies, completely unaware of similar efforts and other resources close at hand. We once belonged to a consortium of in-service educators. We met four times a year to share what we were doing in our institutions with orientation, new graduate programs, and legal issues. Such a consortium would be a very effective adjunct to any community's patient-education efforts. It should consist of inpatient and outpatient representatives, as well as people involved in school health education and self-help groups.

Sharing Programs

Related to the idea of a community consortium is the suggestion that we share resources so that programs are not duplicated. Limited patient-education resources demand that there be no repetition of patient-education programs within a community. Having hospitals and outpatient agencies jump on the patient-education bandwagon has produced a tremendous proliferation of services. We knew of a medical center and a smaller community hospital that successfully shared an enterostomal therapist. The therapist went to the community hospital for particularly difficult cases and also shared her expertise with the staff. This arrangement worked very well until one of the staff surgeons of the community hospital decided that the community hospital had to have its own enterostomal therapist. Nursing service complied with the request and financed a position, and the nursing staff quickly forgot all their learning about caring for ostomates, letting the enterostomal therapist take over instead.

Many patient-education programs such as cardiac rehabilitation, diabetes-patient–family groups, and fresh-air (respiratory) clubs could be shared in one community. The inpatient phase of cardiac rehabilitation could be handled at the hospital where the patient was hospitalized, but once he was ready for discharge and outpatient cardiac rehabilitation, he could attend a center whose facilities were shared by various community members needing health education. Sharing equipment, personnel, audiovisual resources, and other resources seems much more sensible than encouraging the duplication of services. Issues related to territoriality, power, and control have to be solved, however, before such sound practices will be commonplace.

Appendix A: Foundations

The most useful foundation directory is The Foundation Center's *The Foundation Directory,* 8th ed. (New York, Columbia University Press, 1981)

The American Hospital Association, in conjunction with the Centers for Disease Control's (CDC) Health Education Project and Center for Health Promotion, published a very useful booklet entitled *Foundation Funding for Health Education, 1972–1980.* Publication of the booklet was funded by the U.S. Department of Health and Human Services under contract number 200-79-0916 with the American Hospital Association. This publication details organizations that made grants for health-education projects from 1972–1980. For a complete list, obtain the booklet from the following:

U.S. Department of Health and Human Services
Public Health Service
Centers for Dieseae Control
Center for Health Promotion and Education
Community Program Development Division
Atlanta, GA 30333

The three largest independent foundations that are well known for funding health-education programs are the following:

The Robert Wood Johnson Foundation
P.O. Box 2316
Princeton, NJ 08540

The Ford Foundation
320 East 43rd Street
New York, NY 10017

The WK Kellogg Foundation
400 North Avenue
Battle Creek, MI 49016

References

1. McColloch C, Boggs B, Varner C: Implementation of educational programs for patients. Nurs Adm Q 4, No. 2:61–65, 1980
2. Somers A: Consumer health education: To know or to die. Hospitals 50:52–56, 1976
3. Nordberg B, King L: Third-party payment for patient education. Am J Nurs 76, No. 8:1269–1271, 1976
4. Green LW: The potential of health education includes cost effectiveness. Hospitals 50:57–61, 1976
5. James WG: The psychological control of pre-operative anxiety. Psychophysiology 12:50–54, 1975
6. Egbert LO et al: The value of the pre-operative visit by an anesthetist: A study of doctor–patient rapport. JAMA 185:553–555, 1963
7. Egbert LD, Battit GE, Welch CE et al: Reduction of post-operative pain by encouragement and instruction of patients: A study of doctor–patient rapport. N Engl J Med 270:825–826, 1964
8. Schmitt RE, Woolridge PJ: Psychological preparation of surgical patients. Nurs Res 22:109–116, 1973
9. Schwain WS: Patients' rights in decision-making: The case for personalism versus paternalism in health care. Cancer 46:1035–1041, 1980
10. Cousins N: Anatomy of an Illness as Perceived by the Patient. New York, WW Norton, 1979
11. Letton AH, Mason EM: Five-year-plus survival of breast screenees. Cancer 48:404–406, 1981
12. Cancer Patient Survival Report No. 5, DHEW Publication No. (NIH) 77-992. Bethesda, MD, The National Cancer Institute, 1976.
13. Stern MP: The recent decline in ischemic heart disease mortality. Ann Intern Med 91:630–640, 1979
14. Eisenberg M, Bergner L, Hallstrom A: Paramedic programs and out-of-hospital cardiac arrest: I. Factors associated with successful resuscitation. Am J Publ Health 69(1):30–8, 1979.
15. Eisenberg M, Bergner L, Hallstrom A: Paramedic programs and out-of-hospital cardiac arrest: II. Impact on community mortality. Am J Public Health 69, No. 1:39–42, 1979
16. Avery CH, Green LW, Kreider S: Reducing emergency visits of asthmatics: An experiment in patient education. Pittsburgh, President's Commission on Health Education, 1972
17. Miller L, Goldstein J: More efficient care of diabetic patients in a county hospital setting. N Engl J Med 286:1388–1391, 1972
18. Green LW: Evaluation and measurement: Some dilemmas for health education. Am J Public Health 67:155–161, 1977
19. Rutman L: Evaluation Research Methods. Beverly Hills, Sage Publications, 1977

Bibliography

Books

Abdellah FG: Better Patient Care Through Nursing Research. New York, Macmillan, 1979
Bille DA (ed): Practical Approaches to Patient Teaching. Boston, Little, Brown & Co 1981
McCormick RM, Gilson-Parkevich T (eds): Patient and Family Education: Tools, Techniques, and Theory. New York, John Wiley & Sons, 1979
Narrow BW: Patient Teaching in Nursing Practice: A Patient and Family Centered Approach. New York, John Wiley & Sons, 1979

Pohl ML: The Teaching Function of the Nursing Practitioner. Dubuque, IA, William
Brown, 1978

Redman BK: Issues and Concepts in Patient Education. New York, Appleton-Century-
Crofts, 1981

Redman BK: Patterns for Distribution of Patient Education. New York, Appleton-Century-
Crofts, 1981

Sweeney MA, Olivieri P: An Introduction to Nursing Research: Research, Measurement,
and Computers in Nursing. Philadelphia, JB Lippincott, 1981

Journals

Applebaum AL: Who's going to pay the bill? Hospitals 53, No. 19:112–120, 1979

Hyner GC: Bridging the gap: Definition of terms and proposal for patient education. Health
Educ 9, No. 3:19–21, 1978

Jencks SF, Green LW: Establishing a hospital-based patient education program. QRB 4,
No. 10:8–11, 1978

McCarthy JT (et al): Successful grantsmanship. Health Care Manage Rev 3, No. 3:37–43,
1978

McCulloch C, Boggs BJ, Varner CF: Implementation of educational programs for patients.
Nurs Admin Q, 4, No. 2:61–65

Papers

American Hospital Association: Professional, accreditation, and legal statements supporting
patient education. Catalog No. P014. Chicago, American Hospital Association,
1977

American Nurses' Association: Issues in evaluation research. Publ. No. G-124 2M. Kansas
City, American Nurses' Association, 1976

American Nurses' Association: New directions for nursing in the '80s. Publ. No. G-147 2M.
Kansas City, American Nurses' Association, 1980

American Nurses' Association: The Professional Nurse and Health Education. Kansas City,
American Nurses' Association, 1975

American Public Health Association: A Model for Patient Education Programming: Report
of the APHA, Public Health Education Section. Atlanta, Center for Health
Promotion and Education, 1979

Blue Cross Association: White paper: Patient health education. Chicago, Blue Cross
Association, 1974

Deeds SG: Overview of evaluation presented at the national conference on hospital-based
patient education, Chicago. Atlanta, Bureau of Health Education, 1976

Executive summary: Financing for health education services in the United States—Third
party payers. Blue Cross/Blue Shield Associations, American Hospital Association, and Department of Health and Human Services. Atlanta, Center for Health
Promotion and Education, 1981

Financing for health education services in the United States. Blue Cross/Blue Shield
Associations, American Hospital Association, and Department of Health and
Human Services. Atlanta, Center for Health Promotion and Education, 1980,
1981

Health Promotion and Consumer Health Education. A Task Force Report Sponsored by
the John E. Fogarty International Center for Advanced Study in the Health
Sciences, NIH, and the American College of Preventive Medicine. New York,
Prodist, 1976

Lee E: American Hospital Association national patient education survey. In: Annual Arizona patient education conference proceedings. Phoenix, Arizona Department of Health Services, 1979

Newby LG, Spratt JS, Alfieri Z: A conceptual model for evaluation of patient education for cancer. Presented at the annual meeting of the American Educational Research Association, Toronto, 1978

Chapter 4

A Model for Patient Decision Making and Mutual Goal Setting

In the preceding chapters we have examined issues that concern primarily health-care providers. We have focused on issues that arise when they attempt to find complementary roles in delivering patient education but discover they differ over when and how it should be implemented. We have seen these issues surface often even though the nurses, the physicians, and other team members may agree that patient education is important.

The issues considered in this chapter are those the patient faces as a result of a complex variety of factors, including his understanding of health-care recommendations and his attitudes and beliefs. These issues cause each patient to impact on the health-care system in a unique way and influence his decision making as a consumer of health-care services. We discuss situations in which the patient's values are in conflict with those of the health-care provider and in which patient education does not result in the behavioral changes suggested by the provider. Finally, we use the Chatterton Model,* based on the Health Belief Model,[1] as a framework for assisting the patient in decision making. The Chatterton model will be applied to clinical situations to illustrate how issues arising from attitudes, beliefs, previous life experiences, and present life stresses influence the choices the patient makes at different stages in his health care.

Patient Education: A Process of Influencing Behavior

Dr. Scott Simonds, Chairman of the Health Education Department at the University of Michigan, provides us with the following definition:

*An unpublished model developed by Howard Chatterton, M.D., Ph.D., and used with his consent.

Patient education is the process of influencing behavior, producing changes in knowledge, attitudes, and skills required to maintain and improve health. The process may begin with the imparting of information but it also includes interpretation and integration of information in such a manner as to bring about attitudinal or behavioral changes which benefit the person's health status.[2]

Because patient education is a process, it occurs over a period of time and requires an ongoing assessment of the patient's knowledge, attitudes, and skills. The patient's readiness or motivation to change and the obstacles to change are important factors to be considered during the process of assessment. Chapter 6 offers an in-depth discussion of assessment for patient education. Most practitioners involved in teaching patients realize the impact of the family on the patient's behavior. A close, supportive family unit may facilitate the integration of new health behaviors, while the family facing conflict or lacking understanding often poses barriers to behavioral change. Strong religious, ethnic, or cultural beliefs may also prevent change. A Patient–Family-Education Assessment Guide, introduced in Chapter 6, provides guidance in examining factors that may promote or impede the process of patient education. The practitioner can then offer the patient and his family assistance in overcoming obstacles to behavioral change.

Compliance Orientation

We asked physicians and nurses to share with us what they considered to be obstacles in their experiences with patient education. All of them identified problems with either motivating patients or achieving patient compliance. When they were asked to elaborate, it became evident that they saw the two problems as closely related. The implication was that a sufficiently motivated patient would comply with the doctor's or nurse's instructions.

Many of us have justified our involvement in patient education by asserting that it would increase patient compliance or, in other words, convince patients to follow our suggestions. As research in the area of health education becomes more extensive, it becomes apparent that, in spite of teaching, patients frequently do not make the choices recommended to them by nurses, physicians, and other health professionals. This is often termed *noncompliance*.

We are uneasy with the term *compliance*. It implies that we dictate to the patient what is to be done or changed and that the patient is to follow instructions—to obey us. Further soul searching brings us to the realization that our real discomfort stems from the patient's right to choose *not* to follow our advice, even though we know what is best for him.

In sharing our thoughts and ideas on the compliance orientation with Dr. Godfrey Hochbaum,[3] we have developed a broader appreciation of the patient's position in patient education. It is natural for the health professional to want the patient to choose the recommended course of action; however, what we really should strive to enlist is his partnership or cooperation rather than compliance. We want him to *choose* what we suggest.

An orientation toward cooperation rather than toward compliance causes us to think about our own effectiveness in patient education in a different light. Perhaps patient-education successes have more to do with patients' preparation to make informed choices than with their compliance. If, in fact, patient education acknowledges the patient's free will to make choices, it must afford understanding of the importance of his values and wishes and his ability to participate in decision making.

Clinical Situations

During a discussion of patient compliance, a nurse offered the following concern:

When I was a student, I always thought that it would be difficult to deal with the patient's background. Right now, I'm having a lot of difficulty dealing with my own background. It is part of my professional role to emphasize health and the prevention of illness or further complications from illness. But how do I offer my patients education and expect them to accept my values? I'm not sure in some cases if what I offer them would make them happier and healthier or just more like me.

This nurse related a recent experience that she had in a family-medicine center when she attempted contraceptive counseling with a 17-year-old girl who was sexually active. The nurse discovered that the patient did not share her values (*i.e.,* the importance of completing a high-school education or preventing pregnancy until marriage). The nurse discovered that the patient had an older sister who gave birth at the age of 17. The baby was raised by the patient's mother and according to the patient, "it all worked out fine." Several of the patient's friends were also unmarried and pregnant. The patient was not interested in any kind of birth control.

The story is a familiar one. It prompts recollections of frustrating and futile attempts to persuade patients to follow the health-care plans formulated for them, which we felt certain would make them happier and healthier. The obstacles that often prevent us from influencing patients' behavior may be attributed to issues arising from the patient's values, beliefs, and life stresses, which are sometimes in conflict with our own. In the case of the 17-year-old patient, peer influences, sociocultural values, and the lack of alternative role modeling resulted in her cool reception of contraceptive counseling.

On the following office visit one month later, the doctor and nurse persuaded the same patient that she should begin using birth-control pills. The patient obtained the pills from a pharmacy that day. However, four months later when she returned to the clinic she was pregnant. She told the doctor and nurse that she had failed to take the pills "every" day. She was considered by the office staff to be noncompliant.

Another example is that of a 52-year-old woman with adult-onset diabetes, hypertension, and obesity. In well-documented patient-education sessions with her doctor and three of the office nurses, the patient demonstrated she had the knowledge and skills to manage her diet and medications at home. When at home, however, she did not follow her daily management regimen and had several emergency admissions to the hospital. She was experiencing marital problems and had a complicated social and financial situation. She reported that her husband was sexually involved with other women and that she was unhappy with their relationship. It was her feeling that he should take care of her. While making a home visit to follow up on the patient's medical problems, the nurse noted that five of the patient's six children were living at home; the youngest was 23, and only one of the children was employed. The patient's husband worked in a local factory, and their only other income was her disability-insurance check. Her medical care was covered by Medicaid. The family did not have a car and lived in a small, ill-kept, four-room house. Although the nurse felt confident that the patient knew how to manage her health problems at home, it was evident that many other factors influenced the patient in her decision not to carry out her daily management responsibility. After several admissions for a myocardial infarction and cerebrovascular accident, the patient died.

In spite of the health-care providers' ongoing assessment and attempts to influence the patient's behavior through patient education, she chose not to follow their recommendations. It is important to recognize that the patient may ultimately reject health-care services in spite of apparent acceptance of information.

A third example is that of a 65-year-old home builder who referred to himself as a "stubborn Irishman." This patient, who had a history of myocardial infarction and current problems with hypertension, would not consider alterations of his life-style, which was rushed, tense, and dictated by deadlines. He refused to receive a tetanus immunization, which both the nurse and the physician tried to convince him was important for someone in his occupation. He also announced loudly that he was not interested in losing weight. It was important for this overweight "stubborn Irishman" to be in control of his life-style and to present a strong, rugged exterior. He did, however, agree to take an antihypertensive medication regularly and to keep his appointment every six months. On the third follow-up visit he agreed to receive a tetanus shot. He could then be labeled *cooperative*.

The previous examples illustrate the importance of considering the patient's perception of his health needs and his own situation. They show us that effective patient education requires an understanding of those factors that influence the patient in his decision making: values, beliefs, attitudes, current life stresses, religion, previous experiences with the health-care system, and life goals. They also illustrate that patient education involves teaching and learning that must be accompanied by behavioral changes. Patient-education providers may begin with giving information and demonstrating skills, but if the patient is not included in deciding how learning will be applied and the goals of patient education are not mutually agreed upon between the teacher and the learner, behavioral changes usually will not occur.

We must understand that while the health professional tends to view cooperation with the medical regimen as a single choice, the patient's cooperation with the regimen involves many choices every day. The choice to follow the diabetic diet, for example, means not one choice but constant (often inconvenient and painful) choices throughout each day. We expect him to do this every day for the rest of his life, even though we cannot guarantee that he will be free of neuropathies, retinopathies, nephropathies, or other complications. We offer him our guidance and support. We must also be willing to respect the patient's right to choose, although we may not agree with his choice.

We reserve the right to keep trying. In spite of poor cooperation in the past, we remain hopeful that a patient may be more open to patient-education messages during future encounters. We must also respect the patient's right to change his mind. He may choose to take the course of action we suggest or to turn away from it if he judges that the cost or hardship to him outweighs the benefit, as in the case of a terminally ill patient receiving chemotherapy. He initially decided to take the treatment, but later decided to discontinue the chemotherapeutic drugs because he weighed the costly and uncomfortable side-effects against the benefits.

Patient Decision Making

Patient Issues: A Review of the Literature

A review of patient-education literature reveals many of the variables that influence patients' choices not to follow the suggestions of health professionals. Lack of cooperation is common among patients of all economic and educational backgrounds, not just among low-income populations.[4] Rationalization and denial are common problems encountered in patient education and are often seen in the management of chronic illness. They also affect the patient's participation in preventive health care. The Health Belief Model demonstrates that the patient's perceptions about the presence of disease or the likelihood of contracting disease are a predictor of his consumption of health services.[1]

Feelings such as anxiety, depression, and anger influence the patient's understanding and, eventually, his choices.[5] In addition, religion, ethnicity, family problems, and family experiences influence the patient's course of action. Finally, sociological variables (knowledge about disease and prior contact with disease) are identified as modifying factors in the patient's consumption of health-care services.[1]

Patient education thus requires an openness on the part of the health professional, as well as a desire to discover the variables that influence a patient's choices. Working through, rather than around, patient issues helps us to intervene most effectively and to address the barriers that prevent patients from cooperating.

Patient education requires us to take a skilled approach in assessing patient issues and problems and in setting goals with patients. Chapters 6 and 7 help strengthen this approach through use of the nursing process.

The Health Belief Model

The traditional Health Belief Model was constructed to predict health behaviors. It provides a tool for understanding the patient's perception of disease and his decision-making process in the consumption of health-care services. Although the Health Belief Model was originally designed to predict the likelihood of patients' taking recommended preventive action such as obtaining screening tests and annual checkups, it has been the basis for other models adapted to consider the consumption of health-care services in the presence of chronic illness.[6] Although its application as a model in research is often for compliance prediction, it is also useful for gaining a better understanding of the patient's motivation for seeking and obtaining services.

The Health Belief Model predicts that an individual is likely to consume health-care services if he does the following:

1. Perceives that he has a disease or condition or is likely to contract it
2. Perceives that the disease or condition is harmful and has serious consequences
3. Believes that the suggested health intervention is of value
4. Believes that the effectiveness of the treatment is worth the cost and barriers he must confront

The Chatterton Model

Relying heavily on the Health Belief Model, Dr. Howard Chatterton, a family physician, developed yet another model (Fig. 4-1). (In this model, *disease* indicates medically defined disease; *health-care services* include products.) Chatterton's purpose was not to predict patient compliance but to examine more closely the continuous decision-making process the patient experiences as a health-care consumer.

The Chatterton Model encourages us to examine the patient's understanding of his condition as a product of the patient education provided, his values, beliefs, and past experiences in health care, and the present life stresses that may interfere with the desired behavioral changes. It helps us to consider how the patient makes health-care decisions rather than simply whether he is cooperative with the provider's plan for medical management. The model encourages a deeper understanding of patient behaviors and helps us to direct patient education so that we can better prepare the patient to make choices.

For our discussion, we consider once more the situations of the 17-year-old young woman, the 52-year-old woman with numerous health problems, and the 65-year-old home builder. We will discuss health-maintenance situations as well as diseases, and observe each patient through each step of the model. We will emphasize incorporating the patient's understanding, attitudes, beliefs, and life stresses, as well as previous experiences in health-care systems, into patient education. We will examine how patient education is used to influence behavior and we will make suggestions for patient education in each situation. We also will consider barriers to change and the factors that affect either the behavioral change or the lack of it for each patient.

Applying the Chatterton Model to Clinical Situations

Step I

The model first considers whether a disease or condition is present. This assessment is made on the basis of medical judgment. At this point, patient education should include an explanation of the problem and associated symptoms, and the provider should explore the patient's prior knowledge of, or experience with, such a

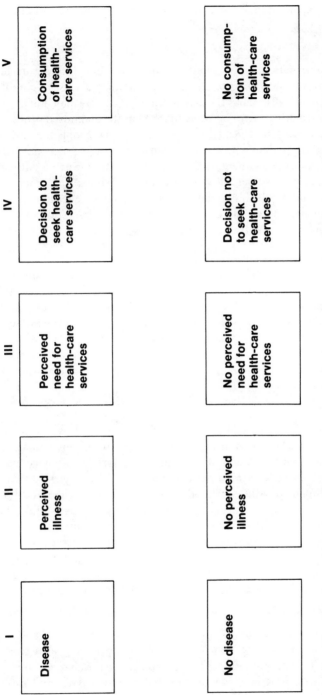

Fig. 4-1.   *The Chatterton Model, based on the Health Belief Model, illustrates patient decision making in the consumption of health-care services. (Courtesy of Howard T. Chatterton, M.D.)*

condition. In Step I it is important to consider anxiety and fear as possible obstacles to understanding.

Step II

Depending on the patient's understanding in Step I and the factors of denial, anxiety, and fear, the individual with a medically defined disease or condition may also perceive that he is ill and has the diagnosed problem. He may, however, despite a medically defined disease, *not* perceive that he has the diagnosed problem; in this case further consumption of health-care services for the problem is unlikely. It is also possible that the patient with no diagnosed disease or problem may perceive, in spite of the provider's assessment, that he *has* a condition. Such a patient usually continues to seek services from the same provider or "shops" for another opinion. Patient education in Step II should include assessing the patient's understanding of, and feelings about, the diagnosis, the symptoms, and the suggestions offered by the provider. It is important to discover how the patient feels this will affect his life.

Step III

The individual's perception of his health needs and his situation is of great importance here. This step corresponds to the Health Belief Model's consideration of whether the patient believes that the condition is harmful to him or has serious consequences. The patient considers at this point whether health-care services are of value. Patient education, in addition to discussion of beliefs and attitudes, should include a review of what may happen, both with the patient's decision not to seek health-care services for such a condition and with a decision to pursue health-care services.

Step IV

The patient decides whether or not to seek health-care services in this step of the model. The patient's motivation to change or "get well," his denial, fear, and feelings of trust in the provider and the health-care system influence his decision and should be explored as part of patient education. The suggested treatment or regimen (including medications) will be discussed by the provider at this time and the patient should be made aware of financial costs and corresponding changes in life-style. Any possible side-effects of treatment or medications, along with an honest explanation of prognoses both with and without intervention, should be discussed. The mutual goal setting that follows involves the patient's decision as to whether the intervention and his behavioral changes are desirable and worth whatever cost or barriers he might confront. Again, the patient education prepares him to make such decisions.

Step V

The individual decides whether he will consume the suggested health-care services. We consider whether the patient is indeed committed to the changes contracted for in Step IV. Family pressures, anxiety on the patient's part, and difficulty in implementing the proposed changes should be assessed. The patient may consume some or all of the services offered. For most patients, Step V involves the most difficult of all decisions in the course of treatment and, in some cases, even after choices have been made to follow the provider's recommendations, the corresponding changes in behavior are not accomplished. This step should not be considered the end point of patient-education responsibilities. As demonstrated in the clinical situations that follow, the educational process is an ongoing one, even after choices have been made. Decisions can be modified on the basis of better understanding and the resolution of issues that initially pose barriers to the consumption of health-care services. Step V frequently involves negotiating goals once more with the patient and his family to work toward the resolution of issues.

Application of the Model to Three Patient Situations

Case Study 1

Reviewing the case of the 17-year-old patient, we recall that she was not interested in contraception despite the wishes of the physician and nurse. On a subsequent visit, she agreed to take birth-control pills after having been "convinced" to do so by her health-care providers. It is unclear from the patient's record how this "convincing" was done or to what extent the patient participated in the discussion or in goal setting. We do know that when she returned to the office four months later and was pregnant she was labeled *noncompliant*. We question the patient's motivation to consume that particular service even when she began taking the oral contraceptive, but surmise that including her in the patient education and decision making might have enabled the health-care providers to foresee problems with the patient's making the daily choice to take a pill. At this time, it is helpful to follow her through the steps of the Chatterton Model (Fig. 4-2).

Step I

Although pregnancy is not a disease, we consider contraception a health-maintenance measure for the sexually active young patient. Both the patient and provider agreed that there was a possibility of pregnancy if no method of contraception was used.

Step II

Again, there was mutual agreement about the perception of pregnancy as an outcome. However, the patient did not see this as a negative outcome, although the providers did. This patient entered the model at Step II because she did not have such a condition initially and did not see such a possibility as being harmful to her.

It appeared that the patient understood and was not anxious or fearful. The provider may have felt that in this situation the patient did not fully comprehend the responsibility and life-style considerations a pregnancy would involve. Patient education should have explored her attitudes, her perception of her sister's and her friends' pregnancies, and her ideas about how a similar experience would affect her life and her life goals.

Step III

It was clear on the initial visit that the patient did not regard contraception as valuable to her and was not willing to pursue the proposed health-care service at that time.

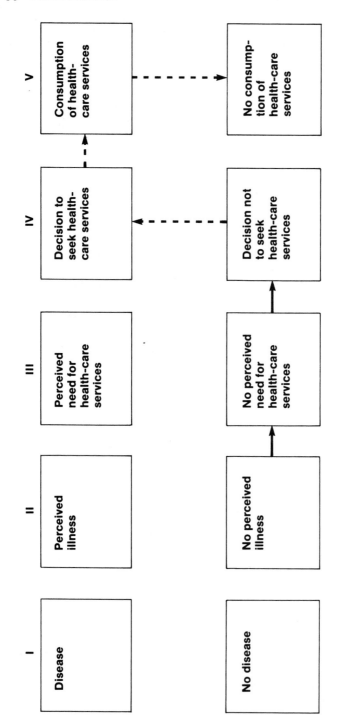

Fig. 4-2. The Chatterton Model, applied to the clinical situation of a 17-year-old patient.

Step IV   The patient decided at the first visit not to consume the service (contraception). Although this decision was not well received by her health-care providers, it was congruent with the patient's own perception of her needs and her life goals.

On the second visit, as a result of persuasion by the physician and nurse, the patient changed her decision of the first visit and chose to seek the health-care service (birth-control pills). It is doubtful that her choice to make a behavioral change reflected a significant change in feelings or attitude, but there is no documentation of the discussion. We do know that the patient's feelings of trust in the provider and the health-care system may have influenced her decisions in this step of the model, and we surmise that the patient may have been trying to please the providers or be a "good" patient. Without documentation of what occurred we cannot make that assessment. We do not know on what basis the patient's decision was made.

Step V   While the patient may have consumed the health-care services for some period of time, within the first few months she rejected those services by stopping the birth-control pills. It appears that the patient had not made a commitment to the behavioral change; she reaffirmed her original choice that she was not interested in preventing a pregnancy.

This patient situation clearly emphasizes the effects of values and peer influences on the consumption of health-care services. It shows that poor cooperation may be predicted when the patient does not consider the intervention to be of value.

Case Study 2   The second situation we consider is that of the 52-year-old woman with a number of health problems, including morbid hypertension, obesity, and adult-onset diabetes. The areas of stress identified at home were financial problems, marital disharmony, five dependent children who were unemployed but able to work, and small living quarters. The patient kept her appointments with her doctor and participated in well-documented sessions of patient education at each office visit. In the course of the patient's treatment, one of the nurses made three home visits to assess problems in the family and to better understand cooperation problems. While the patient was participating in patient education, she was involved in goal setting and demonstrated the skills and understanding necessary to manage her health problems at home through diet, medication, and blood-pressure checks. In spite of the patient's decision to seek health-care services as described, her behavioral changes were not consistent, and she did not take her medications regularly. She was unable to follow her diet and her hypertension was out of control most of the time. She rejected the health-care services in spite of her acceptance of information. As we follow the steps of the Chatterton Model (Fig.

4-3), we see how this patient's problems at home posed stresses and, ultimately, barriers to the desired behavioral changes.

Step I   The assessment made on the basis of medical judgment identified the patient as having adult-onset diabetes, obesity, and hypertension as major health problems. It was also noted that the patient experienced a great deal of stress at home, which may have contributed to her health problems. From the documentation of patient education, it is clear that the problems, the associated symptoms, and the patient's understanding of her condition were discussed and that she recognized the presence of disease.

Step II   Again, the patient seemed to comprehend her problems. The symptoms of hyperglycemia and the dizziness associated with her hypertension reinforced her perception that she had the diseases. In talking with her about how she thought the health problems would affect her life, she began to discuss her relationship with her husband. She reported that he was unfaithful to her, that she was unhappy with the relationship, and that she felt he should take care of her.

Step III   The patient's perception of her health needs dictated her consideration of the services proposed by her physician. The dependency needs highlighted in Step II may also have influenced her decision. The proposed services included antihypertensive medication, insulin, urine testing, and a diet that would be worked out with her by the dietitian. There is documentation describing an explanation that was made to the patient about hypertension and diabetes and what could be expected in terms of prognosis if the patient participated in the suggested treatment plan. The patient's husband was also included in the discussion.

Step IV   The patient decided to take the antihypertensive medication and learn to give herself insulin injections. She agreed to check her urine at home and see the dietitian about her diet. In the documentation of patient education, both the nurse and dietitian referred to her as a pleasant woman who demonstrated an understanding of her health problems and an ability to perform the skills she was taught. Issues that were discussed in this step of the model were the patient's financial problems and her inability to afford the foods suggested by the dietitian. Her physician referred her to the Department of Social Services and a social worker in the outpatient clinic for assistance with buying her medications and with transportation because she did not have a car.

Step V   Although she had participated in patient education and demonstrated understanding and skills, the patient did not manage her care at home according to suggestions. Her emergency admissions and the assessment gathered on home visits by the nurse supported the finding that the patient was not cooperative in spite of her agreement with the treatment plan. During the three years she

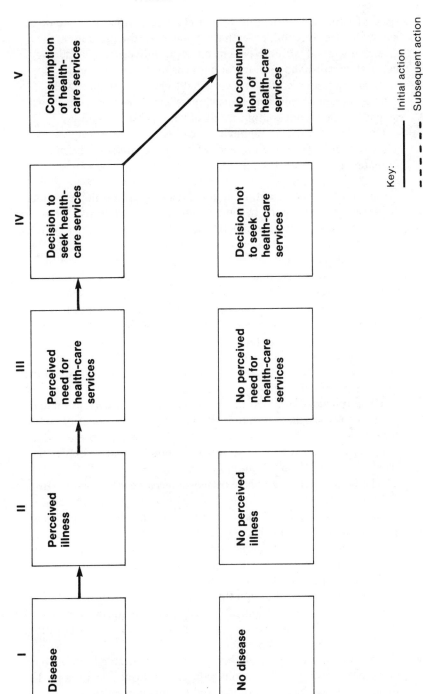

Fig. 4-3. The Chatterton Model, applied to the clinical situation of a 52-year-old woman.

was under the care of the physician and nurses, efforts were made to review the decision making with the patient. At the same time, the physician worked with the patient on her family problems and included her husband and one of her sons in the discussions. Community resources were investigated to help the patient with dietary, transportation, and housing problems. Despite these efforts, the patient died from complications of her disease.

This clinical situation highlights the difficulty in effecting behavioral changes in the presence of other life stresses. The patient ultimately rejected health-care services.

Case Study 3

The third clinical situation involves the 65-year-old home builder described as a "stubborn Irishman." On his first office visit he agreed to take medication for his hypertension but refused to take a tetanus immunization as a preventive measure and would not consider modifying his life-style, which was rushed, tense, and dictated by building deadlines. He had a history of myocardial infarction, but would also not consider ceasing or reducing his cigarette smoking. He smoked three to four packages a day at that time. On subsequent visits, patient education was reinforced and the patient reconsidered his decision to take a tetanus shot. His need to present a rugged exterior and maintain control of the situation was respected by the physician. We will consider his decision-making process through the Chatterton Model (Fig. 4–4).

Step I

The physician diagnosed this patient as having hypertension and a history of myocardial infarction. He saw the patient's obesity and cigarette smoking as risk factors. Although the patient presented a rough and controlling exterior, it is very possible that he experienced fear and anxiety to some extent in this step.

Step II

The patient perceived his hypertension as a health problem. He did not, however, see lack of tetanus immunization, obesity, or smoking as posing health problems or being harmful to him. The patient's need for control, as well as his desire to maintain a rugged image, particularly influenced him in this step. He also used rationalization to deny the importance of his health problems.

Step III

The patient responded in this step by perceiving his need for health-care services, although this perceived need involved only antihypertensive medication. It is clear in the documentation of patient education that he understood the risks of his hypertension, and he decided to seek treatment.

Step IV

The patient took charge in his treatment. He decided to take the antihypertensive medication and requested information about it. In the areas of his obesity, smoking, and tetanus immunization, however, he decided not to seek services.

Step V

In this step, the patient consumed health-care services (medication) for his hypertension but not initially for other health

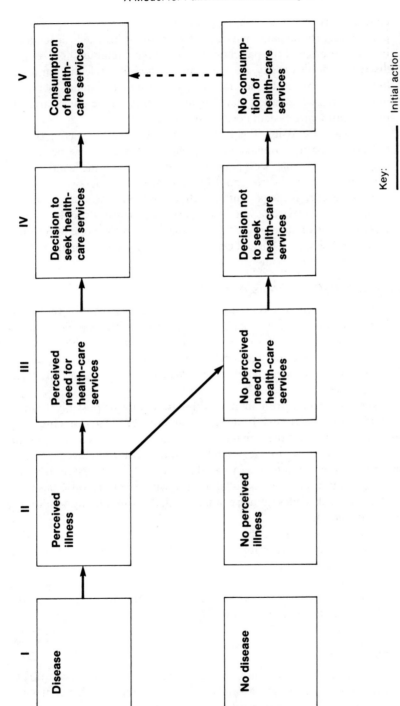

Key:

———— Initial action

- - - - Subsequent action

Fig. 4-4. *The Chatterton Model, applied to the clinical situation of a 65-year-old man.*

concerns. At a later appointment, during a regular follow-up visit, patient education again included a discussion of his need for tetanus immunization, and the patient decided to take a tetanus shot. A discussion of his obesity, smoking, and rushed life-style did not result in any decisions on the patient's part to consume health-care services in those areas. It is noted that the patient's trust in the physician and in the health-care system developed slowly.

This case discussion illustrates the importance of respecting the right of the patient to make his own choices. Changes may be negotiated over time, with patient education for various health problems continued throughout his care. The situation also demonstrates that the patient may choose to consume some of the recommended services and reject others. The provider should honor these decisions but continue patient education in the hope of future behavioral changes. The educational process goes on even after choices have been made.

Contending with Patient Decisions

In every situation, the patient's right to know and right to choose should be respected. The health-care provider is challenged to explore with the patient and his family the information pertinent to the particular disease or problem and its recommended treatment. Mutually acceptable plans for care should be pursued with consideration of the issues the patient faces as a product of his values, life-style, and current life stresses.

The issues patients confront in the health-care setting are possibly the most complex of all the issues we discuss. If physicians and nurses are to deal effectively with these issues, we must meet the demands of individual situations that require an understanding of the patient's vantage point. We should muster whatever resources are available to aid the patient in creative alterations to his life-style that are acceptable to him. This often requires collaboration with other professionals in an attempt to work on the obstacles to such changes, including poor living conditions, poverty, and family conflicts.

The issues the patient faces should be assessed during each encounter with health professionals. Patient education should be seen as an integral part of each patient contact. Documentation of these issues, as well as of information given to the patient and the feelings he expresses about his care, is vital to the work of the health-care team. Suggestions for effective written communication among the members of health-care team are offered in Chapter 9.

Summary

It is often difficult to accept the patient's prerogative to make a decision contrary to the suggestions offered by the physician and nurse. Just as legal and financial issues can deter nurses in patient-education roles, issues related to patient decisions can also leave nurses feeling defeated and unprepared. A broader understanding of the patient's choice can be gained from the applications of the Health Belief Model and the Chatterton Model. Learning why these issues arise and how to deal with patient decisions helps the nurse remain committed to patient education. We recognize that the ultimate role of the health professional is to encourage the patient to make informed choices about his health, rather than to guarantee compliance or obedience.

References

1. Hochbaum GM: Public participation in medical screening programs. U.S. Public Health Service Publication No. 572. Washington, DC, U.S. Government Printing Office, 1958
2. National Task Force on Training Family Physicians in Patient Education, Patient Education: A Handbook for Teachers. Kansas City, The Society of Teachers of Family Medicine, 1979
3. Hochbaum GM: Professor, School of Public Health, University of North Carolina at Chapel Hill. Conference with author, June 1981
4. Marston MV: Compliance with medical regimens: a review of the literature. Nurs Res 19:312–323, 1970
5. Redman BK: The Process of Patient Teaching in Nursing. St Louis, CV Mosby, 1980
6. Kasl SV: The health belief model and behavior related to chronic illness. Health Educ Monogr 2:433–454, 1974

Bibliography

Books

Dalis GT, Strasser BB: Teaching Strategies for Values Awareness and Decision Making in Health Education. Thorofare, NJ, CB Slack, 1977

Green LW, Kreuter MW, Deeds SG et al: Health Education Planning: A Diagnostic Approach. Palo Alto, Mayfield Publishing, 1980

Leininger MM: Nursing and Anthropology: Two Worlds to Blend. New York, John Wiley & Sons, 1970

Leininger MM: Transcultural Nursing: Concepts, Theories and Practices. New York, John Wiley & Sons, 1978

Journals

Becker MH, Drachman RH, Kirsht JB: A new approach to explaining sick role behavior in low-income populations. Am J Public Health 64:205–216, 1974

Marston MV: Variations in interpretation of prescription instructions. JAMA 227:927–931, 1974

Partridge KB: Nursing values in a changing society. Nurs Outlook 26:356–360, 1978

Rosenstock IM: Patient's compliance with health regimens. JAMA 234, No. 4:402–403, 1975

Rosenstock IM: Historical origins of the health belief model. Health Educ Monogr 2:328–335, 1974

Chapter 5
Legal and Ethical Issues

So far, we have examined various issues that the nurse encounters in her delivery of patient education. Although these issues are complex, their complexity does not approach that of the legal and ethical issues that arise in health education. These issues are very difficult and ambiguous. This chapter outlines the legal and ethical constraints of patient education. Nursing's manifesto for patient education, the states' Nurse Practice Acts, is viewed in light of the American Nurses' Association (ANA) Model Practice Act. The effects on the delivery of patient education of physicians' orders, informed consent, and institutional policies are also discussed. Finally, ethical issues that involve not only the patient, but also society at large, are examined with the intent of providing guidelines that the nurse can use in ethical decision making relating to patient and health education.

Legal Issues

Nurse Practice Act

The most important legal basis for patient education is contained within the Nurse Practice Acts, which have been developed by all 50 states. Not only do the Nurse Practice Acts protect the lay public from incompetent practitioners by establishing procedures for licensure, but most also define the practice of nursing. (There are 11 states that have no definition of the practice of nursing contained within the act.)[1] The practice and function of nursing is described within the ANA Model Nurse Practice Act (see Appendix A at the back of this chapter). There are six basic functions covered by most Nurse Practice Acts; the one pertaining to the provision of health guidance and participation in health education establishes the foundation for the professional nurse's involvement in patient/health education.

Although many states have been recently revising their Nurse Practice Acts to define more clearly nursing practice, other states have noticeably vague definitions or no definition at all. It behooves every nurse to become acquainted with her state's Nurse Practice Act and, if necessary, to work for clarification of definitions. Although we admit the shortcomings of some Nurse Practice Acts, we contend that they are, in most cases, the professional nurse's basis for involvement in health education.

Physician's Orders

Another legal basis for the nurse's participation in patient education is physicians' orders. Nurses are recognized as having functions independent of the physician. It is true, nevertheless, that many of the professional nurse's functions are contained in the Nurse Practice Acts in the category of carrying out the legal orders of physicians for medications and treatments.[1] Many physicians, recognizing the importance of patient education and often wishing to ensure delivery of such education to their patients, will write specific orders (*e.g.,* for diabetic teaching or myocardial infarction [MI] rehabilitation). The problem lies not with the physician who writes orders, but rather with the physician who specifies that he does *not* want his patient educated or to receive particular information. Such an attitude may be the result of the physician's experience with an inadequately prepared nurse who attempted patient teaching or with dependent patients who state that they want "to know enough but not too much." The nurse is then placed in an untenable situation, in which the physician refuses to permit patient education and the Nurse Practice Act mandates it. Most nurses resolve such dilemmas by personally discussing the issue with the physician and, if necessary, with the nursing supervisor. If the nurse is unable to gain a satisfactory answer to her problem, she must then decide whether to go ahead and teach the patient what he wants or needs to know in order to manage his life or to abide by the written or oral physician's orders.

It is undoubtedly true that a small minority of patients would not benefit from patient teaching. This is usually evident to nurses—if not, it will become so during the initial assessment to ascertain the patient's readiness for patient education. Examples of this patient population are the patient with organic brain syndrome or severe mental retardation and the patient who, because of situational constraints, would only be more stressed by patient-education efforts. In such situations, the physician and nurse can collaborate and devise other methods of imparting the necessary information.

Another problem for nurses who attempt to provide patient education is designated by nurses in various practice settings as "the authoritarian, omniscient physician." This is the physician who makes all decisions for his patients and who will frequently refuse to let his patients be educated on the grounds that he "knows what is best" for his patients. If the nurse has attempted discussion with the physician and met with resistance, she may decide to go ahead anyway and complete her patient teaching activities. The nurse should attempt this only when she has established a therapeutic relationship with the patient, when she strongly believes that he needs the information, and when she is confident of her abilities to teach the necessary information. Her teaching/learning activities should then be carefully documented in the patient's chart. We know of no attempt by a patient to sue a nurse for patient teaching, and in our judgment it is better to err on the side of giving too much information than to err on the side of giving too little.

This legal issue is subsumed under the area of a patient's "right to know." When the patient enters into a contractual agreement with medical, nursing, and allied-health-services personnel and willingly presents his body for whatever diagnostic and treatment procedures are deemed necessary, he is guaranteed the right to know. The patient's right to know includes the right to know what is wrong with him, the right to know what diagnostic and therapeutic processes will be used, and the right to know what his prospects are for physical recovery.[2] The nature of this contractual agreement guarantees a patient's right to know what he can do to effect his physical recovery and thus would include necessary patient education.

In recent years, a case arose involving a nurse in Idaho who gave a patient too much education in the judgment of the Idaho State Board of Nursing. Ms. Jolene Tuma had her license suspended for six months after she was charged with unprofessional conduct. The charge resulted from Ms. Tuma's telling a patient, who had already given informed consent for chemotherapy, about alternative forms of treatment. The Idaho Supreme Court reversed the 1976 lower-court ruling in 1979, stating that it found nothing in the Idaho Nurse Practice Act that indicated Ms. Tuma was acting unprofessionally by discussing alternative forms of treatment. The main issues involved in Ms. Tuma's case were whether discussion of alternative forms of treatment after informed consent has been given denotes unprofessional conduct, the lack of consultation with physician and lack of documentation by Ms. Tuma, and her presentation of "questionable alternative therapies" (*i.e.,* Laetrile, nutrition, herbs, and touch therapy).[3] It is our opinion that Ms. Tuma did not act unprofessionally and that she was responding to the patient and his family's request for patient education. Her only faults were her lack of judgment in refraining from discussing the incident with the physician and her lack of documentation.

The discussion of these issues is continued in the section of this chapter dealing with informed consent and also in the section on ethics.

Institutional Policies

Because patient education is one of the independent functions carried out by the professional nurse, there have been very few legal problems arising between the nurse and the institution. Many nurses are involved in teaching standard patient-education protocols or programs. Most of these, however, have been developed by nurses and physicians who have given their approval to the content; thus, the institution would not be responsible for problems arising from patient teaching. *Respondeat superior*, referring to a master–servant relationship, is the legal term that holds an employer or institution responsible for the wrongful acts of its employee.[4] As patient education becomes more highly developed within hospital settings, the possibility exists that nurses and other professionals employed by the hospital to develop and participate in patient-education activities could be sued on the basis of their teaching, and the institution could also be sued on the basis of *respondeat superior*.

The possibility, which presently appears dim, of institutional licensure could place legal constraints on the nurse's patient-teaching activities. If nurses were licensed by institutions instead of individually, the institutions would be responsible for defining nursing practice. This could have a great impact on patient education, depending on each institution's definition of nursing. Legal issues arising from institutional policies do not presently seem to pose many problems for nurses, although problems may arise in the future.

Informed Consent

Informed consent is a topic that serves as a useful transition from purely legal issues to ethical issues because it contains elements of each. First and foremost, *informed consent* is a legal term and can be defined as a voluntary act by which one person agrees to allow someone else to do something to him, after he has first received information.[4] Informed consent is part of the contract, mentioned earlier, to which the patient agrees when he presents himself for health care. Informed consent is a specific kind of consent that allows a health professional to perform a procedure or treatment involving touching the patient. Without informed consent, such touching would be considered battery because the intentional touching of another person without authorization is a legal wrongdoing.[5] A written consent, in order to be valid, must be signed by the client and witnesses, must indicate that the procedure done was the one consented to, and must indicate that the consenting client understood the nature of the procedure, the risks involved, and the probable outcome.[4]

Contrary to popular opinion, the only legal involvement the nurse has in informed-consent situations is to witness the signature of the patient. She is not responsible for the explanation of medical care to the patient, nor is she legally responsible for judging the quality of the explanation or ascertaining the patient's understanding of the consent form. She should, however, be able to certify that the patient was mentally competent and signed the form without coercion.

The nurse does have a responsibility to determine that the patient is literate and possessed of his faculties. Chapter 8 presents methods of determining patients' literacy levels. If the nurse recognizes that the patient is unable to read the informed-consent document, then it must be read to him. She must make the physician aware of the patient's lack of reading skills before the patient signs the consent form. Patients who do not understand descriptions of procedures are said to give *uninformed consent*.[6] If the lack of understanding is caused by illiteracy or poor explanation of the procedure, the physician is considered negligent in performing his duty.

The patient should know that he has the right to change his mind after signing the informed-consent form, and if he does so the nurse should report it immediately to the physician. Not only does the patient have a right to change his mind after signing a consent form, he also has the right to decide to withdraw from the treatment or procedure and to refuse involvement in the recommended medical regimen. Some patients remove themselves from the therapeutic regimen when they find that the therapy does not seem warranted by the outcome or that the outcome is not what they were first led to believe. Our experience, however, indicates that the majority of patients are sufficiently intimidated by health-care providers to be fearful of removing themselves from diagnostic procedures or treatment. As health-care providers, we frequently neglect to inform the patient that he may withdraw from treatment. We believe that health-care providers must make this option known to patients, regardless of the fact that the patient may choose something different from what we think is best.

Another corollary to informed consent is that patients must be enlightened regarding the risks and consequences of *not* having diagnostic procedures and therapy performed.[6] For instance, a diabetic patient has the right to refuse to comply with insulin or diet therapy, but he must be made well aware of the probable outcome of noncompliance. When we taught diabetics about management, we found that we avoided telling them about the neuropathies, nephropathies, and retinopathies that could develop because we did not want to frighten the newly diagnosed diabetics. Such knowledge, however, is central to the management of diabetes and should be transmitted to the patient.

The preceding explanation of informed consent sounds fairly simple and straightforward. There are, however, a number of problems that can arise. One situation with which we are familiar involved an obstetrical nurse clinician in a community hospital. Amniocentesis was performed at this hospital and the nurse clinician routinely explained the procedure to each patient before she obtained a signed informed consent. The physician had mentioned to a particular patient that she might need amniocentesis, which "simply involves getting some fluid out of the sac surrounding the baby." The nurse clinician proceeded, as she had in previous situations, to inform the patient completely of the procedure and its attendant risks. The patient, at this point, refused to have the procedure performed. When the physician found out he became very angry with the nurse and refused to let her do any teaching with his patients. The physician had certainly violated the most up-to-date understanding of informed consent, the "reasonable-person standard." This standard, based on three court decisions in 1972, requires the physician to disclose all facts that a reasonable, average layperson would need before deciding to participate in a diagnostic or treatment procedure.[4] The physician obviously did not reveal the material necessary to make such a decision and when the nurse did disclose the risks in the correct fashion, her position was questioned.

The fact that a patient has contracted with health-care professionals should guarantee his right to know the information needed to make decisions regarding his own care. Physicians, however, sometimes out of misguided paternalism and sometimes operating in what they believe to be the best interests of the patient, will often veil the consent form in medical jargon or explain the procedure so simply that the possibility of dangerous ramifications is never communicated.

On occasion, permission may be given to perform a second procedure contingent upon the results of the first. Until recently, informed consents for breast biopsies contained the provision that if the initial pathology report revealed malignancy, a mastectomy would be performed while the patient was still anesthetized. This contingency portion of the informed-consent document effectively removed a woman's right-to-know and revoked her ability to make an informed decision. In one case with which we are familiar, a nurse who was hospitalized for a biopsy refused to sign the informed-consent document because it contained the provision for an immediate mastectomy. She told her physician that she wished to be involved in the decision making regarding her mastectomy, to which he replied that he would not do the biopsy unless she gave him total power to make the decision. Such incidents not only reflect the grossest possible paternalism, but also reflect a complete abrogation of the patient's right to know. The patient is thus deprived of making choices relating to her own health care and her life.

Informed consent in patient education involves a participation of the nurse in the patient's basic right to know. Although the law requires only that the nurse witness the patient's signature to an informed-consent document, the nurse has another legal obligation based on her state's Nurse Practice Act—an obligation to perform patient teaching. The patient's contract with his health-care providers also guarantees the right to such education. The nurse must make decisions in many informed-consent situations. Some of these decisions will rest on legal bases while others will be related to her own ethical code.

Ethical Issues

Ethics, as a branch of philosophy, is a way of thinking that helps us deal with questions of human conduct. To those of us involved in the health professions, *ethics* pertains to the questions asked about what is right or what ought to be done in situations involving moral decisions relating to patients. In the past, nursing ethics dealt primarily with codes of conduct and professional etiquette. Health professionals became sharply aware of ethical issues when the horrors of Nazi medicine were revealed during the Nuremberg Trials following World War II. The American Nurses' Association (ANA) adopted its first Code of Ethics in 1950. The 1976 revised edition is printed below.

American Nurses' Association Code of Ethics for Nurses

1. The nurse provides services with respect for human dignity and the uniqueness of the client unrestricted by considerations of social or economic status, personal attributes, or the nature of health problems.

2. The nurse safeguards the client's right to privacy by judiciously protecting information of a confidential nature.

3. The nurse acts to safeguard the client and the public when health care and safety are affected by the incompetent, unethical, or illegal practice of any person.

4. The nurse assumes responsibility and accountability for individual nursing judgments and actions.

5. The nurse maintains competence in nursing.

6. The nurse exercises informed judgment and uses individual competence and qualifications as criteria in seeking consultation, accepting responsibilities, and delegating nursing activities to others.

7. The nurse participates in activities that contribute to the ongoing development of the profession's body of knowledge.

8. The nurse participates in the profession's efforts to implement and improve standards of nursing.

9. The nurse participates in the profession's efforts to establish and maintain conditions of employment conducive to high quality nursing care.
10. The nurse participates in the profession's effort to protect the public from misinformation and misrepresentation and to maintain the integrity of nursing.
11. The nurse collaborates with members of the health professions and other citizens in promoting community and national efforts to meet the health needs of the public.

(ANA Model Practice Act. Kansas City, American Nurses' Association, 1976. Reprinted with permission of the American Nurses' Association)

The growth of nursing ethics as an independent body of knowledge has been slow. It is interesting to note that, in the five years from 1956 through 1960, the *Cumulative Index to Nursing Literature* contained only 28 entries relevant to nursing ethics.[7] By 1981, there were 98 entries under the title "Ethics," indicating that more individuals were recognizing the importance of ethics in nursing. This portion of the chapter does not try to encompass all facets of nursing ethics, but rather examines the relationship of ethics to the delivery of health education.

Two different types of ethics will be viewed: *individual* ethical issues as related to patient education, and *health-policy* ethical issues as related to health education. For the purpose of brevity, the first area will be called *microethics* because the individual is the smallest system we can examine relative to patient education. The second area will be referred to as *macroethics* because this encomapsses large-scale issues present at the community, state, and national levels. We will demonstrate that the decision-making process in both microethics and macroethics is the same.

Microethics and Patient Education

Anne Davis and Mila Aroskar, in their excellent book *Ethical Dilemmas and Nursing Practice,* define a dilemma as "(1) a difficult problem seemingly incapable of satisfactory solution, or (2) a choice or a situation involving choice between equally unsatisfactory alternatives."[8] An ethical dilemma, then, involves moral claims conflicting with one another. In many situations when moral conflicts exist, what may be considered "good" is not necessarily what is "right." For example, in the patient-education setting, it may be "good" to tell the patient that he should take his antihypertensive medication on a daily basis, but unless he is also warned of the side-effects such as impotence, which may lead to life-style changes, it is not "right."

Patient education can be a morass of ethical dilemmas for the nurse. If the nurse remembers, however, that her primary responsibility is to the patient and her profession and that she is secondarily responsible to the physician and the institution, what is "right" is usually self-evident. An example of a diabetic patient may clarify this point.

As all health practitioners know, the cornerstones of good diabetic control are diet, medication, and exercise. As patient educators, we teach our juvenile-onset and adult-onset diabetic patients that the triad—diet, medications, and exercise—must be strictly controlled and that this will contribute to a longer, healthier life. In truth, close control may or may not contribute to decreased complications and increased life span in those with juvenile-onset diabetes. Even with very strict control, these patients may develop retinopathies and nephropathies in their 30s. Conversely, the adult-onset diabetic may be able to live to an average life span without such rigid, tight control. Not only have patient educators tended to teach all these patients in the same way, but we also have frequently not told them of the complications that may ensue despite measures they take. Rather than try to coerce the patient into compliance, is it not more honest and ethically sound to present the treatment modalities to the patient, suggest that tight control probably means fewer complications, and then let the patient make his own choices?

In many patient-education situations, *we* decide what the patient learns instead of letting him make choices as an autonomous, independent agent. An example of such an attitude is a physician who said, "I've found out that my patients don't act on most of what I tell them so I've decided not to tell them very much in the future. It's just throwing useless information at them." All of us have had this type of experience with patients. It is still, however, our ethical responsibility to give the patient all the information and let him decide what information is useless. Whether we are dealing with a diabetic patient who should maintain better diet control or an emphysematous patient who should stop smoking, the final decision about adherence to our patient teaching is with the patient. As adults, all patients deserve access to all the information we have, whether or not it dissuades them from following our advice.

There are several theories and frameworks for making ethical decisions. Among them are deontology, utilitarianism, Rawlsian ethics, situation ethics, egoism, Firth's "ideal observer," and Frankena's "obligation" ethic.* In actuality, most of us select combinations of theories to use when making ethical decisions. It is not our purpose to distinguish the most useful theories in relationship to patient education. If a nurse is able to clarify her philosophy of nursing, many of her ethical decisions will follow naturally. Most of us believe that the aim of nursing is to foster high-level health and well-being and to enable the patient to perform self-care activities as his abilities allow. The essence of the nurse–client relationship is trust and openness in communication. Ethical decision making is based on mutual respect, trust, and a genuine concern for the welfare of the patient and his family.

Macroethics and Health Education

Most nurses deal with individual patients and are not accustomed to thinking of collectivities and suprasystems. Indeed, one of the problems we have as a profession today is our insularity and an inability to see, much less confront, wider societal issues. The monumental proportions of the health-education issues that we face today are no reason for the nurse to be dissuaded from entry into the larger forum of macroethics in health education.

* For a more comprehensive discussion of ethical theories, see Anne Davis and Mila Aroskar's *Ethical Dilemmas and Nursing Practice* (New York, Appleton-Century-Crofts, 1978) or Shirley Steele and Vera Harmon's *Values Clarification in Nursing* (New York, Appleton-Century-Crofts, 1979).

When we use the term *macroethics* in reference to health education, we are speaking about issues beyond the personal domain. We are referring to health education and its application to problems of poor housing, poverty, environmental pollution, abuse of tobacco and alcohol, automobile-related injuries, and problems of the workplace. If we wish to improve the lot of society as a whole, we can no longer apply only a personal microethic. We have learned that small-scale health education is not a panacea for wide societal health problems; broader campaigns (*e.g.,* antismoking) have proved to be much more effective. We need to view societal health problems from a different vantage point from that from which we view the single patient.

As we look at society's problems in the light of distributive justice, an ethical position that "seeks to distribute benefits and burdens equally throughout society," we can readily appreciate that this approach has not worked.[9] Benefits and burdens are *not* distributed equally; the poor, the underprivileged, and minorities carry most of the burdens and most of the health-care problems. What is needed is a redistribution of benefits—a *re*distributive justice.

In terms of health education, *redistributive justice* means that priorities for health-care education should shift from individualized program planning for a few to a wider, public-health ethic with the goal of preventing premature death and avoidable disabilities for many. It means valuing the previously undervalued, spending more money on minority groups, and generally reordering societal goals.

In applying a macroethics approach to health education, we are saying as nurses that it is time to place greater value on the underserved and the poor. It is time to remember that the poor welfare mother will gain little from our teaching about diet and pregnancy if she has to return to a life-style in which she does not have enough resources to buy food high in iron and protein.

Nursing's understanding of national priorities and their effects on the delivery of health care must be promoted. One impact on health-care delivery of the recently enormous national-defense spending is obvious: the greater the appropriation for armaments, the less the appropriation for health and welfare. This problem is of incredible magnitude and, as nurses, we must educate the public about these issues. In a nuclear arms race, the underserved lose access to health care as it becomes a privilege instead of a right. Another impact on health care of defense spending is that the affluent as well as the poor lose, because they all face the horrors of total nuclear destruction. Rich and poor alike will be annihilated if nuclear war ensues. Because nurses and physicians are respected members of society, we must convey to the public the medical consequences of nuclear war. Physicians for Social Responsibility is a prominent, nonpartisan group with which nurses and other health-care professionals should affiliate to promote public understanding of this risky issue.

As nurses, we are probably more aware than any other group of health professionals about societal health needs. Many of us spend a large amount of time in the community, yet we tend to assuage the needs of only the individual instead of the needs of the entire community. Planning and implementing community health-education programs are discussed in Chapter 11.

Appendix A: Model Nurse Practice Act

Model Act	*Explanation*

Section II

B. Practice of Nursing by a Registered Nurse. The practice of nursing as performed by a registered nurse is a process in which substantial specialized knowledge derived from the biological, physical, and behavioral sciences is applied to the care, treatment, counsel, and health teaching of persons who are experiencing changes in the normal health processes; or who require assistance in the maintenance of health or the management of illness, injury, or infirmity or in the achievement of a dignified death; and such additional acts as are recognized by the nursing profession as proper to be performed by a registered nurse.

The nursing practice act must contain a definition of the practice which it seeks to regulate. This definition must be stated in terms of the acts which persons licensed under the law are permitted to perform, and which in the interest of public health and safety all others are forbidden to perform.

For the purposes of the law, the definition of nursing practice should be stated in terms broad enough to permit flexibility in the utilization of nursing personnel within the bounds of safety. It must also permit changes in practice consistent with trends in the practice of nursing and related health profession.

In order to protect the interests of the public and the practitioner, the definition of nursing practice in licensing must clearly differentiate between those acts which are independent nursing functions, and those which are dependent upon the prescription of or delegation of medical authority.

Also provided are the elements of substantial specialized judgment and skill which characterize the practice of nursing and the nature of the preparation required for the safe practice of registered nursing.

(Excerpted from the ANA Model Nurse Practice Act. American Nurses' Association Publication Code: NP-52M5/76. Kansas City, American Nurses' Association, 1976. Reprinted with the permission of the American Nurses' Association)

References

1. Creighton H: Law Every Nurse Should Know, 3rd ed, p 19., p. 20 Philadelphia, WB Saunders, 1975
2. Regan WA: The patient's right to know. The Regan Report of Nursing Law 16, No. 1:1, 1975
3. News: Tuma case reversed. Am J Nurs 79:1144, 1979
4. Cazalas MW: Nursing and the Law, p. 33, 35, 101. Germantown, MD, Aspen Systems, 1978
5. Rothman D, Lloyd N: The Professional Nurse and the Law, p. 159. Boston, Little, Brown & Co, 1977
6. McCaughrin WC: The case for patient education: An update on recent court decisions affecting physicians and hospitals. Patient Couns Health Educ, 3(1):1-5, 1981
7. Cumulative Index to Nursing and Allied Health Literature. Glendale, CA, Glendale Adventist Medical Center, 1956–1960
8. Davis AJ, Aroskar MA: Ethical Dilemmas and Nursing Practice, p 6. New York, Appleton-Century-Crofts, 1978
9. Simonds SK: Health education: Facing issues of policy, ethics, and social justice. Health Educ Monogr, 6(Supplement):24, 1978

Bibliography

Benjamin M, Curtis J: Ethics in Nursing. New York, Oxford University Press, 1981

Davis AJ, Aroskar MA: Ethical Dilemmas and Nursing Practice. New York, Appleton-Century-Crofts, 1978

Fenner KM: Ethics and Law in Nursing. New York, Van Nostrand Reinhold, 1980

Fromer MJ: Ethical Issues in Health Care. St Louis, CV Mosby, 1981

Lazes PM (ed): The Handbook of Health Education. Germantown, MD, Aspen Systems, 1979

Spicker SF, Gadoro S (eds): Nursing: Images and Ideals: Opening Dialogue with Humanities. New York, Springer-Verlag, 1980

Steele SM, Harmon VM: Values Clarification in Nursing. New York, Appleton-Century-Crofts, 1979

Thompson JB, Thompson HO: Ethics in Nursing. New York, Macmillan, 1981

Chapter 6

Assessment

As nurses, we are aware that there is already a great deal of literature available on patient education. When we first planned this book, we felt strongly that another "how-to" approach to patient education was not needed. Instead, our commitment was to examine issues arising in our own practice environments, as well as issues suggested by our colleagues that posed challenges not dealt with by other authors. The first five chapters, dealing with issues, were thus born.

As we committed our thoughts and strategies to paper, we became aware that despite texts already available, nurses had unanswered questions about "how-to" facets of patient education. We interviewed our peers and asked them to identify pressing problems in patient education. In addition, our publisher conducted a survey of nurse educators across the country, asking them to define the needs of their students in the implementation of patient education. By summarizing these assessments we became convinced that this next section of our book, dealing with principles of patient education, was also needed. We discovered that nurses were looking for practical guidance in integrating patient education into the nursing process. They felt that, while many authors addressed patient education as a responsibility of the nursing profession, few had offered a realistic approach for nurses facing the pressures of time, extensive patient-care responsibilities, and overloads of paperwork.

In the absence of realistic strategies and creative approaches, many of us have looked to committees, policy statements, and health educators for answers to patient-education problems. In some instances, we have depended on clinical nurse specialists and health educators to meet all patient-education responsibilities. We are now beginning to question our own abilities to face the barriers posed by our institutional environments and the barriers of time shortages and nursing-personnel shortages. We also must deal with educational needs by increasing our teaching skills, defining patient-learning needs, and working with patients' families.

Our goal is to help nurses consider their *internal* environments. We wish to review the process of providing patient education and to guide readers in an assessment of their own skills and knowledge. We will apply the principles of patient education to actual patient-care situations to provide practical examples.

The Nursing Process

Since the 1950s, the nursing process has gained recognition as being fundamental to nursing practice. Many nurses have used its problem-solving method to assess problems in our practice areas, to plan new approaches, to implement interventions, and to evaluate both successes and failures. The nursing process is the application of the scientific method to nursing. Table 6-1 lists the steps of the scientific method and the analogous aspects of the nursing process.

Table 6-1. **The Nursing Process as Scientific Method**

Scientific Method	Nursing Process
Recognition of problem area Definition of specific problem Review of related literatures	Assessment
Proposal of hypotheses	Nursing Diagnosis Goals
Testing of hypotheses	Interventions
Analysis of data	Evaluation
Termination or modification of study	Modification

Use of the nursing process prevents the nurse from acting on only an intuitive basis and forces her to think through what she is doing. Another advantage in using this problem-solving approach is that patient care is individualized. Continuity of care is guaranteed by the sharing of the nursing-care plan derived from the nursing process. Still other advantages are that systematically planned care can be implemented by all nursing personnel and that evaluation of the care and the client's response to it can be made. By understanding that problems arise when needs are not met, nurses realize that they may be called upon to intervene when patients, their families, other nurses, physicians, institutions, or communities have unmet needs. When the nursing process is used, we can feel confident that needs will be assessed and problems confronted in a systematic way.

The nursing process is the vehicle by which we deliver goal-directed, person- and family-centered care. An integral part of this care is patient education. When patients are able to define and understand their own needs, they are more likely to make changes in their own health-care behavior. The nursing process is especially useful in meeting patient-learning needs.

In addition, the nursing process helps nurses to gain recognition for the quality of their patient-care management. The knowledge and skills of nurses are better appreciated because of organized and deliberate decision making. The trust and respect professional nurses are seeking as patient educators are enhanced through the nursing process, and accountability is also assured through the documentation of this process.

Learning to Use the Nursing Process in Patient Education

Knowledge of the nursing process itself is not assurance that nurses are fully prepared to deliver patient education. Instead, the nursing process challenges individuals to assess their own learning needs as well as those of their patients. Nurses must be able to define their own continuing-education needs and find resources to meet them. For example, after the diagnosis of a new diabetic patient on her unit, a nurse may recognize the patient's need to learn how to give himself insulin and prevent complications of the disease, but she may be unsure about how to begin the teaching. The nursing process will guide her in considering her own learning needs that must be met in order for her to teach the patient. The questions she asks herself should include the following:

1. What knowledge and skills must I have?
2. What knowledge and skills am I lacking?
3. What resources are available to help me gain the knowledge and skills I am lacking?

In discussing the nursing process (Chap. 6-9), we will consider the relationships among patient education, the nursing process, and patient-care planning. By concentrating on each component in a step-by-step progression, we will present skills or knowledge needed by the nurse to implement the process, consider practical strategies for patient education, discuss documentation and communication among members of the health-care team, and illustrate the content by using one in-depth study that we will follow through the entire teaching/learning process. Other needs are also addressed.

Although many current patient-education publications provide a prescriptive approach to teaching patients and supply teaching guides for patient instruction in specific situations, we wish to emphasize that this book is a different type of resource. Our focus is on the *process* of teaching and learning (Fig. 6-1). Our goal is to encourage nurses to use problem-solving techniques to discover what the patient needs and to help him develop self-care skills within the contexts of his family and his environment. Patient education is much more than imparting information. It involves helping individuals to become active members of the health-care team and aiding them to make informed choices that maintain or improve the quality of their lives.

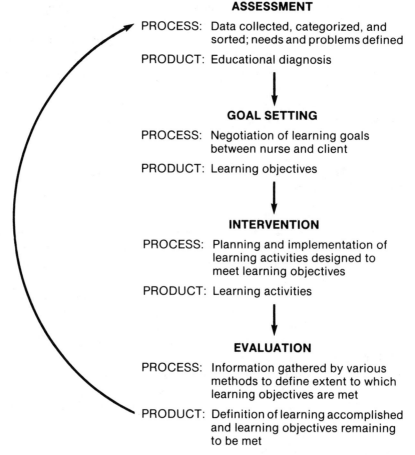

ASSESSMENT

PROCESS: Data collected, categorized, and
sorted; needs and problems defined

PRODUCT: Educational diagnosis

GOAL SETTING

PROCESS: Negotiation of learning goals
between nurse and client

PRODUCT: Learning objectives

INTERVENTION

PROCESS: Planning and implementation of
learning activities designed to
meet learning objectives

PRODUCT: Learning activities

EVALUATION

PROCESS: Information gathered by various
methods to define extent to which
learning objectives are met

PRODUCT: Definition of learning accomplished
and learning objectives remaining
to be met

Fig. 6-1.   *The nursing process in patient education.*

Case studies are examples of courses of action. Just as patient-teaching formats are consulted as valuable resources, the application of our case studies must be individualized by the nurse to meet the needs of each patient. We hope that the reader will consider her own patient-care experiences and use what she reads here to complement her practice of patient education with patients and their families.

The Assessment Process

Looking Back

We interviewed our nursing colleagues about their experiences in patient education. One of them offered the following comments:

> I think that patient education is an important part of the care patients receive. We should be willing to share what we know with patients and help them understand what choices they have.

Sometimes I feel that it really makes a difference and I can tell that the patient understands. But my experiences are not all positive ones and I end up feeling frustrated and angry. After all, patient education takes time out of an already busy schedule of patient care. It requires patience and extra effort to explain procedures and answer questions. I usually have to repeat the information several times or try to explain it in a different way so he can understand. After all my effort, many times the patient still doesn't take his medications or treatments as he should. I end up wondering if he just doesn't want to be well or if he would have taken the information more seriously if it came from a doctor. Then I ask myself, "What did I do wrong?"

Physicians express similar feelings of anger and frustration when patient education fails. Although we all recognize that patients have the right and free will to make choices, we also question our own skills in teaching our patients. We wonder, "Should I have done things differently?"

Where Have We Gone Wrong?

Many health-care professionals describe *patient education* as *giving patients information about their problems and treatments.* The quality of patient education is perceived to have a direct correlation with the availability of audiovisual programs, well-equipped file drawers, and the presence of informative posters in the physician's office. When patients fail to perform the desired behaviors, we assume that they were not given enough information or that they failed to assimilate it. We respond by repeating the information or giving it in a different form.

When the behaviors of patients fail to change, can we assume that they have not learned the facts we have tried to impress on them?

Information Alone is Not Enough

Godfrey Hochbaum suggests that the temptation to give more (or more forceful) information to drive home to patients the possibly dire consequences when they do not exhibit desired behaviors comes from our own assumptions that human behavior is shaped by rationality and sufficient motivation.[1] We assume that one or both must be missing if a person does not act as we expect him to.

The learning of information alone does not assure that behavioral change will follow. To illustrate this point, Hochbaum asks health professionals to compare their own daily behaviors with the behaviors they prescribe for their patients. He reminds us that we tell patients to refrain from smoking, to exercise regularly, to fasten their seat belts, to keep their weight within prescribed limits, to floss and brush their teeth every day, to eat a balanced diet, to have periodic dental and medical checkups, and to follow the physician's instructions accurately. Yet he asks, "How many health professionals comply with all these practices?"

In an attempt to better understand why *patients* do not perform desired health behaviors, Hochbaum asks health professionals to consider why *we* do not practice what we preach. Health professionals are generally more knowledgeable than others about the harmful consequences of not following these practices, and because they see these consequences in their workplace, one would expect them to be "at least as motivated to perform them as the most motivated laypersons."[1]

Identifying Barriers to Behavioral Change

There are many factors that enter into the choices patients make. The integration of learned facts into everyday life is the key to behavioral change. For example, when a patient agrees with the physician that he should lose 20 pounds, that decision alone does not guarantee that he will lose the weight. Upon consideration, we recognize that the initial decision involves making many choices, on a daily basis, that are much more difficult to make than the original decision. These choices involve making sacrifices and overcoming obstacles in day-to-day situations. Patients encounter many strong influences that pose barriers to their maintenance of a medical regimen. Even the most informed and motivated patients have difficult and discouraging experiences where they live, work, and play. Hochbaum suggests that if health professionals can assist patients in identifying these barriers and in finding ways to overcome them, the patients will better cooperate with the medical regimen.[1]

Looking Ahead

We have begun to realize that patient education involves much more than simply sharing the medical information we have with the patient by communicating it in a vocabulary he can understand. We recognize the importance of assessing individual situations to see the patient as he sees himself. Only then can we assist him in recognizing and overcoming obstacles that prevent the desired behaviors. This requires a skilled approach to patients for which health professionals must be prepared. When they are armed with skills in teaching and learning, health professionals are our best resource of patient education. This is not to say that teaching tools such as handouts and audiovisual aids are unimportant, but, if effective learning is desired, they should be individualized for each patient by professionals.

Although nursing programs today include patient-education skills in their curricula, many nurses already working are not well enough prepared to assume patient-education responsibilities. We hope that a review of the process of teaching and learning will help both groups of nurses to respond confidently to the educational needs of patients and their families.

Nursing Policies Can Pose Barriers to Patient Learning

Patient-education skills can be learned, just as we learned to give injections. However, using patient-education skills effectively is dependent on our ability to do things *with* patients, rather than *to* them. Especially in the hospital setting, patients are often put in a dependent position, and their choices are made *for* them by well-intentioned nurses. A learning environment should offer the patient an opportunity to try out new behaviors and receive support and instruction from the staff. What often occurs is that the patient is instructed and shown skills, but he remains in a dependent role. He is discharged from the hospital without having had the opportunity to try out new behaviors.

Health-care settings make heavy demands on professionals, who often respond to their stressful work by categorizing duties and patients. We formulate teaching protocols to assure high-quality care for patients with similar problems. We construct standards and adhere to them. We schedule treatments, medications, and meals. All of this is done in an effort to provide the best of care to patients. If strategies for assuring high-quality care are implemented so rigidly that they stifle the patient's development in a cooperative learning relationship, they may destroy real patient education. As nurses, we must prepare ourselves for the teaching role.

The Nursing Process Model for Patient Education

The nursing process aids the nurse in a reexamination of her relationship to the patient. It offers a reminder that each patient is a person with individual needs and problems. Application of the nursing process encourages the application of protocols and standards that will direct patient care, rather than dictate in a rigid fashion. The components of the nursing process offer a framework for modifying nursing care in such a way that both the nurse and the patient grow in a cooperative relationship. When this is accomplished, the patient is cared for as an individual, and he can learn to participate in his care in a meaningful and satisfying manner.

We will illustrate the use of the nursing process as a model for patient education, highlighting the important skills of assessment, goal setting, intervention, and evaluation. While the principles may appear simple, our intent is not to oversimplify but to provide a vehicle for better understanding and preparation. It is the application of the nursing-process method by our colleagues that promotes patient-education successes.

Enacting the Assessment Process

Assessment is a process of collecting data systematically in order to identify accurately the needs and problems of patients and their families. In the assessment process we continuously collect information from different sources, validate these data, sort and categorize the data, and summarize or interpret the information. The end product of the assessment is a nursing diagnosis—a nursing judgment based on sound data that has been systematically collected and analyzed.[2]

Assessment
- A systematic process
- Collection of information from a variety of sources
- A sorting and categorization of information
- Definition of needs and problems

The practice of nursing is founded on the ability of nurses to carry out nursing interventions based on the assessment of individual situations. Nurses are called upon to respond to patients and their families when they are unable to meet their own needs. The goals of nursing care are to reinforce the client's strengths, assist the client to meet basic human needs, and help the client to regain his own ability to meet these needs to the greatest degree possible. To provide appropriate nursing care we must be able to define strengths and unmet needs accurately and to state patient problems clearly.

Nursing assessment is not guesswork. It is a conscious, deliberate process, consisting of four steps. We make assessments every day in our personal and professional lives, often without realizing it. While driving to work, we quickly note that the fuel gauge reads *E* and drive into the closest gas station. We take inventory in the pantry and make a list before grocery shopping. We walk into a patient's room, notice his shortness of breath, and elevate the head of the bed. All of these actions are based on *assessment*—the ability to collect and sort information and define areas of need or problems. It is vitally important in patient education for the nurse to make an accurate assessment of strengths and problems so that learning may be tailored to the specific situation. This assessment is based on the collection of specific data from a variety of sources, a sorting of the data, and a written summary statement of problems or needs (a nursing diagnosis), which we call the *educational diagnosis*. The assessment should be documented to assure accountability.

Four Steps in Assessment

1. Select area(s) to be assessed
2. Gather data
3. Sort and categorize data
4. Write a summary statement

In patient education, the goal of the nurse is to assure that the patient is guaranteed his right to know and that he is given the necessary professional assistance to acquire knowledge and skills that will help him to meet his basic human needs. It is obvious, then, that taking the time to make a thorough assessment is essential for accomplishing nursing goals. We now look at each step in the assessment process as it is applied to patient education.

Step 1: Selecting the Area to be Assessed

Working nurses are especially aware of the need to make data collection as organized and efficient as possible. Because data collection is time consuming, it is imperative for the assessment process to collect only useful information. The nurse must avoid the common mistake of gathering too much data because she overlooks how the information is to be used.

Learning needs are defined when a nurse assesses the patient. The assessment for patient education does not have to be separate from other patient-assessment activities. Information about the learning needs of the patient and his family is gathered with other data about the patient's condition. In order to collect information vital to an assessment of learning needs, the nurse must keep the following questions in mind:

What information does the patient need?
What attitudes should be explored?
What skills does the patient need to perform health-care behaviors?
What factors in the patient's environment may pose barriers to the performance of desired behaviors?

The Use of Assessment Instruments

Data should be gathered using a guide or a set of criteria that will direct the nurse to the areas to be assessed. There are many such instruments, published in the literature, that nurses will find helpful in assessing the learning needs of patients and families. Many guides are directed toward a particular patient population such as diabetic patients, stroke patients, patients with ostomies, and so forth. Some nurses choose to construct their own assessment tools, which may better meet individual situations. The important point to remember about assessment tools is that they should guide the nurse in a holistic view of the patient within the contexts of his family and his environment. The instrument should help the nurse to focus on the total person and direct her in collecting data in specific areas related to what the patient needs to learn.

The assessment instrument may be in checklist form. It may be a standard form with space included for responses or it may be in guide form with an accompanying flow sheet for summary in the patient's chart. The tool that seems most helpful to the nurse is the one she should choose.

We constructed our own guide for assessment in patient–family teaching and demonstrate its application in this chapter. This guide is applicable to a wide variety of situations and prompts a thorough consideration of those factors that will either promote learning or pose barriers to behavioral change. We also constructed a patient-care plan (Fig. 6-2) to use with the guide. The care plan emphasizes problem solving in the documentation of the assessment and is found on page 116. We have developed this format as a useful means of putting nursing-process data into a concrete, written form. The case study presented at the end of this chapter will be condensed and used to illustrate the advantages of this form. As the nursing-process chapters (Chap. 6–9) continue we will add more data so that assessment, goals, interventions, and evaluations will all be illustrated using the same case study.

The guide uses a systems-theory framework for assessing the patient and his family. Systems theory encourages an assessment of the total family as the client, rather than dealing with only the patient himself as the client. Because most patient education has ramifications for the entire family, we feel it is important to focus from the beginning on the family system.

Systems theory has gained prominence among family therapists as a method of understanding the effects of family members on one another during their ongoing interactions. The product of the interactions of the individual members, or *subsystems,* are the beliefs, goals, roles, and norms that form the *family system.* One of the corollaries of systems theory is that the system is *more* than the sum of its parts. To the patient educator, this means that the family system must be assessed and intervened with if the patient (subsystem) is to internalize and act upon the information imparted. For example, if the spouse and children of a hypertensive patient are unwilling to prepare and eat low-sodium, low-triglyceride, low-cholesterol meals, the hypertensive patient is going to have difficulty complying with the medical regimen.

Another aspect of systems theory that is important to the patient educator is the concept of the *suprasystem.* We have so far discussed systems and subsystems. When we consider the family as a system, the *suprasystem* is the community to

Patient and Health-Team Assessment	Factors Affecting Behavioral Change for Health Promotion	Educational Diagnosis

Fig. 6-2.   *Nursing-care plan for documentation of patient-family education: Assessment.*

which the family relates. It includes schools, churches, and economic, legal, and health institutions. Assessment of the suprasystem is important in patient education because it affords the patient educator information about support systems that may be mobilized to aid in rehabilitation and financial assistance.

Patient-Family-Education Assessment Guide

   I. Family profile: A word picture of the family
     A. Household composition
     B. Sex and age of members
     C. Occupations of family members
     D. Health status of family members; physical limitations
     E. Genogram
  II. Resources available to the family
     A. Ability to provide for physical needs
       1. Home: Has it space, comfort, safety?
       2. Income: Is it sufficient for basic needs and important extras?
       3. Health insurance: Is it available to the family?
     B. Neighborhood/community resources: Are friends, neighbors, church, and community organizations helpful and involved?
 III. Family education, life-style, and beliefs
     A. Educational backgrounds and attitudes toward education
       1. Do all adult family members have basic reading and writing abilities?
       2. To what extent is education, formal or informal, valued? How much education does each family member have?
       3. Are there language barriers to verbal communication among the patient, family members, community, and medical personnel?
     B. Life-style and cultural background
       1. Does the family subscribe to folk-medicine beliefs?
       2. Is there a conflict between cultural/life-style approach and the health professional's teaching?
       3. What are the normal diet patterns of the family?
       4. What are the family's sleep habits?
       5. What are the activities, exercises, occupations, and hobbies of family members?
     C. Learning abilities of family members
       1. Do they assimilate information easily?
       2. Are they able to apply what is taught?
     D. What is the family's self-concept?
       1. Are family members lacking in self-esteem?
       2. Do they have feelings of powerlessness, as a result of either life situation or patient's sick role?
 IV. Adequacy of family functioning
     A. Ability to be sensitive to the needs of the family members

   1. How is the identified patient perceived?
   2. What are the relationships of other family members to the identified patient and each other?
   B. Ability to communicate effectively with each other
   C. Ability to provide support, security, and encouragement, especially pertaining to the learning environment
   D. Ability for self-help and acceptance of help from others when needed
   1. How open is the family to the health professional's teaching?
   2. How likely are family members to request help in the future if needed?
   E. Ability to perform roles flexibly
   F. Ability to make effective decisions
   G. Ability of the family to readjust ideas about family status, goals, and relationships
   H. Ability of the family to handle crisis situations
   1. Has the family been confronted with chronic illness in the past?
   2. How has the family reacted to situations such as accidental injury or death? Who helped them through it?
 V. Family understanding of the present event
   A. Current knowledge about the problem
   1. Does the family know others with the same problem?
   2. What does the family feel that it needs to know about the illness or problem?
   3. Has the family accepted the illness or problem?
   4. How do they perceive its effect on their lives?
   B. Point in the life cycle of the family at which the problem occurred
   C. Type of onset of the illness or problem: gradual or sudden?
   D. Prognosis for survival and/or prognosis for restorative training
   E. Nature and degree of limitations imposed on the patient's functioning
   F. Level of the family's confidence in the health system with which they affiliate
VI. The identified patient, health problem, and educational needs
   A. The patient's educational and cultural background, especially if different from the family's
   B. The patient's self-concept and reaction to stress
   C. Physical limitations that are barriers to learning or self-care
   D. Information base of the patient
   1. Does he understand the health-team management and the health team's advice?
   2. Does he know others with the same problem and have knowledge of their treatment?
   3. What are his position and his role in the family?

4. Has he had past illnesses?

5. What kind of physiologic feedback is he using?

E. Are the patient and his family members willing to negotiate goals with the health-care team?

F. Are the patient's perceptions and expectations congruent with his family members'?

Patient–Family-Education Assessment Guide

Philosophy. Our opinion is that patients who have the support of family members in the learning process will cooperate better with the medical regimen. In our clinical experiences we have witnessed such a correlation. As patient education clearly becomes recognized as being within the domain of the nurse, questions arise as to who will be taught.

In the past, the nursing profession centered its interest on the hospitalized patient. Any teaching that was done with a patient's family members tended to be peripheral or due to a particular necessity (*e.g.,* if the patient was blind and unable to draw up his insulin or if the patient had sensory aphasia). With the growing recognition of the importance of families and a view of man as "an interrelated, interacting, and interdependent part of a significant network," many health professionals are now beginning to include families in the process of patient education.[3] We are discovering that a systems approach to patient education mandates the inclusion of family members and that teaching one isolated subsystem without dealing with the important family system can, in some instances, negate all teaching efforts.

We believe that educating the patient without including his family will frequently result in poor rehabilitation and poor cooperation with self-care measures, whether the patient is acutely ill or whether he and his family face life with a long-term chronic illness. We feel strongly that patient education should be conducted with the family present, whether in the hospital or at home.

We developed the Patient–Family-Education Assessment Guide to set the stage for such a teaching environment. It was first used for an adult patient and his family who were dealing with a chronic illness. With some minor changes, the guide can be adapted to a family dealing with a patient who has just suffered an acute illness or to a family, such as one with a newborn, trying to establish everyday health maintenance.

Perspective. Using a systems perspective, this guide moves from the family system, its structure, function, and processes, and how the family relates to education, to the patient as a subsystem of the family, and to some of his educational needs.

Theoretical Basis. Families, like other social systems, have structures and functions. The structure of the family is important in assessment for patient-education purposes. The effectiveness of a family's organization can affect the extent to which new health behavior is assumed. Problems with family organization and role definition often pose obstacles to learning.

Differentiation and specialization of roles are important in assessment. For example, the patient's roles may have to change with the onset of a chronic illness, and the provider needs to recognize this in order to assist the family to adapt. Parts I and II of the guide cover some aspects of structure and were partly adapted from MacVicar and Archbold.[4]

Family functions are closely related to family structure, as pointed out by Horton. The functions that remain in the family " . . . are the maintenance of the household and the intimate personal relations of the family members."[3] The criteria developed by Otto for assessing family strengths relate closely to family functions, and some (but not all) are important in assessing the family for patient-education purposes. These are covered in Part IV of the assessment guide. If the desired family strengths are absent, the wisdom of including the family in patient education must be reconsidered or planned in a careful way because the family may be more destructive than beneficial, posing barriers to the patient's learning process.

The family processes of adaptation, integration, and decision making are important to patient–family education. A family faced with the illness of one of its members must be able to adapt and change in a healthy fashion. The ability of the family to handle a crisis situation is a strong indication of family adaptation.[4,5] Boundary maintenance, or the ability to meet needs by obtaining, containing, retaining, and disposing of resources, reflects important data about the ability to adapt. Assessment questions pertaining especially to obtaining and containing resources are found throughout the assessment guide. Dealing with neighborhood and community resources is of special importance. Human resources outside the family are necessary during illness or stress, and they are also indicative of the family's ability to form trusting, caring relationships with others outside of the family. As Lewis points out, this ability is one of the most significant variables in optimally functioning families.[6]

The family process of integration is covered mainly in Parts III and V, and chiefly refers to the family norms and beliefs that help to form the bonds in well-integrated families. It should be noted that a high degree of family integration, built through cultural beliefs and life-styles, may complicate the learning process if the beliefs and values differ widely from those of the health-care provider. Guidelines for Parts III and V were expanded from the works of Gragg and Rees and Redman.[7,8]

Decision making in the family during events of stress or illness can affect the family's future. If decision making is not organized adequately, the family may be unable to make important choices related to health-care plans or unable to assume responsibility in health-care practices. When patient education is involved, it is frequently necessary for the family to decide, whether by consensus, accommodation, or *de facto* decision making, who is going to learn, for example, how to irrigate a colostomy or give an insulin injection.

The importance of assessing the patient as a subsystem of the family is covered in Part VI of the assessment guide, drawn partially from Robinson.[9] The patient's perception of his relationship to the family, whether realistic or unrealistic, can alter the educational process and should be determined before the teaching plan is begun.

Additional Comments. There have been various guides drawn up for assessment of individual learner's needs, and family assessment guides are abundant in the literature as well. Our guide is based on material contained in educational, nursing, psychological, and sociological writings. The guide considers the patient and his family as a system in a potential learning environment. It also illustrates the importance of evaluating the family as a system while considering the impacts of the community, the health-care system, and sociocultural influences as suprasystems.

This assessment guide has worked well for us in our patient-education roles. It has helped us in assessing strengths and weaknesses that influence the ability of patients and families to adapt health behaviors. Later in this chapter, we present a case study that illustrates the use of the Patient–Family-Education Assessment Guide. A model of patient–family education was constructed to help the reader visualize the related components that influence learning (Fig. 6-3). The model is presented and explained.

Figure 6-3 illustrates the components of assessment found in the Patient–Family-Education Assessment Guide. This model represents a healthy educational situation, in which the family has reasonable resources and an assessment of family functioning demonstrates strengths. Two-way arrows

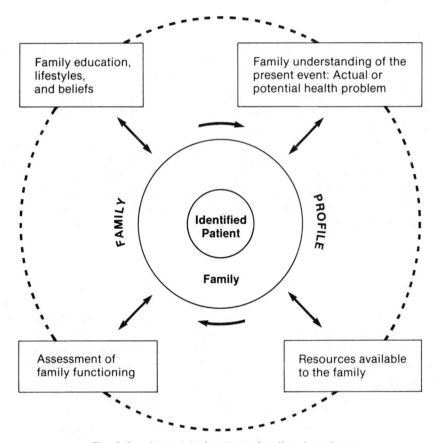

Fig. 6-3. *A model of patient–family education.*

between each component and the family system demonstrate their dual effects on each other. Finally, the entire model is encircled by a broken line to indicate the interactions among all of the components and the family.

Step 2: Gathering Data

Data should be as objective as possible. Collecting these data (using fact or measurement, rather than reflecting feelings or judgments) will guide the nurse to define needs or problems accurately. Words such as *seems, appears, acts,* and *looks* should be avoided. More useful data would note direct observations or actual behaviors. Whenever possible, note what the patient said in his own words. Describe what you hear, smell, see, and feel. Share your observations with the patient in order to validate what you observe. Note the source of the information.

There are several methods of gathering data. The most effective follow:
1. Observation
2. Interviews with patient, family, and significant others
3. Review of patient records
4. Review of the literature: continuing education
5. Collaboration with the health-care team

Observation

A significant amount of information can be collected by the use of the senses. Assessments can be made of the patient's ability to perform self-care activities, his physical appearance, and his affect. The nurse can gather valuable information in the home by observing the interactions of family members, the comfort and safety afforded by the patient's dwelling, and the facilities available to meet his basic needs. Observation will also provide information about the patient's literacy level, his leisure activities, and the role he assumes within the family. While the most common method of observation is through sight, the nurse also relies on information from things she hears, feels, and smells. Verbal and nonverbal cues gathered by observation provide us with valuable information about what the patient thinks, feels, and believes. Questionnaires and tests are often used to assess a patient's knowledge of facts and to explore his attitudes.

The Interview

Taking a patient history or performing a patient–family interview is the most reliable method of obtaining data. When the patient is unable to supply information, owing to his physical or emotional condition, family members are asked to supply as much information as possible. Whether the nurse finds herself interviewing the patient or one of his family members, there are guidelines and suggestions for interviewing effectively; some of those we have used follow.

Establish a trusting environment. The patient must feel a sense of security and trust in order to confide information. He needs to feel that his concerns are taken seriously, and that his needs are important and respected. Communicate trust and respect to the patient by concentrating attention on him, maintaining eye contact, and being an active listener. The necessity of establishing a trusting environment is illustrated by the situation that develops when a nurse deals with a venereal-disease patient. The nurse must assure the patient that his case will be held in strict confidence. After the nurse has assured the patient of confidentiality, she must then explain the importance of notifying the patient's sexual contacts so that they can be treated. Such situations are very delicate, and if the client does not trust the nurse it will be impossible for the nurse to assist the client.

Use open-ended questions. Help the patient to provide more complete information by using the principles of active listening. Use phrases such as "Go on" or ask, "Can you tell me more about that?" and repeat the last words of what the patient has just said. This communicates an interest in what he has to say and a desire to understand how he feels. Open-ended questions that ask for descriptions rather than a "yes" or "no" answer help the patient to give information about how he perceives his needs. If we continue with our example of the client with venereal disease (gonorrhea), the nurse can use open-ended questions such as, "Can you tell me a little more about what you know about gonorrhea?" If the nurse states to the client, "You know how you got this, don't you?" the client will probably simply respond, "Yes," because he is embarrassed, he does not want to admit his ignorance, and he feels generally uncomfortable in the presence of the nurse. It is important in such situations, and in many other patient-education settings, to avoid judgmental behaviors. The use of open-ended questions allows the client to present what he knows so that the nurse can assess what else she needs to teach.

Choose the right setting and timing. Effective interviewing takes place in a setting where the patient and interviewer can be free of distractions and where information can be shared privately. Obstacles to effective interviewing arise when the patient is too tired or too ill to share his thoughts comfortably or when the interviewer is distracted. Extremely lengthy interviews are difficult for both the patient and interviewer. Plan the interview so that critical information is obtained first; perhaps it will be necessary to have several short interviews. For example, counseling related to venereal disease must be accomplished discreetly and without family members or anyone else present. In the outpatient setting, the client should be alone with the nurse in a private room where there will be no interruptions.

Let the patient "tell his story." Allow the patient to tell you how *he* perceives his needs and problems. Maintain objectivity about what he says and try not to make judgments about his perceptions of his pain or his needs. Speak to the patient using language he can understand, rather than medical terminology and abbreviations. Speak slowly and clearly, allowing him time to think about your questions before he answers. If he wanders off the track, gently lead him back by repeating your question. Explain the purpose of the interview to the patient. Let him know that you want to get to know him better in order to care for him in the best manner possible. For example, let the chronic obstructive pulmonary disease (COPD) patient with asthma explain his perception of the problem. He may believe that his recent onset of severe symptoms is related to a specific activity such as walking or sexual intercourse when, in fact, his theophylline blood level is not in the therapeutic range. Once we find out what the patient believes, we may be able to correct some important misconceptions.

Tips on note taking. Notes from the interview will make documentation more accurate and more efficient. It is important, however, that you avoid writing too many notes during the interview because this may disturb the patient. Facts, symptoms, times, names, and short quotes from the patient may be recorded quickly and can be used when you are ready to document the results of the interview. Before beginning to record data during an interview, it is imperative to say to the patient, "I am going to write down a few things you say so that I don't forget anything important." Taking notes during an interview frequently makes clients uncomfortable; an explanation can alleviate such discomfort and prevent misunderstandings.

Review of Patient Records

The patient's medical records are often the nurse's first source of information. Although information can be gathered quickly from the patient's chart, it should be supplemented by information from other sources. Medical records supply data about the patient's health history, his previous hospitalizations, his past experience with the health-care system, and observations others have made about him. They can give us clues to finding additional sources of information, such as a public-health nurse or community agencies that have worked with the patient. Information gathered from the patient record should be validated by observation and the patient interview.

Review of the Literature: Continuing Education

In the nursing field, which is becoming increasingly specialized and advanced, reading texts and journals to update knowledge and skills is a professional responsibility. Basic nursing education is a foundation for practice, but the ability to anticipate and intervene in areas of need depends on willingness to increase that original knowledge base through continuing education.

In order to intervene responsibly with patients and their families, be prepared with an understanding of the disease or health problem, its medical management, and its impact on life-styles. Textbooks and manuals such as *The Lippincott Manual of Nursing Practice* are valuable resources.[10] Many journal articles describe new approaches to teaching patients and their families or increase our awareness of self-help groups and other resources that assist in preventing, resolving, or coping with health problems. Workshops and other continuing-education programs offer good opportunities for learning about patients' problems, and the causes and management of these problems, from experienced colleagues.

Collaboration with the Health-Care Team

Data gathered by other nurses, and by physicians, dietitians, pharmacists, physical therapists, and social workers, can validate and supplement information gathered from the sources previously mentioned. Whenever possible, team members should contribute to planning the care of the patient and his family. Patient education is a concern of the team. Coordination of learning goals and activities is important for ensuring that the time of the professional and the patient/family is used productively.

Collaboration is facilitated by good verbal and written communication, team conferences, updated nursing-care plans, and effective use of such opportunities as physicians' rounds to discuss the patient-teaching plan. For example, the hospital social worker who interviews the family is frequently given lists of medications that the patient has received from various physicians. The social worker will then give this list of medications and prescribing physicians to the nurse, whose responsibility it is to share the list with the patient's admitting physician.

Step 3: Sorting and Categorizing Data into Problem Areas

Data gathered from a variety of sources must be carefully considered, validated, and grouped into problem areas. Under optimal circumstances, the health-care team sits down together and agrees upon assessment of patient problems and learning needs, factors affecting behavioral change for health promotion, and a summary statement, referred to as the educational diagnosis.

Step 4: Writing a Summary Statement: Educational Diagnosis

The formulation of a summary statement and documentation of the assessment are critical points in the assessment phase. They mark the conclusion of the initial phase and prepare for a negotiation of learning goals among the provider, the patient, and his family. In addition to helping to assure the quality of the patient's care, conscientious documentation clearly notes patient-care planning and reinforces communication among members of the health-care team, the patient, and the family. This final step in the assessment process is a good opportunity to validate the provider's perceptions of the needs and problems with the family.

An effort to prioritize the identified needs and problems will help the provider to counsel the patient and his family in setting learning goals. The summary statement should reflect the prioritizing of educational needs. The summary statement and nursing diagnosis are synonymous. Because we are discussing nursing diagnosis and patient education we call this statement an *educational diagnosis*. The nurse analyzes the assessment data and the factors affecting behavioral change and develops a concise educational diagnosis that is a synthesis of the first two assessment steps. An educational diagnosis identifies the patient's learning needs and suggests a plan of action.

It is often difficult to set priorities when faced with problems in several areas. A consideration of a hierarchy of human needs will aid the nurse in a prioritization of problem areas and offer guidance in how and where to begin patient teaching.

Prioritizing Needs and Problems

As human beings, all of us have common needs that must be satisfied. The ability of patients and their families to survive depends on their effectiveness in meeting these basic human needs. When they are unable to meet basic needs, problems arise that they often cannot resolve alone. At that point, health professionals are called upon to intervene. Our goal is to help clients regain the ability to meet their own needs and to foster their maximum development, both as individuals and in their relationships with others.

Maslow suggests that needs exist in various levels and that these groups of needs can be visualized as a hierarchy in which lower needs must be at least partially met before a person can meet higher-level needs.[11] A consideration of these needs helps us to prioritize needs in nursing care and in patient teaching. Many of us have discovered that learning is hampered when the family faces problems with housing, finances, or threatened self-esteem. Because the assessment process involves not only a listing of needs but also a consideration of priorities, it is helpful to use Maslow's hierarchy of needs as a guide in doing so. The five levels are briefly presented here and are discussed in more detail in Chapter 7. Figure 6-4 illustrates examples of nursing interventions related to patient education in each of the levels for the individual; Figure 6-5 illustrates nursing interventions for families and communities at each level of the hierarchy.

Maslow's Hierarchy of Needs

Physiologic and Survival Needs
Oxygen; food; water; elimination; sleep; sexual satisfaction; physical and mental comfort

Safety and Security Needs
Physical safety; housing; economic security; job security; emotional security

Affection and Belongingness Needs
Giving and receiving of kindness, consideration, love; feelings of acceptance by others, prestige; membership in a family; opportunity to give and receive; interaction with others

Esteem or Recognition Needs
Expression of ourselves and being understood by others; sharing of hopes, dreams, fears, desires; others' recognition of our personal development; status; accomplishment; the desire to be "somebody"

Self-Actualization: Self-Determining Needs*
Achievement of potential; independence; ability to meet one's own needs; self-fulfillment; creativity; the process of becoming.

*This is the highest level of needs. This measurement is different for each person.

Learning Takes Place During the Assessment Process

When the patient and his family have an active role in defining their problems, family learning occurs. Self-care activities are dependent on the patient and his family's abilities to solve problems by gathering information and categorizing signs and symptoms into problem areas. We can help them build these skills by verbally sharing our thoughts during the assessment process. Let the patient and his family witness and contribute to a systematic collection of data and definition of problems. Inform them about the rationales for collecting certain kinds of data and the best ways for discovering and documenting them. The promotion of learning during assessment builds problem-solving skills, encourages validation of data with the patient and his family, and serves as a motivator for future learning. Adults

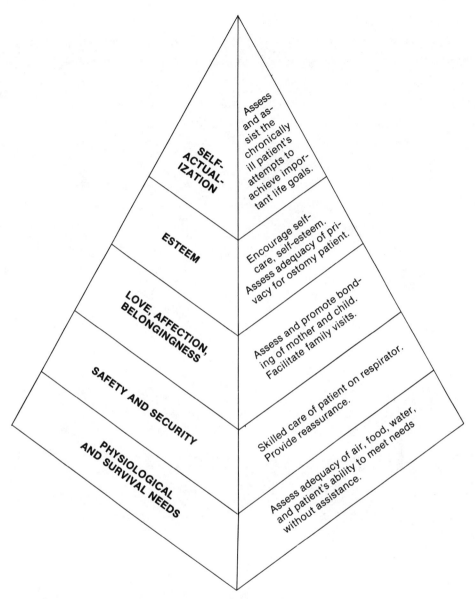

Fig. 6-4. *Using Maslow's Hierarchy in nursing assessment of the patient.*

are more motivated to learn when they have been able to identify their own needs and to contribute toward planning a program that is tailored to their particular circumstances.

A Thorough Assessment May Be a Time Saver

Time-management issues are often mentioned as impediments to the assessment process. It seldom seems feasible to dedicate an hour to collecting information in an

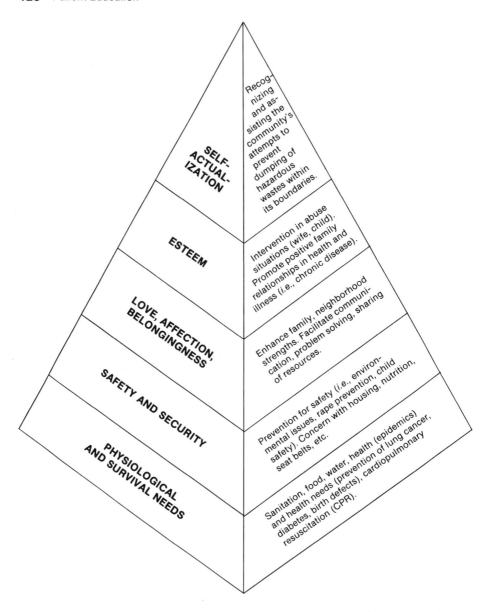

Fig. 6-5. *Using Maslow's Hierarchy in nursing assessment of the family and community.*

interview or to making a detailed assessment. We would like to emphasize a few points related to time issues.

1. Assessment requires spending time in astute observation and active listening. Much time is lost when the care plan is constructed without input from the patient and his family; interventions in such cases are often

ineffective and we spend additional time going back to the assessment process to discover barriers to change that were preventing our progress all along.

2. The patient and his family have a need to tell their story. They must be given time to offer their perceptions of their own problems. We must take time to help them understand what is expected of them if they are later to take charge of self-care activities.

3. Assessment can be made anytime we interact with patients and their families. Gathering information need not be restricted to a one-hour interview. Bathtime, mealtime, rounds, visiting hours, and medication times are all potential opportunities for assessment.

4. Patients are sensitive to the time pressures of health professionals. They often do not know what is expected of them, whether (or for how long) they will have your attention, or how to contribute important information. We can teach them to help us with time restraints by offering statements like the following: "Mrs. Wise, I have set aside 15 minutes this morning at about 10:00. I will be asking you and your husband to answer some specific questions for me about your health problems so I can better plan your care with Dr. Jones and the nursing staff." This gives the patient an idea of what is expected of her and informs her that she will be asked specific questions instead of being put in the position of not knowing what information is important. In some instances, a questionnaire can be given ahead of time to collect initial data, which will be discussed during the interview. Whatever we can do to minimize interruptions and distractions during the interview will help to maximize productivity. Fifteen minutes of well-planned, well-used time accomplishes more toward assessment than does an hour with interruptions and lack of direction.

Although some might argue that the Patient–Family-Education Assessment Guide is too lengthy and time consuming, we wish to emphasize that its criteria offer a comprehensive tool for identifying barriers to learning and clues for individualizing the teaching plan. Clearly, even with such a tool, it is seldom possible to gather all this information at one time, and we are sometimes unable to cover every aspect. The more information to which we have access, the better able we are to understand and influence patient behaviors. The guide offers direction for discovering such information during the initial assessment and throughout ongoing assessment as part of the provider–patient–family relationship.

Case Study: Mrs. Dawe   We met Mrs. Dawe when she came to the outpatient clinic for her regular appointment. She told us she had come to the clinic "to keep check on my sugar and have my blood pressure checked." She offered the information that she was a diabetic and needed help with her "weight problem." Her physician shared with us some of his frustration in caring for Mrs. Dawe. He referred to her as a "delightful lady" who was just "not compliant" in spite of numerous patient-education efforts. We suggested making one or two home visits as a means of identifying factors that might be influencing Mrs. Dawe's cooperation with her medical management. The physician agreed that this was a good idea and together we suggested to the patient that we make a home visit.

The following information was collected using the Patient–Family-Education Assessment Guide.

Family Profile   Mrs. Dawe was a white, 73-year-old, grossly obese woman. At five feet eight inches, she weighed 280 pounds. Her manner in the outpatient clinic was matter-of-fact and when we requested some urine for testing, she immediately asked, "Clean-catch or not?" We had known that the patient was a retired registered nurse. She was not going to lose any time making certain we recognized her status and competence.

An appointment for the first home visit was made during the visit in the outpatient clinic. The following information was obtained during two home visits.

Mrs. Dawe met us at the door when we arrived for the home visits. She was much more casually dressed than she was in the clinic. She wore a housedress with sandals and no hose. Her white hair was neatly combed. Mr. Dawe was ready for the first visit. He was dressed in denim overalls. He was smaller in stature than his wife and was considerably outweighed by her. He was slightly deaf, but made every effort to keep up with the conversation although he was neither as verbal nor as articulate as his wife. Mr. and Mrs. Dawe were both born in the South and both had lived there all their lives, except for a short time when Mrs. Dawe was still single and she lived in New York City working at a large city hospital.

Mr. and Mrs. Dawe were both retired. Their last jobs were at a medical center, where Mrs. Dawe worked as an RN floater and Mr. Dawe was a maintenance worker. Before their children were born, Mrs. Dawe did private-duty nursing, until the Depression made such work unavailable. Mr. Dawe's occupational history included various skilled and semi-skilled jobs; he had worked for railroads, textile mills, and during World War II, for the Army at a military camp.

The household had once included the Dawes' four children, born between 1932 and 1937. The oldest child (and only daughter) was presently employed at a local governmental agency. This daughter had been educated at a local private university, and then she was married and widowed within four years. A daughter from this first marriage, now 20 years old, was presently a freshman in a local state university. The Dawes' daughter had remarried, and this second marriage was an unhappy one, with physical abuse and separations involved. The Dawes' second child had married, had three children, and lived and worked in the same county as his parents. He was employed in the electronics industry. The third child seemed to be the "fair-haired boy." This son graduated from a local state university and then went to work for a large insurance company, which had steadily promoted him and transferred him around the country. This son, his wife, and three of their four children were living in Arizona and were greatly missed by Mrs. Dawe. Living nearby, with his wife and son, was the Dawes' fourth and youngest child. He worked as a painter and had recently painted the exterior of his parents' house.

The health status of the Dawes is important to consider at this point in assessment because it influences other areas in the analysis. Both of the Dawes were in robust good health well into their 50s. At that point, however, Mrs. Dawe's genetic heritage and the effects of Mr. Dawe's physically demanding work caught up with them.

In 1963, at age 56, Mr. Dawe had a power-tool accident that resulted in permanent loss of function of his left hand. Ten years following surgery, Mr. Dawe suffered a myocardial infarction (MI) from which he fully recovered. Two years following the MI, emphysema developed and persisted, limiting Mr. Dawe's ability to engage in yard work or gardening. Mr. Dawe smoked about a pack and a half of cigarettes per day. Eight years ago, Mr. Dawe had been hospitalized with a bleeding ulcer, but had not been similarly affected since. Three years ago he had had a herniorrhaphy performed at the local medical center for an inguinal hernia. Glaucoma had been a problem, but was arrested by medications. Mr. Dawe was amazingly spry, considering his ailments.

Mrs. Dawe's health history was not as long and complicated, but its implications for the future were probably more negative. Mrs. Dawe's diabetes was first diagnosed in 1965, at age 56, and she was placed on insulin at the time of diagnosis. Her insulin requirements had steadily increased; at the time of the home visit she was on a daily dose of 55 units of U100 NPH insulin. Her weight had steadily increased from 170 pounds to 280 pounds and her attempts at weight reduction using an 800-calorie-a-day diet were fruitless. Retinopathies and a cataract needing removal had developed since the onset of diabetes. Mrs. Dawe's written records of urine sugar and acetone levels showed very few periods of diabetic control. Hypertension had been diagnosed about eight years earlier. It was poorly controlled by 100 mg hydrochlorothiazide daily. Mrs. Dawe had exercised progressively less as she had grown older, and the combination of obesity, diabetes, and hypertension had left her in very poor physical health. The slightest amount of exertion made her short of breath and she stated that she could not participate in any guided exercise program. Mrs. Dawe was at risk for both a stroke and a myocardial infarction.

Resources Available to the Family

The Dawes' seven-room, completely owned home was situated in a small rural community and had aged comfortably over its 30 years. The interior of their home had been well kept, with additions such as carpeting and a new furnace added since they had first built the house themselves, "piece by piece," in the 1940s. The interior was clean, the furniture was comfortable and in good repair, and there was a homey feeling, accentuated by a pleasant clutter of family photographs, trophies, and knickknacks. Prominently displayed on a table was a photo of their second oldest son and his family, who were now located in Arizona. Photos of other children and grandchildren were in less prominent places. Mrs. Dawe gave us a tour of the home, pointing out the large size of the rooms and explaining that the candy in the dining room was not for her but for the visiting children. We also noted with interest three boxes of cake mix in Mrs. Dawe's kitchen cupboards and a cake plate sitting out in the dining room. The home was larger than necessary for their present needs because separate bedrooms had been promised to each child when the house was built. The Dawes' past lack of financial resources seemed to have been surmounted.

Income for the family was derived mainly from Social Security benefits. The two pensions from the medical center amounted to only $36/month. Although the Dawes' income was limited, it did allow for travel; the previous summer they had driven to Arizona to visit their son and his family. Limited financial help was received from their children in the form of home improvements and money for traveling. Recognizing the limitations of Medicare, Mr. and Mrs. Dawe paid insurance premiums that amounted to $348/year, a rather large expenditure for them.

Neighborhood and community resources were informal but supportive. Neighbors watched the homes of one another and they all kept keys to one another's homes. In the summer and fall the Dawes enjoyed their neighbors' garden produce. The family faithfully attended a local Methodist church because it was convenient and they liked the parishioners, but both hastened to add that they were not members of the church. When questioned about involvement in community organizations, Mrs. Dawe spoke with pride of her work in the local school system when they were both employed. She told us about her initiation of an immunization program at a local elementary school in 1947. She remarked that she still had a feeling of accomplishment every time she saw the school. This was a family with informal and unstructured interface with community agencies and resources. In times of personal need, however, they had obtained services from the church, which had also helped their daughter through some difficult times.

Family Education, Life-styles, and Beliefs

Education was highly valued by this family, especially by Mrs. Dawe. She stated, "One of the reasons we moved to this area was that there are four universities nearby." Mrs. Dawe had finished a nurses' training program in 1927 and opted for a year at a large

hospital in New York City in advanced medical–surgical nursing.
Mr. Dawe had graduated from high school, but had no further
formal education. All four of the Dawe children had graduated from
high school; two had completed college. Revealing that her own
mother had valued education highly, Mrs. Dawe said that her mother
had taught herself to read and write and then encouraged her 12
children to get education beyond high school, which some did.
Books, magazines, and newspapers were evident in the household.

Mrs. Dawe denied that she held folk-medicine beliefs. If
Mr. Dawe subscribed to any folk-medicine beliefs, it seemed certain
his wife did not share them. She prided herself on keeping current
with medical matters, gaining most of her knowledge from *Family
Health* magazine, to which she subscribed.

The learning abilities of Mr. and Mrs. Dawe were adequate,
although Mrs. Dawe was unable to follow her 800-calorie diet. The
self-concept of this couple appeared healthy. Together they expressed
the view that they had worked hard in life, "but had come through in
good shape." As a couple, they both seemed to have achieved
Erikson's various stages and were in the eighth developmental stage,
completing the tasks of ego integrity.[12] Erikson's developmental
stages are defined in Chapter 7.

Adequacy of Family Functioning

The adequacy of family functioning had to be assessed on the
basis of the husband–wife dyad and self-report. Mrs. Dawe appeared
to be viewed by her husband with a fondness and warmth that had
developed over 47 years of a marriage marked by economic and
personal tribulations. Mrs. Dawe was quick to say that the marriage
had been good, and that they were very happy together now.
Mr. Dawe laughed in a somewhat embarrassed fashion, but
nonverbal clues such as nods of agreement and appropriate smiles
indicated that he agreed with her assessment. Relationships with their
children seemed healthy and supportive on the basis of Mr. and Mrs.
Dawe's reports. Three of the four children lived in the same county
and, although there was no constant interchange ("We don't get
involved in their business"), there was a feeling of closeness. Both
Mr. and Mrs. Dawe had been worried about their oldest child, a
daughter, who was involved in an unhappy second marriage and
had recently been separated. Mr. Dawe however, indicated overall
feelings of pride in their children.

Communication between husband and wife was adequate. As
mentioned earlier, Mr. Dawe was not as verbal as his wife and he
tended to let her finish his sentences for him. These communication
patterns had probably developed in the past and had tended to be
reinforced by his deafness and her manner of taking charge of
situations. Also to be considered was the fact that our first contact

was with Mrs. Dawe alone; Mr. Dawe may have felt that his presence was somewhat peripheral to the visits. Support and encouragement for one another were communicated in important nonverbal ways, such as Mr. Dawe's willingness to take his wife to the outpatient clinic to talk with us and his willingness to be available when we arrived. Another sign of mutual support and security was the fact that they still slept in the same double bed together. Mr. and Mrs. Dawe maintained their emotional and financial resources carefully, sharing them mainly with their children. Mr. Dawe had a more obvious desire than his wife to prevent sharing of family-system information with us.

The family's ability to accept help, especially in areas of health care, was limited. This was mainly because of Mrs. Dawe's background as a nurse; she had a need to feel competent and self-sufficient in all medical areas. Other family members placed proscriptions and expectations on her that made it difficult for her to follow her health-care plan. This was the area that caused the greatest difficulty in patient–family education. Because Mrs. Dawe was not following her 800-calorie ADA diet, she was placed in a constant state of jeopardy—she knew what she should do but could not, or would not, comply. As a result, her weight continued to increase and Mrs. Dawe was left in the rather untenable position of having to justify her situation by claiming she had "a strange case of diabetes." Unfortunately, Mrs. Dawe's choices would have negative outcomes for the family system in the future.

Role flexibility was not of imminent importance to this family in its life cycle. In the past there had been some flexibility (*i.e.,* Mrs. Dawe had worked during the 1930s through 1950s, when women were not a large part of the labor force and were expected to stay in the home). During the time of our contact with the family there was a fairly traditional delineation of work: Mrs. Dawe did the household chores and Mr. Dawe worked outside in the yard.

Decision making in this family tended to fall primarily to Mrs. Dawe, as had discipline of the children in the past. Although some of the decisions were made in a *de facto* manner by Mrs. Dawe, there were also instances when decisions were made by the process of accommodation (*i.e.,* a process of begrudging compromise and a questionable commitment to the decisions).[3]

In the Dawes' viewpoint, family status, goals, and relationships were not seriously impaired by chronic illness. Adjustments to Mrs. Dawe's diabetes and to Mr. Dawe's emphysema had been smooth. The concurrent onset of chronic illness and onset of aging had, perhaps, made acceptance of the illnesses easier. Relationships had been changed as children grew up and moved out but, overall, this family seemed to have adjusted very well.

Crisis situations, especially serious injury or death, had been responded to by the Dawes with an immediate mobilization of energies. Because of Mrs. Dawe's background as a nurse, she immediately was called upon in times of illness or injury. Besides caring for the ill or injured family member, she also carried messages from the rest of the family. Mr. and Mrs. Dawe both indicated that although they became very distressed in such situations, they felt they were able to respond appropriately.

Family Understanding and the Present Event: Chronic Illness

This family had had a long association with diabetes through relatives on both sides of the family. The Dawe family genogram (Fig. 6-6) shows the remarkably high incidence of diabetes and diabetes-related deaths on both sides of the family. Both partners seemed to accept the presence of diabetes philosophically—even fatalistically. When asked how he had felt 17 years before about the diagnosis of his wife's diabetes, Mr. Dawe stated, "It's just something that happens." He felt that the only way her diabetes had affected him had been in her cooking: "It's not as good as it used to be."

The fact that this chronic illness was not diagnosed until late middle age and the relatively few restrictions imposed on the family's ability to function at a pre-illness level had probably accounted for the relative ease with which they had handled it. Although Mrs. Dawe had to contend with a limited menu, insulin injection, urine testing, and other medically prescribed guidelines, her role within the family was initially undisturbed. Also, the prognosis for adult-onset diabetes is generally favorable and there is now little, if any, stigma attached to diabetes—it is a very common and acceptable chronic illness.

The complications of diabetes (retinopathies and hypertension) that were found in Mrs. Dawe were of more concern to the family and did interfere with daily activities. Mrs. Dawe was no longer able to drive, and this made her more dependent on her husband. Her hypertension was not well controlled. As her activity level declined and her weight went up, she was increasingly unable to move around easily. This limited the mobility the couple had enjoyed during the past few years. Mrs. Dawe's role as provider of nursing care and child care for grandchildren and other family members also was restricted, and would become more so.

The children of Mr. and Mrs. Dawe recognized the hereditary nature of diabetes and had their blood checked every so often for sugar, Mrs. Dawe reported. As far as the parents knew, however, their children had no pervasive fear of diabetes.

The Dawes had confidence in the nearby medical center, and both of them had chosen to be hospitalized in the medical center rather than in the local county hospital. Mr. Dawe exhibited less faith in

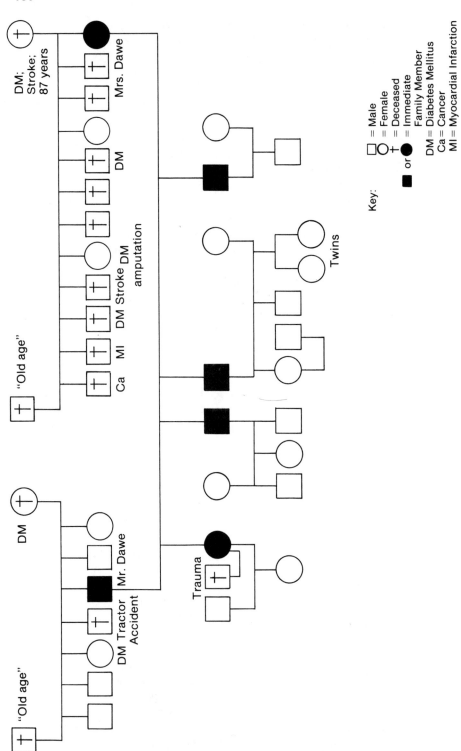

Fig. 6-6. *Genogram: The Dawe family.*

medical care than did his wife; he felt he had received bad treatment from a local physician. His approach to dealing with health-care agencies was basically to allow his wife to make decisions and negotiate for him.

The Identified Patient, the Health Problem, and Educational Needs

Educational and cultural background was similar for all family members so that no further assessment of this area for the identified patient, Mrs. Dawe, was needed. As stated earlier, Mrs. Dawe's educational background as a nurse occasionally became problematic. Her self-concept involved an image of herself as one who should be able to cope with diabetes-management problems and at times she hesitated to ask for support or advice: "I just don't feel I can ask these young guys about things the way I used to when I knew them from working with them." Superimposed on the problem of daily diabetes management was her hypertensive situation. The physiologic feedback she received (headache, occasional nausea) was symptomatic for both and, therefore, confusing.

The principles of diabetic self-care (diet, exercise, medication, response to hypoglycemic and hyperglycemic reactions, prevention of complications) were outlined for us by Mrs. Dawe. She was proud of her medical knowledge and skills. It became clear, however, that in this case (as with many other health professionals under medical care themselves) knowledge and skills were often not enough to promote healing behaviors. To assess Mrs. Dawe's learning needs accurately, it was especially important to understand the barriers to desired behaviors outlined in Mrs. Dawe's care plan (Fig. 6-7).

A helpful resource in this assessment was an article in which Betty Richardson offers an assessment tool designed to confront problems with the diabetic's self-care regimen.[13] It deals with the following areas of concern: diet, activity and rest, blood glucose levels, finances, and skin condition and care. We included parts of this tool to encourage Mrs. Dawe to talk about problems with her treatment plan and her life-style. Her responses to questions defined the following areas that Mrs. Dawe saw as problems:
1. Diet of 800 calories too restrictive; cannot eat "normally"; "always hungry"
2. Unable to follow exercise program due to fatigue, shortness of breath
3. Takes blood pressure medication but without good control; unable to follow low-sodium diet; salt substitute "tastes awful"; husband likes salt used in cooking
4. Poor control of diabetes—hyperglycemia, retinopathies

Mr. Dawe displayed a lack of knowledge about diabetes and its management when he was questioned. He left it "up to her"

PATIENT AND HEALTH-TEAM ASSESSMENT	FACTORS AFFECTING BEHAVIORAL CHANGE FOR HEALTH PROMOTION	EDUCATIONAL DIAGNOSIS
1. OBESITY Recent weight gain due to the following: a. Inability to follow 800-calorie ADA diet b. Inability to follow exercise program	1. OBESITY + knowledge about health problem + patient cooks + patient makes decisions – self-concept – environment (sweets around house) – feels hungry – feels diet is too restrictive	1. OBESITY Negotiation and behavior modification related to diabetic diet needed
2. SHORTNESS OF BREATH 2° obesity	2. SHORTNESS OF BREATH + interferes with role of caring for others, grandchildren + decreasing mobility and independence; patient wants to be independent – obesity – increasing dependence on husband – inability to follow diet	2. SHORTNESS OF BREATH Negotiation and behavior modification necessary to increase exercise
3. HYPERTENSION	3. HYPERTENSION + knowledge about health problems – poor cooperation with diet, exercise – husband likes food cooked with salt	3. HYPERTENSION Learning needs related to management of hypertension. Negotiation of plan for medication, diet, weight reduction
4. DIABETES Poor control Hyperglycemia Retinopathies	4. Diabetes + family history + symptoms bothersome + knowledge about disease/management – self-concept, role conflict (care-giver vs. patient) – husband not impressed with seriousness of problem	4. DIABETES Self-care attitudes and commitment should be explored. Plan for behaviors to be negotiated with patient/family

Key:
+ = Positive factors affecting behavioral change
– = Negative factors affecting behavioral change

Fig. 6-7. *Nursing-care plan for documentation of patient–family education: Assessment.*

(Mrs. Dawe) to know what to do because she was a nurse.
Mrs. Dawe did not talk about her diet with him, but he noticed that
her "cooking had changed some."

We concluded the assessment for patient education by discussing
and validating the problem areas with Mrs. Dawe. We then
documented the assessment using the nursing-care-plan form
presented earlier in the chapter (Fig. 6-2). This included the
following:

1. Assessment of patient problems and learning needs
2. Factors influencing behavioral change—positive and negative
influences
3. The educational diagnosis

Figure 6-7 shows this nursing-care plan for Mrs. Dawe.

References

1. Hochbaum G: Patient counseling versus patient teaching. Top Clin Nurs 2:1–8, 1980
2. Bower F: Nursing Assessment. New York, John Wiley & Sons, 1977
3. Horton T: Conceptual basis for nursing intervention with human systems: Families. In Hall J, Weaver B (eds): Distributive Nursing Practice: A Systems Approach to Community Health, pp 101, 104, 105, 112. Philadelphia, JB Lippincott, 1977
4. MacVicar M, Archbold P: A framework for family assessment in chronic illness. Nurs Forum 15, No. 2:180–194, 1976
5. Otto HA: Criteria for assessing family strengths. Fam Process, 2:329–337, 1963
6. Lewis J: No Single Thread, pp 206–207. New York, Brunner-Mazel, 1976
7. Gragg S, Rees O: Scientific Principles in Nursing, pp 66–72. St Louis, CV Mosby, 1980
8. Redman B: The Process of Patient Teaching in Nursing. St Louis, CV Mosby, 1980
9. Robinson L: Patients' information base: A key to care. Can Nurse 10, No. 12:34–36, 1974
10. Brunner LS, Suddarth DS: The Lippincott Manual of Nursing Practice, 3rd ed. Philadelphia, JB Lippincott, 1982
11. Maslow A: Motivation and Personality. New York, Harper & Row, 1970
12. Erikson E: Childhood and Society, pp 247–274. New York, WW Norton, 1963
13. Richardson B: The real world of diabetic noncompliance. Nursing '82 12, No. 1:68–73, 1982

Bibliography

Abdellah FG et al: Patient Centered Approaches to Nursing. New York, Macmillan, 1960
American Hospital Association: Implementing Patient Education in the Hospital, AHA Publ No. 1488. Chicago, American Hospital Association, 1979
Bower FL, Bevis EO: Fundamentals of Nursing Practice: Concepts, Roles and Functions. St Louis, CV Mosby, 1979
Christensen PJ (ed): Nursing Process: Application of Theories, Frameworks, and Models. St Louis, CV Mosby, 1982
Edinburg GM, Zinberg NE, Kelman W: Clinical interviewing and Counselling: Principles and Techniques. New York, Appleton-Century-Crofts, 1975
Ellis JR, Hartley CL: Nursing in Today's World: Challenges, Issues, and Trends. Philadelphia, JB Lippincott, 1980

Green LW, Kreuter MW, Deeds SG et al: Health Education Planning: A Diagnostic Approach. Palo Alto, Mayfield, 1980

Kron T: The Management of Patient Care. Philadelphia, WB Saunders, 1981

Lamonica EL: The Nursing Process: A Humanistic Approach. Menlo Park, CA, Addison-Wesley Publishing Co, 1979

Leonard BJ, Reland AR (eds): Process in Clinical Nursing. Englewood Cliffs, NJ, Prentice-Hall, 1981

Long L, Prophit P Sr: Understanding/Responding: A Communication Manual for Nurses. Monterey, Brooks-Cole, Wadsworth Health Sciences Division, 1980

Murray RB, Zentner JP: Nursing Assessment and Health Promotion through the Life Span. Englewood Cliffs, NJ, Prentice-Hall, 1979

Rogers ME: An Introduction to the Theoretical Basis of Nursing. Philadelphia, FA Davis, 1976

Roy C Sr: Introduction to Nursing: An Adaptation Model. Englewood Cliffs, NJ, Prentice-Hall, 1976

Urosevich PR (ed): Assessing Your Patients. Horsham, PA, Intermed Communications, 1980

Yura H, Walsh MB: The Nursing Process: Assessing, Planning, Implementing and Evaluating. New York, Appleton-Century-Crofts, 1978.

Chapter 7

Client Goals in Patient Education

Using Data from the Assessment

In Chapter 6, we discussed the process of assessment. The next step is a negotiation of learning goals among the patient, his family, and the health-care team. The more comprehensive the assessment, the more aware we will be of the needs and problems involved. This awareness facilitates our counseling of clients and helps us to provide them with learning experiences through which they may gain knowledge, attitudes, and skills to promote health.

Assessment provides us with information about what the patient and his family know and what they want or need to know. The learning needs we identify relate to their right to know and prepare them to make informed choices. The definition of learning needs also involves dealing with barriers to behavioral change and expanding knowledge, attitudes, and skills related to diagnosis, complications, management, prognosis, prevention, and resources for assistance. We encourage the active involvement of patients and their families in assessment. Our task is to help them articulate their perceptions of their needs and problems.

The Importance of Goal Setting

We address the importance of goal setting with the patient and his family and offer tips for working together in planning patient education. We demonstrate how learning objectives are constructed and how they determine the entire learning process. Finally, we outline the components of a learning contract and discuss its use as a motivator for learning, a mechanism for communication, and a source of standards for evaluating the teaching/learning process (Fig. 7-1).

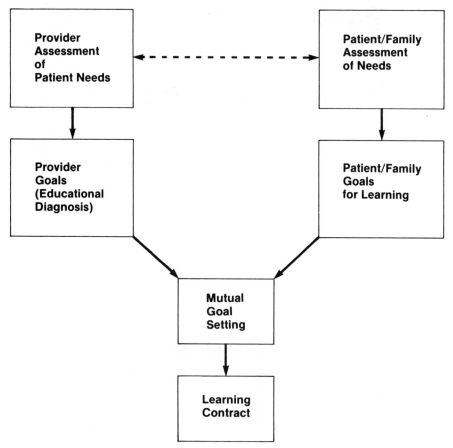

Fig. 7-1. *Designing a Learning Contract based on client goals for patient education.*

The negotiation of goals is essential to the success of learning. It is, however, a step of the learning process that is often ignored. The importance of goal setting is better appreciated in light of the principles of adult learning. We begin by discussing the characteristics of an adult learner and considering how a negotiation of learning goals sets the stage for learning activities.

Characteristics of the Adult Learner

The question most commonly asked by nurses attending workshops we have conducted on patient education is, "How can I motivate patients to learn?" They realize, from their experience, that the learner must play an active role in the teaching process—that they cannot *make* him learn, but they can *help* him learn. What, then, prompts learning or a change in behavior? A discussion of how to motivate patients is offered here. Additional tips are presented in Chapter 12.

There are several sources we can tap to arrive at a better understanding of the adult learner. We have chosen two that we have found to be most helpful in the patient-education area. One of these is our own experience as adult learners and the second is the work of Malcolm Knowles, the father of *andragogy* (adult learning).[1]

Many nurses teach patients and their families in the way they were taught as children. The learner assumes a passive role and the nurse lectures and demonstrates to him, as her teacher did in the grammar-school setting. If the nurse tries to imagine herself as an adult student seated in a fifth-grade classroom, she will understand why the adult patient needs a different environment. She might imagine herself feeling anxious about what the teacher expects, concerned that the material may be repetitious and boring, and that the class schedule is rigid and her chair uncomfortable. She knows that she is not allowed to speak without permission. She feels that her past experience is not important and that she may have to learn things that are not relevant to her interests.

When the nurse considers her own positive learning experiences as an adult, she is likely to recall an environment of physical and psychological comfort in which she felt accepted, valued, and encouraged to contribute her thoughts, ideas, and past experiences. The subject matter was of interest to her and would help her in her job or her role (*e.g.,* as a spouse or parent). With help, she defined her own learning goals and then evaluated the result of the learning activities. There were opportunities for role playing or trying out new behaviors. She felt free to ask questions without fear of embarrassment. Adult patients have similar needs as learners. Physical and emotional comfort and active participation in defining their own needs and goals motivate patients to learn. Nurses who are aware that adult patients and their family members learn best in the same kind of environment that would be personally comfortable for the nurses themselves tend to provide such an environment for patient education.

Malcolm Knowles contributes four reasonable assumptions about adult learners that distinguish them from children (see page 144). Readers are strongly encouraged to read his book, *The Modern Practice of Adult Education,* for more information on the role of the adult educator and on strategies for helping adults learn.[1] We outline his four basic assumptions and some major points that apply to the patient–education process. In Table 7-1 (page 145), applications of each of the four assumptions to patient–family teaching are made.

Because, as Knowles suggests, the adult's readiness to learn (and, thus, his motivation to try out new behaviors) is influenced by developmental tasks, the patient educator will want to be familiar with Erik Erikson's writings on the *eight stages of man.*[2] Briefly outlined in Table 7-2 (page 146) are the eight stages as Erikson identifies them.

In Erikson's first stage, trust *vs.* mistrust is the development issue; this stage lasts from birth to one year of age. Meeting the child's needs for physical care and for receiving love influences his future trust of people and the world.

In the second stage (age one to two), children strive for autonomy, building mental and motor skills and gaining a feeling of independence and control.

From ages three to five, in the third stage, children continue to master skills and take initiative. They need freedom to gain independence without guilt.

From age six to puberty (Erikson's fourth stage), the child learns how things are made and how they work. He needs encouragement of this industry and a sense of accomplishment as opposed to feelings of inferiority and failure.

Knowles's Assumptions About the Adult Learner

As a person matures . . .

1. His self-concept moves from dependency to self-direction. He sees himself as capable of making his own decisions, taking responsibility for their consequences, and managing his own life.

2. He accumulates life experiences that are an increasing resource for learning.

3. His readiness to learn is increasingly oriented to his developmental tasks and social roles.

4. His time perspective changes and his orientation to learning shifts. He needs immediate application (rather than postponed application) of knowledge and his learning is problem-centered rather than subject-centered.

The following points made by Knowles offer additional guidance in goal setting with the patient and his family:

• The adult sees himself as a producer or doer and derives self-esteem from his contributions.

• The adult has a need to be perceived by others as self-directing.

• The adult responds in an environment that is informal and friendly, where he is known by name and valued as an individual.

In the fifth stage, during adolescence, identity emerges with the integration of roles as a student, son or daughter, wage earner, athlete, and so forth. Role models and peer pressure are strong influences in this stage.

Early adulthood (stage six) is a time when intimacy, courtship and beginning one's own family are issues. Roles as a spouse or parent are developed.

In the seventh stage, adulthood, productivity and contribution to society are valued. A sense of accomplishment from caring for others is pursued.

Maturity is Erikson's eighth stage. It is a time of reflection, looking back on life's accomplishments. Pride in family and children adds to self-esteem. Dealing with death and dying is characteristic of maturity.[3]

Goals and Objectives

Adult learners are motivated to learn when they recognize a gap between what they know and what they want to know.[1] Assessment provides us with information about where the patient stands with respect to the knowledge, attitudes, and skills important to self-care. Goal setting is an activity whereby the patient educator contracts with the patient for what he want to accomplish. The readiness of the patient and his family to learn is especially important to consider. Their ability to participate in this step is influenced by their degrees of physical discomfort, denial, grieving, and dependency needs. At no time should the teacher force her own goals on the patient and his family. She should instead try to meet them on their own

Table 7-1. **Application of Adult Learning Theory to Patient–Family Education**

Assumptions About Learner	Applications
Self-concept moves from dependency toward self-direction; sees self as capable of making own decisions, taking responsibility for consequences, managing own life	Acknowledge learner's desire to articulate own needs, make choices, and gain respect for own ability to manage life; create psychological climate that communicates acceptance and support; help learner to feel comfortable taking chances, expressing his thoughts and ideas without fear of shame or embarrassment; remember that adults are motivated to learn when they realize that they have a need to learn
Growing reservoir of life experience is a resource for learning	Use past experiences as a resource for learning; remember that adults experience positive feelings of support and recognition when their experience is acknowledged; relate new learning to old; have adults teach other adults in a group setting; be aware that negative past experiences may pose barriers for learner and teacher
Readiness to learn is strongly influenced by social roles and developmental tasks	Recognize social role of patient (*e.g.,* father, mother, husband, wife, worker) and developmental tasks; relate learning to ability to become, to succeed in these roles
Time perspective changes; orientation to learning shifts; needs immediate application of new knowledge and problem-centered learning	Give adults practical answers to their problems; help them to apply new knowledge immediately through role play or hands-on practice (*i.e.,* return demonstration); remember that adults are particularly motivated to learn at times of crisis or when problems arise; prioritize learning activities by immediacy of need and patient–family perception of need; reinforce learning and promote problem-solving skills

(Content adapted from Knowles MS: The Modern Practice of Adult Education. New York, Association Press, 1970).

Table 7-2. **Erikson's Eight Stages of Man**

Stage	Issue
Oral–Sensory	Trust *vs* Mistrust
Muscular–Anal	Autonomy *vs* Shame
Locomotion–Genital	Initiative *vs* Guilt
Latency	Industry *vs* Inferiority
Puberty, Adolescence	Identity *vs* Role Confusion
Young Adulthood	Intimacy *vs* Isolation
Adulthood	Generativity *vs* Stagnation
Maturity	Ego-Integrity *vs* Despair

ground, encourage whatever participation she can, and consider ways to support and reinforce strengths.

The learning experience is directed by goals and objectives. Goals are the desired outcomes of learning. An example of a goal might be *Mrs. Jones will lose ten pounds by March 2.*

Objectives are specific statements related to the goal. They describe in more detail the behaviors that will be performed to meet the goal. The following are sample objectives: Mrs. Jones can outline breakfast, lunch, dinner, and snack menus for one day using a 1200-calorie ADA diet plan; Mrs. Jones will keep weekly clinic visits with the nurse for weight checks and review of daily food intake; Mrs. Jones will record the foods she eats in a notebook each day and bring this notebook to clinic visits.

Both goals and objectives must be clearly stated and agreed upon by the patient, his family, and the teacher if patient education is to have a focus.

Rationale for Using Goals and Objectives in Patient Education

We have stated several times that patient education is a process of influencing behavior, rather than of only giving information. For instruction to be successful, it must be directed toward accomplishing behavioral change. We must justify that what we teach will help the patient to perform the desired behavior.[4] The setting of specific goals for patient education assures that the learning interventions will be tailored to the situation and to the client's needs. Goals also offer criteria for evaluation of patient education. Did the patient and his family successfully meet the goal? Mager highlights other outcomes of goal setting that can be applied to patient education.[4]

When goals and objectives are clearly stated, the learner knows what his role is and what is expected of him. He can organize his energies toward accomplishing the goal. Occasionally, goal setting itself is the only intervention necessary to motivate the patient to change his behavior. He is motivated by articulating what he can presently do and what he wishes to be able to do.

The teacher also knows her role when goals and objectives are stated. Both teacher and learner know how the results will be measured. Written documentation of goals ensures the patient's straight-forward communication with the health-care team.

What happens when objectives are not clearly stated? There is then no sound basis for nursing intervention. We do not know which learning activities are appropriate or what the roles of the teacher and learner will be. A common result is that the patient and his family receive information but fail to understand how to use it in their own environment and individual circumstances. They may acquire information, but they do not learn new skills.

Many health-care professionals have not had experience in writing behavioral objectives and, therefore, have difficulty with constructing objectives even though they understand the rationale for doing so. Learning to articulate behavioral objectives is not difficult and is outlined in this chapter. With practice, skill in writing objectives increases.

Another concern identified by health professionals is the problem of setting priorities for what is to be taught first. The following section considers the setting of teaching/learning priorities.

Considering Teaching/Learning Priorities

A common mistake made by health professionals is that of trying to teach too much during a short period of time. We have seen this occur most often in the inpatient setting, where patients are overwhelmed with instruction before discharge. Reinforcement and evaluation of learning are often neglected. We contend that, for a number of reasons, patient and family learning needs should be carefully prioritized and creatively met in a variety of settings. Although teaching about chronic illness often takes place in the hospital setting, it must be followed up and reinforced in the home or in the outpatient clinic. This shows the importance of the efforts of nurses to use telephoned or written communication to inform nurses and physicians in health departments, offices, clinics, and nursing homes about the teaching plan and the patient's progress. Learning overload also occurs in outpatient settings, where patients are given many instructions related to self-care and prevention. Review and reinforcement are often lacking when the patient attempts to integrate the learning into changes in his daily behavior.

The following four points support the importance of prioritizing learning needs and setting attainable goals in each patient situation. They also highlight the need for cooperation among professionals in many health-care settings.

1. Length of hospitalization has shortened dramatically in recent years due to rising health-care costs, bed shortages, and improved technology. Patients are discharged when they are physiologically stable, rather than when teaching is completed. Patients are often acutely ill during most of the hospital stay and have physical and emotional restrictions that prevent learning. They may leave the hospital having had little opportunity to practice skills, review information, or articulate questions. Nurses are often informed of the patient's discharge with only a few hours' notice, and they worry that the client has not been taught enough to manage his care.

2. Patients who are overloaded with learning materials and activities feel a sense of frustration and failure when they cannot perform all behaviors

successfully. This causes them to feel powerless, defeated, and dependent on others. Many adults would rather deny failure than admit to it, and they will revert back to old behaviors instead of asking for assistance.

3. Patients need to know what self-care activities are most important in their individual situations. When time and energy are at a premium, they need to know what learning must be achieved for survival.

4. Health professionals also have limited time and energy. Setting priorities for teaching helps to structure their time for its best use and ensures that acute learning needs are met. Professionals can discharge patients more confidently when they know that learning will be continued and reinforced.

The prioritization of learning needs is helped by considering the individual within the context of Maslow's hierarchy of needs (Fig. 6-5). Because five different levels of needs exist, we recognize that needs lower on the hierarchy must be at least partially met before needs on the next level can be satisfied. This helps us to order learning needs and to recognize the patient's reliance on others to help him satisfy higher needs.

1. Physiologic and Survival Needs
    Examples: Care and use of oxygen
    Recognition of health problem, danger signs, and how to respond to them
    Nutrition and hydration
    Sexuality
    Pain management
    Recognition of depression and how to deal with it
    Administration of insulin and other medications or treatments
    Care of ostomy or Foley catheter
2. Safety and Security Needs
    Examples: Poison prevention
    Ability to hold job
    Ability to deal with hazards on job or in environment (*e.g.,* toxins, dangerous machinery, stress)
    Family violence
    Financial abilities in meeting basic needs of food, shelter, medication
3. Affection and Belongingness Needs
    Examples: Adaptation to peer pressure
    Family role maintenance
    Ability to "contribute"
    Need to feel lovable and desirable in spite of illness or problem
    Ability to deal with body image, disfigurement

4. Esteem or Recognition Needs
   Examples: Need to succeed
   Need to make choices, control own destiny
   Need to be recognized as a valuable individual
   Need for privacy, dignity
   Ability to deal with lack of respect, abuse, ill treatment on job or in family
5. Self-Actualization: Self-Determining Needs
   Examples: Success through own definition of what is desirable
   Ability to meet developmental milestones
   Independence in meeting lower needs

In acute and chronic illness, patient education is often limited to physiologic and survival needs. Prioritization of these learning needs involves asking the following questions:

1. What are the most acute needs of this individual?
2. What does he already know? What behaviors can he perform?
3. What learning needs are unmet? Which are life threatening? Number accordingly.

The scope of learning in level one (physiologic and survival needs) for acute and chronic illness encompasses knowledge, attitudes, and skills related to the categories in the following list.

Scope of Patient Education in Acute and Chronic Illness

1. Diagnosis (problem)
   a. Etiology
   b. Contagiousness, malignance, premalignance, heredity
   c. Anatomy, physiology involved
2. Complications
   a. Causes
   b. Prevention
   c. Early signals
3. Management
   a. Surgery
   b. Radiation
   c. Diets
   d. Exercise, relaxation programs
   e. Medication
   f. Behavior modification and controls
   g. Environmental control
   h. Counseling
   i. Appliances (*e.g.,* pacemaker, braces, crutches, traction)
   j. Consultation and referral
   k. Soaks, hot packs, dressings, treatments

4. Aggravating factors
   a. Foods
   b. Tobacco
   c. Drugs, alcohol
   d. Schedule of work and rest
   e. Interpersonal relationships
   f. Environmental aspects
5. Prognosis
   a. Short term
   b. Long term
6. Prevention of Recurrence
7. Resources for Assistance
   a. Psychosocial
   b. Economic
   c. Audiovisual
   d. Printed
   e. Specialized (*i.e.,* patient groups)

(From Society of Teachers of Family Medicine: Patient Education: A Handbook for Teachers. Kansas City, Society of Teachers of Family Medicine, 1979)

Stating Goals and Objectives

Learning connotes a change in *knowledge, attitudes,* or *skills* as a result of an educational experience. Behavioral objectives guide the planning of learning activities and the measurement of learning outcomes. They should state what the learner will *do* as a result of patient teaching (Fig. 7-2).

A behavioral objective has three components: performance, conditions, and criteria.[4]

Performance states what the learner will do. It uses an action verb and denotes an activity that can be measured. Examples of action verbs follow:

choose	*locate*
collect	*measure*
compare	*name*
compute	*practice*
define	*prepare*
demonstrate	*recognize*
describe	*record*
discuss	*report*
identify	*test*
list	*use*
	write

Verbs such as *believe, understand, value,* and *know* are not measurable and should be avoided when performance is being described.

When choosing an action verb, the teacher should ask, "Can I measure whether or not the learner is able to do this?" The verb should be simple enough that the learner will be able to understand how he is expected to show his competence.

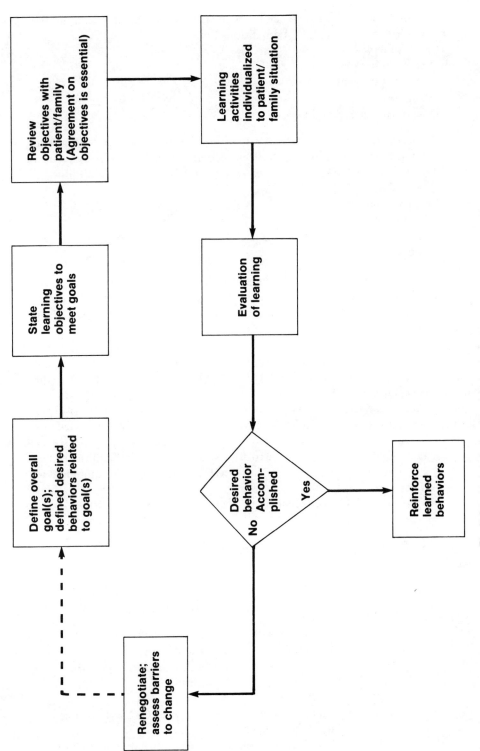

Fig 7-2. Using behavioral objectives in the learning process.

Conditions state what special circumstances will be included in the learner's performance. Examples of conditions follow:

Time of day
Sterile technique
Use of equipment, tools
Place
Use of calorie restrictions

Criteria offer a component of evaluation. They state *how* the teacher and learner will know when the learning has been accomplished. A criterion states how long or how well the behavior must be performed. Examples of criteria follow:

Score or speed
Weight, quality
Number of times
Accuracy
Frequency

Sometimes it is difficult to distinguish between a condition and a criterion. For example, consider the following behavioral objective: Mrs. Jones will draw up and administer 22 units of U100 NPH insulin using sterile technique at 7:00 a.m. on three consecutive days.

The criteria used in measurement include the number of units of insulin, the time, and the frequency of administration. Yet the time of day, 7:00 a.m., is a condition as well as a criterion because it describes a circumstance under which the behavior is performed.

Mager states it is important for both the teacher and the learner to answer the following questions related to the behavioral objective. These are intended as a help to the writer designing an objective.[4]

1. What does the learner have to do to show he has achieved the learning?

2. Under what conditions will he do it? (Will he use special equipment or do without an aid?)

3. How will he know when it is done well enough? What is the performance standard?

Three Components of a Learning Objective

1		2		3		
Performance	+	Conditions	+	Criteria	=	Behavioral Objective
What is the learner able to do?		Under what conditions will he do it?		How will we know when he has accomplished it? How well must it be done?		

For example, the patient will

1. Draw up and administer 22 units of U100 NPH insulin,
2. using sterile technique,
3. from 7:00–7:30 a.m. on three consecutive days.

Making Learning Objectives Specific, Measurable, and Attainable

A well-constructed behavioral objective is specific and the learner knows what is expected. The behavior is measurable, achievement can be evaluated, and the standard is attainable. This requires an understanding of the patient's view of what he wants to achieve. Although the learner's ability should not be doubted, it is important that goals are not set too high. Learning should be a positive, supportive experience in which the learner gains confidence and self-esteem. Learning should begin with activities in which the patient will succeed and should move from simple behaviors to those that are more complex.

Getting the Patient and His Family Involved

The involvement of the patient and his family in setting learning goals affirms their willingness to participate. Criteria for evaluation should be acceptable to them and valued by them. For example, working an hour in the garden without breathlessness or being able to care for a grandchild may be more meaningful outcomes to them than 22 respirations per minute or a ten-pound weight loss. The behavioral change involved for these, however, may be the same and could satisfy both the provider and the patient. It is important that patients express their own goals verbally or in writing. The patient educator should encourage them to talk about the changes they would like to make and help them to state these in objective form.

Health professionals must honestly share with the patient their goals for him. We must be willing to revise these goals and objectives if they are not agreeable to him. The patient may understand the hazards of smoking but may not be willing to give up his evening cigarettes. The patient may understand the need for weight reduction and want to lose weight but be unwilling to sacrifice ice cream. A measurable reduction in smoking, or a measurable weight loss using a modified diet plan, may be a workable compromise.

Some strategies for getting the patient and his family involved include asking them for their perceptions of their problems and what they would like to change. Share your view of the problem and ask the patient if he would like help in working on the identified problems. Discuss the priority of needs with the patient and write behavioral objectives using his input. Together, contract for what is taught, what the patient is to learn, and your respective responsibilities.

The Learning Contract

A learning contract is a tool used to formalize the agreement between the teacher and learner. It clearly states learning behaviors, the responsibility of the teacher and the learner, and the methods of follow-up and evaluation. The contract is renegotiated as learning is accomplished and new goals are defined. If the patient changes his mind or finds the goals too difficult to achieve, the objectives can be revised. We have used learning contracts with a high degree of success in the hospital, home, and clinic settings.

Designing a Learning Contract

Figure 7-3 illustrates the essential components of a learning contract. We have found it helpful to type a standard contract form on hospital or clinic stationery and complete it with the patient. We keep a copy in the nurses' station or in the patient record and give a copy to the patient. A bonus clause has been used to denote additional resources available to the patient, (*e.g.,* self-help groups, classes, and other health professionals). As behaviors are accomplished, we find it essential to include a *reinforcement* as an intervention to support the patient when the contract is revised. The reinforcement may be weekly weight checks in the clinic, an occasional home visit, a telephone call, or a referral to the public-health nurse or office nurse.

Benefits of the Learning Contract

The contract is often a *motivation for learning* for both patient and staff. Through the contract, goals and objectives are specific, achievable, and clearly defined. The contract provides a *mechanism for communication* by formalizing conversation. There is a time limitation for renegotiating the contract, which outlines the responsibilities of members of the health-care team and the community resources that may be of assistance to the patient. It provides *standards for evaluation* of learning by specifying desired behaviors, conditions, and criteria, and also provides opportunity for measurement of behavioral change.

Documentation

Documentation of assessment for patient education clearly states problems and their related learning needs. We have referred to this as the *educational diagnosis.*

Learning Contract

Goal:

Learning Objectives:

Provider/Teacher Actions:

Patient/Family Actions:

Method of Measurement:

Length of Contract:

Bonus Clause:

Signatures:

Date:

Fig. 7-3. *Sample learning contract used in patient education.*

Goals to Promote Knowledge, Attitudes and Skills	Teaching/Learning Formats and Activities
1. GOAL: To lose ten pounds by 6/1/82 OBJECTIVES: -Outline food exchanges for break-fast, lunch, and dinner using a 1200-calorie ADA diet plan. -Describe how one-half cup of ice cream is worked into the weekly meal plan. -Record in notebook all foods eaten during the week. -State why weight control is especially important in the management of diabetes. 2. GOAL: To achieve systolic blood pressure below 160 points and diastolic blood pressure below 90 points by 6/1/82 OBJECTIVES: -State name, dose, and frequency of hypertension medication. -Record in notebook when hypertension medication is taken each day. -Omit salt in cooking. -Name ten high-sodium foods that should be avoided. -Eliminate canned foods from the diet during the week. Substitute fresh fruits and vegetables, recording them in notebook.	

Fig. 7-4. *Mrs. Dawe's nursing-care plan for patient education.*

Problems are prioritized and goals and objectives corresponding to each problem are constructed. These contribute to the documentation of patient education in the medical record. A copy of the learning contract may be included in the record.

The nursing-care plan for patient education was first introduced in Chapter 6. A *Goals* column is added in this chapter to illustrate the mutual development of patient goals (Fig. 7-4). The *Teaching/Learning Formats* column will be completed in Chapter 8. The Dawe family will again be discussed to present the goal-setting process.

Case Study: Mrs. Dawe   Mrs. Dawe identified her greatest problems as her weight and her high blood pressure. She agreed that she would like to work on these problems. She stated that her shortness of breath would decrease if she lost weight and she felt that she would "get out more" if she lost ten pounds. She described her 800-calorie ADA diet as "too restrictive," but agreed to a 1200-calorie ADA diet, which included one-half cup of ice cream each week. She felt that her weight increase and blood-pressure problem were closely related. She also saw her shortness of breath as a problem and stated, "I would be happy if I could keep my granddaughter for the day without getting sick."

We shared our perceptions with Mrs. Dawe. They were similar to her own about her obesity, hypertension, and shortness of breath. We reinforced her knowledge of her health problems and her positive behaviors of checking her urine and examining her feet regularly. We complimented her dependability in keeping her appointments and

FAMILY MEDICINE CENTER

Learning Contract

OBJECTIVES:

To lose 10 pounds during the next two months (present weight, 280 lb).
To achieve systolic blood pressure below 160 mm of mercury and diastolic blood pressure below 90 mm of mercury by two months from now (present BP, 190/102).

LEARNER ACTIONS:

Record in notebook all foods eaten each day. Follow 1200-calorie ADA diet. Limit ice cream to half-cup servings per week. Take 100 mg hydrochlorothiazide daily and record in notebook. Eliminate salt in cooking and at meals. Record intake patterns in notebook. Eliminate canned foods this week. Return for clinic visit next week.

TEACHER ACTIONS:

Supply diet outline for 1200-calorie ADA diet.
Check weight and BP weekly.
Label reading models—will review with Mrs. Dawe at clinic visit 4/7/82. Instruction in reading labels on canned foods done today in the home.

METHOD OF MEASUREMENT:

Weight
BP
Patient record in notebook

LENGTH OF CONTRACT:

2 months

BONUS CLAUSE:

Diabetic luncheon at County Hospital
1200-Calorie ADA diet plan and instructions
Booklet: "Your Diabetic Diet"
Appointment with dietitian scheduled for 4/7/82

SIGNATURES:

_____   _____

_____   _____

Date: 3/31/82

Fig. 7-5. *Learning Contract with Mrs. Dawe.*

taking her medications. A diet was planned to help her lose weight and lower her blood pressure. She was in agreement with our suggestions. We postponed a discussion of her diabetes management until her clinic visit scheduled for the following week.

Learning goals and objectives related to her problems with obesity and hypertension were mutually negotiated. By 24-hour recall, Mrs. Dawe's current intake was estimated at approximately 2200 calories per day. She agreed to a 1200-calorie ADA diet on the condition that she could have ice cream once a week as a treat. She agreed to limit her salt use in cooking, and her husband agreed to use it only at the table. Mrs. Dawe was willing to keep specific records in a notebook, which she would bring to her next office visit. We wrote up and signed a contract, which she kept at home (Fig. 7-5). When we returned to the office, we documented our agreement in the progress-notes section of her chart and made an appointment for her with the dietitian; this had been suggested so she would have an opportunity to explore variations on her diet and receive cooking suggestions. Mrs. Dawe would return to the family practice clinic for a visit one week later.

Prioritizing problems was not difficult because the problems were closely interrelated physiologic needs. An effort to set achievable goals increased the probability of attaining success and developing a positive self-image. Mr. Dawe was willing to help by supporting Mrs. Dawe's renewed effort to follow her diabetic diet and to limit her salt intake. He remarked, "It would help me to cut down on my salt, too, and I can use some at the table."

References

1. Knowles MS: The Modern Practice of Adult Education. New York, Association Press, 1970
2. Erikson EH: Childhood and Society. New York, WW Norton, 1950
3. Kaluger G, Kaluger MF: Human Development: The Span of Life, St Louis, CV Mosby, 1979
4. Mager RF: Preparing Instructional Objectives. Belmont, CA, Fearon Publishers, 1975

Bibliography

Books

American Hospital Association: Implementing Patient Education in the Hospital. Catalogue No. 1488. Chicago, American Hospital Association, 1979
Blevins DR: The Diabetic and Nursing Care. New York, McGraw-Hill, 1979
Bower FL, Bevis EO: Fundamentals of Nursing Practice: Concepts, Roles and Functions. St Louis, CV Mosby, 1979
Douglass LM, Bevis EM: Nursing Leadership in Action. St Louis, CV Mosby, 1974
Kron T: The Management of Patient Care. Philadelphia, WB Saunders, 1981
Long L, Prophit P Sr: Understanding/ Responding: A Communication Manual for Nurses.

Monterey, Brooks-Cole, Wadsworth Health Services Division, 1980

Redman BK: The Process of Patient Teaching in Nursing. St Louis, CV Mosby, 1976

Yura H, Walsh MB: The Nursing Process: Assessing, Planning, Implementing and Evaluating. New York, Appleton-Century Crofts, 1978

Journals

Riddle MC: A strategy for chronic disease. Lancet 2, No. 8197:734–736, 1980

Shaw LM: The patient as an adult learner. AORN J 33, No. 2:233–239, 1981

Tarnow KG: Working with adult learners. Nurse Educ 4, No. 5:34–40, 1979

Zemke R, Zemke S: Thirty things we know for sure about adult learners. Training 18, No. 6:45–52, 1981

Chapter 8
Interventions

Individualized goals set the course for patient-education interventions. Between the time goals are agreed upon and the time learning activities begin, decisions must be made about content, staff, teaching methods, and teaching tools. The nurse often coordinates this planning and refers some learning needs to other members of the health-care team. She is the facilitator of team-planning conferences, she has contact with the patient's family, and she has a significant knowledge of hospital and community resources.

This chapter addresses decision making about the design and implementation of educational interventions. Characteristics of a learning environment are outlined, teaching and learning styles are discussed, and the selection of instructional methods and media is explored. Included are a tool for evaluating patient-education materials and appendices suggesting resources for free or low-cost teaching aids, such as printed literature and films.

Scope of Teaching and Learning

Planning interventions that assist the learner in achieving his goals involves making decisions about setting, content, resources, and instructors. Although learning interventions must be tailored to each patient, teaching programs planned for target populations (*e.g.,* patients with newly diagnosed diabetes) provide guidance and standards for care. We strongly support the development of these programs within hospitals and other health-care agencies. A patient-education coordinator may organize task forces composed of physicians, nurses, dietitians, pharmacists, physical therapists, and so forth, to derive teaching plans for special groups. This approach tends to gain support from physicians and other health educators who will feel confident about the quality of the intervention and the preparation and knowledge of staff. Established teaching programs encourage a consistent approach among staff, facilitate a planned interdisciplinary format, and provide populations to be studied so that we may gauge the effectiveness of patient education. We encourage nurses to investigate programs that have been developed in their institutions and to become involved in promoting them. Such programs often provide written and audiovisual teaching tools for the learner as well as teaching guides for health professionals.

In institutions where teaching programs are not developed, the nurse may wish to consult with other health-care agencies to see what approaches they have applied to specific populations. Information about teaching programs may also be obtained from organizations such as the American Hospital Association, the National Institutes of Health, the American Cancer Society, and the American Diabetes Association.

Determining Content

Many nurses feel confident about what the content should be that they teach patients and their families who have a variety of health problems and needs. Other nurses find themselves lacking this confidence and may cover only that material with which they are familiar. Consequently, essential content may be missed, incorrect information may be given, or learning activities may be inappropriate. Some nurses also tend to react to their lack of preparation by avoiding teaching situations and hoping that someone else will meet the patient's learning needs.

A wealth of resources is available to assist nurses in identifying the content to be taught in order to meet learning objectives. The hospital librarian, local nursing-school librarian, patient-education coordinator, and hospital staff are among these. Textbooks, reference books such as the *Lippincott Manual of Nursing Practice,*[1] drug handbooks, nursing journals, and books addressing special patient groups provide valuable pointers in determining content.

Setting Priorities

Consideration of the patient's ability and readiness to learn will help the teacher to set priorities in initiating learning activities. Priorities in the teaching plan are influenced by what the patient and his family see as important, the level of their anxiety about a particular topic or skill, the level of need (*e.g., survival skills*), and the time period available for implementing teaching/learning activities. In general, learning should progress from familiar to unfamiliar and from simple to complex. Printed materials intended for patients to use often lend guidance in introducing concepts and relating these concepts to self-care.

Selecting Instructional Methods and Instructional Media

Instructional methods encompass the format chosen for teaching (*e.g.,* self-directed, individual, small group, large group) and the learning activities used (*e.g.,* lecture, demonstration, discussion, role play). *Instructional media* are tools used by the teacher to help the learner to retain, compare, visualize, and reinforce learning. There is often too much emphasis placed on media, while instruction is insufficiently personalized. An excuse often offered by health professionals for lacking patient-education interventions is the lack of funds to purchase films, videotapes, television equipment, and so forth. Although the effectiveness of instructional media's contribution to learning has been emphasized in patient-education literature, and expensive equipment impresses the public, media must be tailored to individual situations in planned intervention. If there is a lack of funds allocated for investments in software (*e.g.,* videotapes, films, filmstrips) and hardware (*e.g.,* television monitors), effective learning still continues to take place in inpatient and outpatient settings. A wealth of free or low-cost teaching materials may be obtained, and equipment can often be borrowed from state libraries and local businesses. Appendix B at the end of this chapter supplies the names and addresses of organizations that make teaching materials available at little or no cost.

Later in the chapter, we also offer suggestions for obtaining current information about the availability and costs of audiovisual media. Resources are offered for nurses who are in a position to negotiate equipment purchases as well as for those on limited budgets who wish to rent or preview media or make their own audiovisual aids.

Creating a Climate for Adult Learning

The adult learner has special needs as he engages in teaching/learning activities, just as he had in the goal-setting process. When these needs are met, learning becomes satisfying and effective. If the teacher fails to acknowledge the learner's needs, barriers arise that slow down or prevent the learning of new behaviors.

A climate that promotes adult learning takes into account the physical and emotional needs of the learner. It uses problem-centered learning, in which the nurse relates material to the patient's life situations and addresses his concerns. The learning activities include opportunities for an exchange of ideas between the teacher and learner and for applications of learning in simulated or real exercises. We will discuss these needs in more detail and offer tips for fulfilling them.

Physical Comfort

Obvious barriers to learning exist when pain or anxiety interferes with the exchange of ideas or the ability to listen. Patients who are in the hospital or bedridden in the home may depend on others to assist them with bathing, elimination, dressing changes, medication, and ambulation. The thoughtful teacher will be sensitive to these needs and help the patient to be as comfortable as possible. She will take into consideration whether the patient is physically able to tolerate an hour-long teaching session, for example, or to participate in group learning. She will encourage the learner's participation by making certain he has his eyeglasses or dentures and is positioned comfortably. The teacher should be mindful of the basic human needs of all patients and recognize that they may become hungry, thirsty, restless, or uncomfortable, and that they need to be recognized and treated as individuals. The nurse may capitalize on the time she spends helping patients to meet their basic needs by teaching content and skills related to their care. She might teach the patient and his family members about medication while administering it and then ask them to repeat the information to her the next time she administers it. She may talk through the procedure while changing a patient's dressing and ask him to direct her the next time she changes it. She may discuss the function of insulin with the patient at the time he administers his insulin, or discuss insulin reactions with him after he experiences one.

Emotional Needs

Many patients perceive a mystique surrounding the roles of doctors and nurses. Especially in times of illness or change, patients often desire to be taken care of, to find someone who will perform "magical" acts to restore a previous state of health, erase pain, or remove conflict. Too often, health-care personnel have perpetuated this desire by encouraging dependence or by not taking the time to encourage patient learning and patient participation in medical management. Patients may therefore be hesitant to participate at a later time, feeling incapable of learning the proper skills or of managing aspects of their own care. Later, they may worry that they will be deprived of necessary help and unable to meet their own needs.

It is important in patient education to acknowledge each patient's need for support and his anxiety about learning new health behaviors. The patient should know that he will receive necessary help and teaching until new skills are mastered and that he will be supported by medical personnel. The patient may be afraid to disclose his lack of knowledge or to make mistakes. The patient educator can confront these barriers by remaining mindful of the patient's need to be recognized as capable and as an individual. She will structure learning to proceed from simple to complex, so that the patient will feel successful, and she will make herself available for support and advice as the patient tries out newly learned behaviors. She will understand that in times of crisis or stress the patient may need greater support and may test her willingness to help him.

Two examples illustrating emotional needs in patient learning follow.

The first patient, Mr. B., was a 53-year-old man who had been an insulin-dependent diabetic for six years. He made frequent visits to the clinic with a variety of minor complaints but left the clinic much improved after each visit. He lived alone and depended on the clinic staff to support him. He called the nurses' station almost daily, occasionally stating, "I just can't seem to get going, give myself my insulin, and get to work." Through our teaching and review, we knew that he had mastered the necessary skills to do so. The clinic's social worker was called upon to help Mr. B. get involved in the American Diabetes Association, thus increasing his support system. In addition, the clinic's nurses scheduled regular, monthly, one-half hour visits during which they would support Mr. B. and occasionally ask him to share his expertise in insulin injection with patients who had newly diagnosed diabetes.

The second patient, Mrs. H., had received prenatal care at the clinic and was looking forward to breast-feeding her baby. She had read many books on infant care and attended prenatal classes. Although the classes stressed the importance of being flexible in planning labor and delivery, Mrs. H. was determined that she would have a natural childbirth. A breech presentation, however, necessitated cesarean section. Mrs. H. successfully nursed her baby in the hospital and had good support and teaching from the hospital staff. Two days after discharge, Mrs. H. called the clinic's nurse. She was crying, stating that she felt like a failure because the baby "would not take her milk." After supporting her on the phone, the nurse suggested that Mrs. H. come to the clinic and feed her baby in the examination room, where the nurse could offer assistance. The patient happily agreed. When she arrived, the nurse realized that Mrs. H's anxiety was causing her difficulty with nursing. Together they reviewed the progressive muscle-relaxation exercises done in prenatal classes. Mrs. H. then became relaxed before nursing her baby, and the baby nursed successfully. The nurse complimented Mrs. H. on how well she was caring for the baby, weighed the baby so the patient could verify that he was gaining weight, and offered additional visits of this nature if needed. Mrs. H. agreed to call the nurse the next day and let her know how the breast-feeding was progressing. When she did, the report was a positive one. Mrs. H. remarked, "It was just so good to know I could call you if I needed help."

Problem-Centered Learning

Learning activities should be centered around potential problems that the patient may face. The teacher will want to assist the learner in recognizing the problem, knowing what to do, and feeling competent in performing the necessary behavior. Patients often bring problems or concerns with them to the learning session. Breast-feeding problems are a good example. Similarly, expectant parents may express the following concerns: "How can I deal with the pain of labor?" "How will I know if the baby is sick?" and "What do I do if the baby doesn't stop crying?" Preoperative patients also want information: "What will it be like in surgery?" "What will they do to me?" "Will I be in pain?" or "What will it be like when I wake up?" Diabetic patients and their family members also often have questions: "Why are the shots needed?" "How should the shots be given?" and "What is an insulin reaction?"

Some patients will mention their problems and concerns freely, while others hesitate to do so. Occasionally, patients with newly diagnosed problems do not know what to ask. It is the teacher's job to encourage the patient to verbalize concerns and then to address those concerns in learning activities. If the patient and his family need help describing concerns, the teachers may begin by offering, for example, "Patients who are pregnant often have questions about labor and delivery and want to know what to expect. I wonder if you might have concerns about that?"

Application of Learning

Learning activities are structured to provide opportunities for the application of learning. While teaching may include lecture and discussion, it should also propose problems and give the learner a chance to react to them. Application should be as immediate as possible and the learner should be able to receive support and ask questions when trying out new behaviors. Simulated situations aid in resolution in the health-care setting of life problems. An example of this would be a mock labor and delivery used in prenatal classes.

Participative Learning

Participation must be encouraged at the onset of learning activities if the learner is expected to build confidence. Some patients are more comfortable than others in voicing concerns and attempting new skills. Others are reluctant and anxious and may need special attention to prepare them for learning activities. Participation can be gained from even the most reluctant learner with adequate support and realistic learning goals.

Nurses are frequently unable to evaluate patient learning because participation has not been accomplished and they have not observed the application of learning. This problem may arise when adequate time is not allowed for teaching and learning, when learning activities are restricted to lecture and demonstration, when the nurse is not comfortable with the teaching role, or when the nurse does not like to teach. These problems are alleviated by careful selection of learning activities and of staff members who will serve as teachers.

The Teacher–Learner Relationship

Learning is a shared experience requiring openness on the parts of both the teacher and the learner. The teacher must be willing to establish a relationship with the individual learner, to be dependable, to encourage the learner until goals are met, to be flexible enough to negotiate, and to provide support and reinforcement. She commits herself in an agreement, a *learning contract,* whether verbal or written. She is responsible for recognizing her own learning needs and is willing to admit it when she does not have an answer.

As in all therapeutic relationships, the teacher–learner relationship takes time to develop. The teacher gives the learner an opportunity to "tell his story," and the nurse and patient become acquainted. Assessment and problem identification begin. The learner begins a testing phase, in which he considers the willingness and ability of the teacher to understand his needs, to help him, to support him, and to commit herself to mutual goals. Eventually, the teacher and learner establish a working relationship and engage in activities together. The teacher provides experiences through which the learner tries out new behaviors.[2]

Styles of Learners

Patients approach learning in a variety of ways determined by individual life-style, personality, and past experience. The patient educator will want to identify characteristics of the learner's style in planning teaching interventions. While one patient may read extensively about his health problem and vocalize many questions, another patient may want only the basic facts, saying, "Just tell me in a few sentences what is wrong with me and what I need to do." Some patients are comfortable in classroom lectures and others are not. Although one patient may be anxious to perform a return demonstration or a procedure, another may hesitate and ask the nurse to perform the procedure several times first. One patient may freely discuss his own difficulty and confusion, while another denies problems unless he knows they are observed. The patient may play the informed expert and offer the nurse a challenge as she assesses his learning needs. Still another patient may hold back what he knows, wishing to be taken care of rather than assume responsibility in his health management. Patients also learn at different rates depending on age, intelligence, motor skills, degree of impairment, anxiety, and past experience. Each teaching/learning activity must be adapted to the style and need of the learner.

Styles of Teachers

Just as learners have characteristic styles, the nurses who teach them also have particular teaching styles. Some are very comfortable with an "expert" role in telling or showing, while others encourage constant involvement from the patient in a give-and-take fashion. Some may have difficulty dealing with the patient who sees himself as an expert; others may feel comfortable allowing the patient to direct the teaching while they clarify, correct, and supplement knowledge. These same nurses may have problems working with a passive, dependent, or depressed patient.

The approach of the nurse in patient education must be a flexible one because she must respond to the style of the learner in spite of her own preferred style of teaching. For example, a nurse with high control needs as a teacher may compete with the expert patient, in which case the learning experience will become a frustrating, unproductive one. A passive, dependent patient, however, will also learn little if he is only taught according to the needs he verbalizes. For these reasons, a nurse involved in teaching patients should consider her own teaching style and may require training to overcome difficulties adapting to particular learning styles. In addition, the compatibility of the teacher with the learner is an important consideration when selecting patient-teaching staff.

We are familiar, for example, with a situation in which a controlling nurse was assigned to teach tracheostomy suctioning to a patient who had had a radical neck dissection and glossectomy. The patient was attempting to control his environment in response to his multiple losses and refused to accept any teaching from the nonempathetic nurse. His discharge from the hospital was delayed until a new nurse, who understood his attempts to exert control, was assigned as his primary nurse.

Selecting Staff for Teaching

It is important to provide a planned, consistent approach in patient education. We wish to avoid unnecessary repetition and confusing presentation of material. We do not want to overload the patient and his family, but we want to include ample opportunity for review and practice. We should incorporate the contributions of other members of the health-care team (*e.g.,* physical therapists, dietitians, pharmacists) into the teaching plan.

In the midst of other patient-care planning, few of us are afforded the luxury of time needed to construct such approaches. We have discovered, however, that teaching protocols may be established in cooperation with other members of the team and then adapted to patient situations. The protocols are targeted toward specific patient groups, such as those with newly diagnosed diabetes. Provider responsibilities are outlined and staff members are trained in the use of the protocol and teaching activities. This type of planned team approach saves time, alleviates confusion, and directs the selection of staff.

Responses to the following questions will also aid in selecting staff members best suited to carry out patient-education interventions:

1. Does the staff member have ample opportunity to interact with the patient and his family?

2. Does the staff member understand the goals, objectives, and learning style of the patient?

3. Does each staff member understand his role and the other providers' roles?

4. Does the staff member have adequate preparation and knowledge to perform patient teaching?

5. Who will coordinate the teaching plan?

Instructional Methods and Instructional Media

We referred in Chapter 7 to three types of learning behaviors: *cognitive* (knowledge and information), *affective* (attitudes and values), and *psychomotor* (skills and performance). Learning in each of these three areas contributes to behavior change.

For example, in education of a patient with newly diagnosed diabetes, the following patient behaviors are desirable:

Cognitive

1. Can describe what diabetes is and how the involved body systems of a diabetic patient function differently from those of a nondiabetic

2. Can state that insulin reactions may be caused by the following:
   a. The wrong amount or kind of medication
   b. Late or omitted meals or snacks
   c. Failure to follow diet plan
   d. Increased activity

Affective

1. Can discuss why it is important for the diabetic patient, his family, his physician, and other health-care professionals to work together in his medical management

2. Can state why he should tell his friends and coworkers that he is a diabetic and explain to them the signs and symptoms of insulin reactions and what to do if they occur

Psychomotor

1. Can select food exchanges to plan one breakfast, one lunch, and one dinner within guidelines of 1200-calorie American Dietetic Association (ADA) diet

2. Can demonstrate proper technique for daily washing and checking of feet

Learning objectives must be categorized into these three areas to prepare for the selection of teaching/learning formats, methods, and media best suited to patient-education needs.

Teaching/Learning Formats

Teaching/learning formats are chosen to accomplish patient-education objectives. The teacher considers, for example, whether learning can be accomplished in a large group or whether it is better suited to an individual teaching situation. In many instances, a combination of formats can be used to provide learning experiences, add variety, and meet different types of objectives. We will look at three teaching/learning formats (individual teaching, group teaching, and established teaching protocols to be used in hospitalwide programs).

Individual Teaching

Often called one-to-one teaching, individual instruction is ideal for continued assessment of the learner and technical-skill training such as urine testing, insulin injection, and self-catheterization. It promotes the sharing of confidential information and problems, the tailoring of teaching plans, and the learning of persons hindered by a low literacy level, physical impairment, cultural barriers, anxiety, or depression. Individual teaching is often used as an initial intervention through which basic knowledge and skills are achieved and the patient's confidence in self-care is increased. Advantages of this format include an active learner role, which builds motivation, an opportunity for consistent and frequent feedback, and flexibility to create an unstructured, informal atmosphere. "Teachable moments" can be capitalized upon with one-to-one learning. The teacher can respond to the learner's problems and needs in a timely fashion and can help the learner to build problem-solving skills. Preoperative teaching, initial diabetic teaching, and diet teaching are often performed using the individual format. The obvious disadvantages of individual teaching are a lack of sharing and support with other patients and their families and the high cost of staff time for instruction.

Group Teaching

A group-teaching format may be selected for patient education. There are three distinct advantages to group learning: it is economical, it helps patients learn from one another and teach one another through their experiences, and it fosters positive-attitude development. Even though group members may have slightly different learning goals, a needs assessment can be done within the group by asking patients what they want to learn. Teaching content can be tailored to meet learner objectives. Small groups (two to five patients) may be able to offer some of the advantages of individual teaching. Medium-sized groups (five to thirty patients) may be effectively used for prenatal care, pediatric care, stress reduction, safety, diabetes review, or self-help and support groups. Large groups (thirty patients or more) are appropriate for lectures and films, but should be interspersed with small-group experiences or discussion. A medium-to-large-group format is generally unacceptable for skill training and reduces patient–teacher feedback. It is difficult in these groups to evaluate whether individual learning goals have been met. Patients who are physiologically or emotionally unstable are poor candidates for group teaching. The teacher of a group must be aware of the characteristics of patients who are present and must be flexible in her approach. The group format is ideal for teaching patients and their families together.

Self-help groups are gaining the recognition of professionals and patients. They offer mutual assistance to patients with common health-related learning needs. The groups are often led by patients themselves and may be sponsored by community agencies or health-care organizations. Some self-help groups, however, are begun on the grass-roots level by laypersons who recognize the need for mutual support in dealing with prevention, management, and adaptation to chronic illnesses. Physicians are often uncooperative or indifferent toward the self-help movement, demonstrating reluctance or refusal to refer patients to such groups. However, as health-care costs rise and hospitals face increasing barriers to providing free services, health-care professionals, especially physicians and nurses, are reconsidering their attitudes toward self-help groups. They are beginning to recognize that many active self-help support groups play an important role in educating patients and their families, and that they encourage appropriate use of health-care services.[3] We have found that nurses are generally more aware than physicians of community groups and that nurses tend to make more referrals to them.

Hospitalwide Programs

Many hospitals and health-care agencies have developed systematic plans or protocols for educating patients with specific diseases or problems. They use individual and group formats, including self-instruction, and prescribe specific approaches and teaching roles. Patients and their families are taught by a standard outline, including basic information components that are then tailored to the individual situation. Some items may be deleted, for example, and others may be expanded upon to address the patient's personal barriers to behavioral change. Such protocols generally include teaching about pathophysiology, about treatments such as medication, and about diet, diagnostic tests, procedures, activity prescription, and self-care skills. The benefit of using such protocols is that hospitals can tailor patient instruction to the specific procedures that are relevant to that institution.

Staff members are trained through classes and tutoring to use the teaching formats and strategies. The roles of various providers are outlined according to subject matter and areas of expertise. Specific provider responsibilities are described with respect to the teaching/learning process. While nurses often perform the initial assessment, all providers are involved in intervention, evaluation, and documentation of teaching and learning.

Teaching protocols define a target audience and patients should meet these target criteria before they are enrolled in a program. Time required for teaching segments of the protocol is estimated and resources are suggested to help patients meet the learning goals. Content, teaching strategies, and activities suitable to meet the goals are preselected and defined by a planning committee when the protocol is established. Teaching aids such as audiovisuals and printed matter may be purchased by the health-care institution to enhance patient teaching. In addition, the protocol specifies what types of information should be documented in the medical record and where they will be located. Measures for evaluation of patient learning are offered.

We believe that teaching protocols are useful formats for systematic patient-learning experiences. Additional discussion of their benefit is offered in Chapter 1. We do caution that all teaching plans must be individualized to meet patient needs and that an assessment of readiness and barriers to learning is an essential preliminary step in any patient-education approach. The use of formalized protocols also offers a systematic method of evaluation because variables such as teaching methodologies and content are constant.

Learning Activities

Learning can be enjoyable. Knowing how to use a variety of learning activities to meet educational objectives can make patient-education more interesting, challenging, and effective for both the teacher and the learner. The patient educator will want to choose learning activities thoughtfully, so that they will be suitable for particular patient objectives. Below, we offer a guide for selecting activities conducive to cognitive, affective, and psychomotor changes. Notice that some learning activities are appropriate for more than one type of learning objective. Brief descriptions of the major types of learning activities are offered with suggestions for effective and appropriate application.

Selecting Learning Activities for Patient Education

    I. Cognitive (Knowledge)
       A. Learning Facts
         *Lecture
         *Demonstration
         *Independent-Study Format
         *Tests
          Discussion—Questions and Answers
          Practice
          Simulation
       B. Visual Identification
         *Demonstration
         *Simulation
         *Tests
          Practice
          Independent Study
       C. Understanding and Applying Knowledge
         *Demonstration
         *Practice
         *Role Play
          Discussion—Questions and Answers
          Independent Study

Simulation
Tests
II. Affective (Attitudes and Appreciations)
*Discussion—Questions and Answers
*Role Play
Simulation
III. Psychomotor (Skills and Performance)
*Practice
*Role Play
*Simulation
*Demonstration
*Tests
Independent Study

*Very effective

Lecture

Lecture is the method most often used by nurses instructing or transmitting information to patients. It is a very effective method of teaching cognitive behaviors and is more efficacious when used with discussion. Lecture is also enhanced by projected visual aids such as overheads and slides to promote identification. Material presented in a lecture should be prepared according to the learner's level of understanding, and the learner should have an opportunity to ask questions. Lengthy lectures may cause loss of attention if the patient becomes bored, distracted, or anxious about the material presented. Learners may become eager to contribute or to try out or apply knowledge; this eagerness may be stifled by a formal lecture approach in which the teacher is the expert. It is important to remember that lectures can be highly effective for influencing cognitive behaviors but will not be effective in achieving affective or psychomotor learning objectives. For example, lecture is often used to give initial knowledge about pathophysiology to diabetic patients but is ineffective when used alone to teach insulin injection. Lectures may be given in person or by radio or television broadcast.

Group Discussion

Discussion requires two or more people to exchange ideas. It differs from lecture in that it is an excellent method of actively involving patients in the learning process. This learning activity promotes understanding and application of knowledge (cognitive behaviors), as well as developing certain attitudes (affective behaviors). It is frequently directed by the teacher, who asks specific questions or proposes problem situations. Discussion facilitates learning from the experience of others, fosters a feeling of belongingness, and reinforces previous learning.

Demonstration

Demonstration is useful for cognitive and psychomotor learning. It is most often used to teach skills and to present standards for performance. Demonstration may be done in person or by films and videotapes. The sense of sight is used in learning from demonstration, but hearing, smell, and taste may also be stimulated. Demonstration should be performed slowly and the teacher should be certain that the learner can see and hear well. This strategy shows the learner that the behavior is possible and increases his confidence that he will be able to perform it. For example, when teaching insulin injection, the nurse may demonstrate injection on herself using sterile water before the patient actually performs an insulin injection.

Role Play and Return Demonstration

Both role play and return demonstration involve doing or practicing. They help the learner to apply knowledge or skills, usually after demonstration. When used appropriately, role play and return demonstration tailor the learning to the patient's past or present life experiences while the teacher is there to offer guidance and feedback.

In role play, the learner acts out his own situation or that of another person. This is highly effective in meeting affective objectives. It is a type of demonstration. Return demonstration usually follows exhibition of a skill one or more times by the teacher. In both cases, clear instruction must be given to the learner about what to do and how to do it. Enough practice time should be allowed for the learner to repeat the exercise until he has mastered it. Role play and return demonstration are effective strategies for teaching cognitive, affective, and psychomotor behaviors.

Tests

Tests may be valuable learning experiences, as they relate where the learner is and where he wants to be to the progress that has been made toward meeting his goal. Tests are helpful when used to guide patients and give feedback. They are effective in meeting cognitive and psychomotor objectives, but are obviously inappropriate for affective learning because attitudes and values are not measured with a "right-*vs*-wrong" approach.

Patients may become anxious about testing due to school experiences. The nurse should introduce tests positively in patient education and should use the results to reinforce progress toward the learning goal. Tests may use a written, oral, or skill format. They may be used in assessment, to determine the patient's initial level of understanding or skill, and in evaluation after the lecture or demonstration.

Programmed Instruction

Patients can learn by independent study or by using specially prepared workbooks, textbooks, filmstrips, and computer programs. There are many commercially prepared programs on the market, although the teacher may prepare her own rather easily. Programmed self-study units allow the learner to work at his own pace for mastering cognitive and psychomotor behaviors. Frequent testing and review are offered during instruction. Knowledge about chronic illness and management, health-prevention topics, and diet teaching are commonly offered in programmed instruction packets. The teacher should be aware of the level of motivation or readiness of the learner, as well as of his literacy level and his visual and hearing abilities because these factors are crucial in evaluating the appropriateness of such programs for individual clients.

Media

Media are usually used to enhance one of the previously mentioned learning activities. They should not be used in place of the teacher, but can effectively promote all three types of learning when used in combination with other strategies. A health-care professional should be available to discuss, demonstrate, and clarify concepts introduced by media. This role should not be neglected or left to lay volunteers. Media should be carefully selected and should be consistent with instructional objectives.

Media Uses in Teaching and Learning

Having cautioned our readers that media should not be used carelessly in patient education, a question that may arise is, "What is the advantage in using media?"

Media help to deliver a message. A variety of media can be creatively used to help patients learn more, to help them retain better what they have learned, and to encourage the development of skills.[4] Nurses seldom have formal training in media selection and application, and they consequently look for guidance in these areas. We attempt to provide an overview of the types of media that are well suited to patient education. We begin by offering guidelines for media use so that nurses may avoid some of the common pitfalls of inappropriate or unsuccessful use of media.

The teacher must follow three steps when using media in instruction: *preparation, presentation,* and *review. To prepare,* it is necessary to preview the material to be used. A plan for using a medium is constructed including how it will be introduced, followed up, and related to other learning experiences. The environment also needs to be prepared. This includes obtaining physical facilities and equipment needed to display the medium. The learner must be informed of what to expect from the medium, (*i.e.,* significant points or upcoming discussion). *Presentation* of media requires care so that projection and materials are clear, sound is adjusted, and, in general, the message can be received. *Review* involves follow-up of the learning experience and evaluation of whether learning objectives were met.[4]

There are several generalized principles that can be applied to all types of media:[4]

1. No one medium is best suited to all purposes. For example, in some instances visual identification is best accomplished with a picture, cartoon, or slide, while in others three-dimensional images, such as films or videotapes, are most effective.

2. The application of media should be consistent with learning objectives. Just as learning activities promote certain types of behaviors, media are also chosen to coincide with objectives.

3. The teacher must be familiar with the content of the media. A common mistake made by nurses is to use materials unknowingly that are inappropriate in message, presentation, or educational level. Media must be previewed and evaluated.

4. Media must be compatible with learning formats. To illustrate this point, films may be used in a large group, but videotapes and audio-cassettes should not.

5. Media must be selected with the capabilities and learning styles of the audience in mind. Printed booklets with few illustrations are poorly suited to the patient who is unable to read or who dislikes reading, and the message will fail to reach him.

6. Physical conditions influence the effectiveness of media. Improper acoustics, lighting, or seating, distractions, and room temperature may all interfere with the delivery of the message.

Chalkboards, Displays, Flipcharts, and Bulletin Boards

Visual displays using drawings and illustrations do not have to be works of art to deliver a message. They do need to be aesthetically appealing, using contrasting colors and large lettering. There are many advantages to choosing chalkboards, displays, flipcharts, and bulletin boards. They are inexpensive, they require little time to prepare, and they attract attention and interest. They clarify information, simplify concepts, and summarize teaching. Contributions from participants can be written on flipcharts or chalkboards during the teaching session. Bulletin boards in waiting rooms or hospital corridors can spark interest or curiosity in health-care issues and problems.

Use of these types of media is inappropriate in large groups unless the displays are enlarged. They are not well suited to teaching in which movement needs to be demonstrated.

Graphics

Graphics include graphs, charts, diagrams, cartoons, posters, signs, and maps. They can be used to show proportions and relationships that are difficult to understand when presented only by spoken or written material. They emphasize the most important points of a presentation. Posters, signs, and cartoons can deliver a message to patients with limited reading and vocabulary levels as well as to children. For example, picture pages are often used to teach insulin-injection techniques to newly diabetic patients. Cartoons can make learning fun and present thoughts in a humorous but effective fashion. Graphics highlight sequence and also convey general information and key concepts. Some of the main advantages of using graphics for patient education are their abilities to attract attention and to deliver information economically. The graphics may be prepared by the patients themselves or by patient educators, or they may be produced commercially.

Overhead Projection

Overhead transparencies are popularly used for teaching in both large and small groups. They require an overhead projector and a screen. Overheads encourage verbal and visual creativity and allow the teacher to control the materials shown and their timing. They can present ideas in a colorful sequence and help the learner to focus on thoughts and ideas. The instructor can add interest by writing or underlining on the transparencies during the presentation. Overhead transparencies are easy to make and can be prepared ahead of time. Overhead projectors are relatively light in weight and can be easily transported. When preparing or purchasing commercial transparencies, the teacher will want to consider whether the message comes across clearly and encourages learner participation. Two cautions are offered when using overheads. First, print should be large and details kept to a minimum. Second, the teacher should not write on the overhead transparency as much as she would on a chalkboard. This often causes learners to become confused or distracted.

Photographs and Drawings

Patients enjoy pictures and learn from them. Visual images promote understanding of facts and ideas by helping the learner to imagine real situations and reflect on past experiences. Still pictures may be presented in printed matter, on slides, or on filmstrips. They may encourage discussion when the learner is asked to describe what he sees.

Pictures can attract and maintain the patient's interest. They also help the patient to remember what has been said. Generally, color pictures appeal to learners more than do black-and-white pictures. The color should be accurate and portray a realistic image.

Slides can be prepared rather easily and portray situations related to actual patient experiences. They may be commercially prepared as well. They require only a projector and screen and can be easily transported.

Thirty-five-millimeter filmstrips are series of still pictures that can be used in a variety of teaching formats. Filmstrips offer the same advantages as other types of still pictures (*e.g.,* printed photographs, slides) and have several other positive features. Presentation of pictures in a series illustrates sequence and lends structure to the message. Filmstrips require an inexpensive projector that can be easily transported and set up. If, at a later data, the teacher wants to omit part of a filmstrip or add content throughout the program, it can be made into slides very easily.

Filmstrips are easy to store and the sequence of pictures always remains the same. Other still pictures may fall out of sequence owing to frequent use. The patient can use this medium at his own pace and can move through the program by controlling it in a self-study format. Filmstrips are usually sold with a written script or an audio recording.

Sound filmstrips offer a tape or disc recording to accompany the filmstrip. The recorded message explains the picture and magnetically imposed sounds direct the synchronized program of still pictures and speech. An inexpensive cassette-tape player or a sound-filmstrip projector is used to project this medium. Sound filmstrips are ideal for self-instruction as well as for group teaching. Filmstrips on many subjects are produced commercially and are well suited to teaching illiterate patients.

Films

Sound–motion pictures are popularly used in patient-teaching situations, especially to deliver basic information to a group. They present experiences, places, and situations that can recreate life situations, thus encouraging attitude appreciation as well as cognitive learning. Films can display motion. This is helpful in presenting sequenced concepts and skills. Patients and their families usually enjoy films as part of the teaching process. They are often a good introduction, or springboard, for discussion. Films are particularly effective for patients with limited reading abilities.

Sixteen-millimeter films are available on a variety of subjects and may be offered in Spanish. Some are produced in super-eight format. Films are well suited to group teaching when a darkened room and film projector can be provided. Films must be carefully previewed and selected. The teacher will want to evaluate the film with consideration of the patient group's actual life situations, levels of understanding and literacy, and learning needs. Fifteen- to twenty-minute films are ideal for most situations; those longer than one hour are difficult for many patients to sit through. Discussion time should be planned and the presentation reinforced. Additional pointers for film evaluation are offered in Appendix A at the back of this chapter.

Drawbacks to using films as opposed to media such as slides and filmstrips are that films are expensive, the projectors required are expensive, and threading the projector occasionally causes problems. Films are generally not used for individual teaching because of the time required to set them up and the necessity of constant teacher attendance to operate the projector.

Audio Materials

Audiotapes, usually cassette tapes, offer a distinct advantage for some patient-teaching occasions. They are small and easy to transport, and they require only an inexpensive recorder for use. They are available on a variety of topics, are economical, and can be used almost anywhere. Audiotapes can be made by the teacher and tailored to the individual situation to reinforce facts, directions, and support. Patients may use them in the home or office as well as in the hospital or clinic. Study kits with printed text or pictures are available to accompany the audio component.

While cassettes are the audio materials most often used, other audio forms include disc recordings, reel-to-reel tape recordings, and recording cards.

Audio materials are helpful in delivering a message to patients who enjoy radio and who benefit from repetition and reinforcement. Relaxation and stress-reduction exercises are also well suited to delivery by audiotape. Illiterate patients can be taught by audiotapes with accompanying sequenced pictures. For patients suffering from retinopathies secondary to diabetes, audiocassettes are the only practical media.

Videotapes and Television

Television's popularity and pervasive use among American households promotes learning in many spheres and influences knowledge, attitudes, and skills. It is entertaining as well as educational.

The use of television and videotaped recordings has also become an attractive teaching/learning activity in the school, office, and health-care setting. Many groups have made significant investments for the purchase of programs (software) and equipment (hardware). Before making such investments, it is important to consider how suitable this medium is for specific learning objectives and to understand how television is best incorporated into patient education.

Television offers a combination of pictures, sound, and motion. It can transmit programs by cable into homes, into patient rooms in the hospital, or into the classroom. It is best used when the program is carefully selected (see Appendix A), introduced, and followed up as part of patient teaching. It should not be expected to replace the teacher. While the costs of tapes and equipment are often prohibitive to financially restricted groups, hospitals that have cable distribution systems may wish to concentrate on video patient-teaching programs because these programs can be broadcast hospitalwide and reach more people.

Videotapes may be purchased commercially or prepared by audiovisual departments and teachers. To produce videotapes, a videotape recorder (VTR) must be purchased. This can also be used for playing back tapes for viewing. If all programs are purchased, a videotape player (VTP), which is less expensive because it does not include recording features, may be considered. For production of videotapes, a television camera, microphone, and blank tapes must be purchased.

Videotape formats may be described using such terms as *half inch, three-quarter inch, VHS,* and *Beta.* This terminology is often confusing to nurses and other professionals who are considering the use of television in patient teaching. These tape formats are not interchangeable, and selecting compatible hardware and software is crucial. Suggestions are offered later in this chapter for selecting the video equipment best suited to particular needs.

Objects, Models, and Demonstrations

Having actual objects available during patient teaching helps the learner to become actively involved and to apply knowledge and skills immediately. The patient may observe, handle, manipulate, display, discuss, assemble, and disassemble objects while the teacher provides feedback.[4] For example, breast models are often used to teach patients to examine their breasts and pelvic models are used to show patients how to insert a diaphragm. The teacher usually demonstrates the uses of the objects or models and the patient repeats the performance. Some models, such as the Resusci-Annie used to teach cardiopulmonary resuscitation (CPR), are very expensive. Others, such as the plastic female pelvic area, are supplied free of charge by pharmaceutical companies. Through creative experimentation, many nurses find that they can make their own models for teaching a variety of skills. One nurse who was unable to purchase an expensive breast model made her own from a nylon stocking stuffed with cotton socks. She simulated a breast mass in another stocking by adding Styrofoam particles and used the two "breasts" to teach breast self-examination.

Displays can be accompanied by models to encourage patient participation. For example, teaching about infant safety becomes more effective when it is accompanied by a display of actual infant car seats. In one-to-one encounters, demonstration and return demonstration can often be performed by the patient without the use of models. Examples of this are urine testing, breast examinations performed in the privacy of the patient's room, dressing changes, and baby bathing.

Furthermore, these teaching/learning opportunities can take place even if funding for teaching aids is lacking.

Community Resources

Health departments, health agencies, businesses, and professional groups such as fire and police departments offer learning experiences for patients. Valuable support and information can be gained through such resources as diabetic groups, ostomy clubs, hospital health nights, bicycle safety programs, and communitywide infant-car-seat programs. The patient educator can benefit from knowledge of, and referrals to, teaching programs that offer skills training. In one outpatient clinic we saw many patients and their families in the rehabilitation phase after myocardial infarction. We wanted to give family members CPR training but were unable to do so because we did not have enough staff to offer the teaching or the finances to purchase equipment. Many of the family members were unable to pay registration fees for CPR classes at local schools. We discovered that a local fire department offered CPR classes free of charge and we referred our patients to them.

Games and Simulations

Games can be used to involve the patient in teaching and learning. Instructional games can introduce information and offer practice in simulated situations. One of the advantages of using games as learning experiences is that actual situations can be viewed in a condensed time span. During a game, the patient can take a course of action and look at the consequences in a nonthreatening way. Problem solving can be incorporated into the game. Commercially prepared games should be evaluated for use with individual patients. The patient should be able to succeed, yet be challenged in the exercise. Games may use flash cards, pictures, or computer programs. They may be modifications of popular games such as Bingo or crossword puzzles. Games are relatively inexpensive to purchase or make, with the exception of computer games. Simulations include planning meals with the exchange system, using food models, and shopping for low-sodium foods in a mock supermarket.

Printed Materials

Pamphlets and information sheets are among the most common teaching tools. Printed materials can help to explain common health problems and their management, as well as to make the public more aware of health risks and prevention. Some printed materials are ideal teaching tools because they have large print, use language appropriate for the patient audience, emphasize important points, and reinforce learning. Distributing written information seems, at first glance, to be a quick and easy way to teach without requiring the time of health professionals' engaging in verbal exchanges with the patients. This is a misconception held by many physicians and nurses. Handing out written materials does not ensure a transfer of knowledge. Many patients are anxious about the information contained in the literature or are unable to understand it. Even when printed matter is evaluated and used appropriately, the message may not be received.

Printed patient-education materials may be used effectively to enhance participative learning. An individualized teaching plan, designed to use patient-assessment data, will guide educators in the appropriate use of books, pamphlets, and information sheets. Specific suggestions for evaluating printed patient-education materials are offered in Appendix A to this chapter. Appendix B to this chapter suggests resources for free or low-cost printed matter.

We have found printed materials especially helpful in contraceptive counseling. Free booklets from the Department of Health, Education and Welfare have reviewed the various types of contraception, weighing benefits, risks, and precautions, and outlining directions for use. After receiving basic teaching in the office, patients may take the booklet home to consider the various methods of contraception. They frequently return for the next visit prepared to ask questions and willing to take responsibility for choosing a method. Although many patients initially come to an office visit with a particular method in mind, we have discovered through assessment that the decision has usually been based on the experience or on the advice of friends. A combined approach of one-to-one counseling and written patient-education materials promotes enlightened choices.

The use of written materials requires assessment of the readability of each booklet, pamphlet, or handout. We must be certain that the wording and sentence complexity are compatible with the patient's level of understanding. There are many formulas that can be used to predict readability or the grade level at which patient-education materials are written. The most popular formulas include the SMOG formula[5] and the Frye formula.[6] Use of these formulas requires time to count words, sentences, and syllables and to do simple computations. Another method we have used when time has been limited involves having the patient read aloud the first paragraph in the booklet and then tell us, in his own words, what it means. In this manner, we learn whether eyesight and ability to read are adequate and whether the content is understood. We have discovered that patients frequently display less comprehension than would be expected from their highest grade of school completed.

Designing a Patient-Education Program

This section is designed to answer questions about choosing from among the possible options in teaching formats, learning activities, and media. Nurses involved in patient education are called upon to make these choices every day, whether they are answering to individual patient–family situations or designing larger, hospitalwide programs.

Many variables influence the design of a patient-education program. Among these are the numbers and types of staff, monetary resources, types and needs of patients, type of health-care setting, proximity to instructional-design and audiovisual experts, and the availability of hardware and software suitable for use in patient teaching. There is thus no one prescription we can offer for designing interventions (patient-education programs) that is practical for every situation. Instead, we look at the questions asked by nurses as they select instructional formats, learning activities, and media and we offer suggested courses of action.

Selecting an Instructional Format

Group teaching seems to be a good way to provide economical patient education, yet doctors and patients often tell us they prefer individual teaching. How can we encourage clients and physicians to accept the value of group teaching?

Provided that an assessment of the patient–family learning needs is made, group teaching can be tailored to be as effective as individual teaching for cognitive and affective learning. Skills are best taught in small groups (two to four people) or in one-to-one formats. Important considerations in offering group classes include whether transportation and time are convenient and whether patients and their families are physically able to attend. Physicians may be more supportive of group teaching if they are introduced to the class's objectives, content, and staff. Some physicians are interested in participating as teachers; this was our experience in the prenatal classes described in Chapter 11.

Hospitalwide programs seem to be the best way to teach patients. Can this concept also be used in an outpatient clinic? If so, with which target populations should we begin?

Such programs are equally effective in an outpatient clinic. They direct the coordination of the health-care team through teaching protocols. Evaluating common learning needs of patient populations requiring ongoing teaching can be accomplished by using computer statistics that list the most common diagnoses. Nurses may also keep a log of patient-education encounters for a six-month period and make their own comparisons. We used this method in an outpatient clinic and discovered that the following situations are ideal for group teaching: weight reduction, hypertension, diabetes, prenatal care, and neonatal care.

Selecting Learning Activities

How does the nurse decide what learning activities are best for the situation? Frequently, it seems that lecture is the only learning activity employed, although others would be equally effective.

Remember, lecture can be a very effective way to deliver the patient-education message. The important point to remember is that a combination of learning activities works best in each situation. It will help the patient and his family to assume active roles in learning and to enjoy patient education if we keep the following points in mind:

1. Learning activities should be compatible with learning objectives. Refer to the list on pages 169–170 for learning activities best suited to cognitive, affective, and psychomotor learning.
2. Keep the patient and his family involved through discussion, role play, games, and media.
3. Tests can help the patient to feel a sense of accomplishment. Try to build success and reinforcement into patient education.
4. Learning can be fun. Humor and support decrease the learner's anxiety and help him to learn at his own pace.

5. Skills training and attitude development cannot be accomplished by lecture alone.

Selecting Media

Are there general guidelines that can be used to evaluate different types of media, whether they are written materials, videotapes, slides, or filmstrips?

Yes. Appendix A in the back of this chapter is a checklist for evaluation of patient-education materials. It is provided by the Society of Teachers of Family Medicine, a group actively involved in promoting patient education. We have found it very helpful with all types of media.

Where are patient-education materials found?

Appendix B at the back of this chapter provides sources of materials, including low-cost and free media, useful in patient education. We encourage nurses to talk with hospital-supply and pharmaceutical representatives. We have found them quite willing to supply written materials and teaching models and to loan films.

What help can the hospital or nursing-school library provide in locating patient-education materials?

Many medical and nursing libraries participate in an interlibrary program that circulates videotape and film programs, including those on patient-teaching topics. Taking the time to discuss patient-education interests with the librarian often results in acquiring media on loan at no cost. State libraries conduct a similar film program, which we used to acquire the film used in the prenatal classes described in Chapter 11. Many hospital and nursing-school libraries subscribe to the National Library of Medicine's MEDLINE and AVLINE systems. These systems use computerized information-retrieval programs that can contribute to the development of bibliographies and to the collection of materials on patient education.

We are involved in writing a budget proposal for AV equipment and would like to know what specific models to request. What is the best type of video equipment to purchase for patient education?

The video field is rapidly growing and changing. We have found two approaches useful for the media novice involved in patient education. First, *purchase a book* and learn about the basics of video. We recommend *The Video Guide* because it offers, in easy-to-follow language, the state of the art in video systems and advice for selecting the system for your needs.[7] It includes an appendix of video and television magazines, video-program sources, video-equipment manufacturers, and video books. Second, *rely on local experts.* Video experts can be found in the centralized education departments of local hospitals, the audiovisual departments of local universities, and the large audiovisual department of the American Hospital Association in Chicago. They are all willing to listen to your needs and make recommendations. Video dealers are usually willing to send salesmen out to talk about potential purchases of equipment and to demonstrate the equipment. Keeping current on video is difficult for most practitioners. We suggest that you acquire a basic preparation through reading and talking to others but rely on the experts to counsel you before you select video equipment. A final reminder is that there are many learning needs that are not suited to use of videotape programs. In these cases (*e.g.,* teaching in the home or reviewing step-by-step diet instructions), it may be cheaper, easier, and more effective to use other types of media, such as slides or filmstrips.

Can media programs be revised if they become out of date, if the patient audience changes, or if they become damaged?

Slides and filmstrips are easily revised. When slides are used, some may be deleted from the original program and replaced, if necessary, with up-to-date slides made in-house or commercially. Filmstrips are similar to slides. If one frame has been badly cut, the program can be saved by using slide mounts to separate the remaining frames. The filmstrip then becomes a standard slide program. It can still be used with the accompanying written or audiotaped component.

What are the advantages of making your own media programs?

Larger hospitals often decide to make their own videotape programs once they have invested in an in-house cable-television system. If the hospital already owns videotaping equipment and has target populations that would benefit from a tailor-made program, video production may be beneficial. Smaller hospitals may have less expertise and different audiences, and would therefore be better suited to commercially produced programs and less expensive video-playback monitors. Slide programs can be produced easily and economically in large and small hospitals and other health-care settings. A good camera and slide projector are necessary. Practitioners can take their own slides and construct the program. They can personalize learning by using scenery, equipment, and people familiar to the patients. Programs can be accompanied by pulsed audiotape if a cassette recorder with a built-in synchronized pulse capability is purchased. Printed patient-education materials, such as booklets and information sheets, are easily made in-house and may offer specific instructions for emergency care or hospital and office policies. We have coauthored several booklets, with physicians and dietitians, that were better suited to our patient's needs than those commercially available.

Documentation

The nursing care plan for patient education can be updated in two ways (Fig. 8-1). First, code each of the patient-learning objectives, using *C* (cognitive), *A* (affective), *P* (psychomotor). This helps in choosing learning activities compatible with the objectives. Second, complete the column labeled *Teaching/Learning Formats and Activities* with those selected to help the patient meet the learning objectives.

Goals to Promote Knowledge, Attitudes and Skills	Teaching/Learning Formats and Activities
1. GOAL: To lose ten pounds by 6/1/82 OBJECTIVES: C—Outline food exchanges for breakfast, lunch, and dinner using a 1200-calorie ADA diet plan. C—Describe how one-half cup of ice cream is worked into the weekly meal plan. P—Record in notebook all foods eaten during the week. A—State why weight control is especially important in the management of diabetes.	Individual and small-group lecture, discussion, demonstration, return demonstration, and role playing with nurse, using 1200-calorie ADA diet booklet and patient notebook. Referral to dietitian. Discussion with husband and nurse. Referral to Diabetic Luncheon at the county hospital.
2. GOAL: To achieve systolic blood pressure below 160 points and diastolic blood pressure below 90 points by 6/1/82 OBJECTIVES: C—State name, dose, and frequency of hypertension medication. P—Record in notebook when hypertension medication is taken each day. P—Omit salt in cooking. C—Name ten high-sodium foods that should be avoided. P—Eliminate canned foods from the diet during the week. Substitute fresh fruits and vegetables, recording them in notebook.	Individual teaching with husband. Lecture, quiz, and demonstration. Discussion and simulation. Label reading in the home. Role playing of shopping for groceries.

Key:
    C—Cognitive learning objective
    A—Affective learning objective
    P—Psychomotor learning objective

Fig. 8-1. *Mrs. Dawe's nursing-care plan for patient education.*

Case Study: Mrs. Dawe   Mrs. Dawe was taught one-to-one and in a small-group format with her husband. This initial intervention included lecture, discussion, demonstration, and return demonstration, as indicated by the nursing-care plan. We referred Mr. and Mrs. Dawe to the Diabetic Luncheon conducted by the county hospital. This group program offered a review of the principles of self-care, including diet, as well as discussion with patients and health professionals. The program was well suited to meeting the objective of attitude development toward recognizing the importance of weight reduction.

Because we were in the home, media for teaching were not readily available. We did use an ADA diet booklet for diet instruction and used the patient's kitchen cupboards to teach label reading and the avoidance of high-sodium foods. Activities and teaching materials are noted in Figure. 8-1.

In each of the learning activities (lecture, discussion, demonstration, and return demonstration) specific patient variables identified in assessment were addressed. We proposed everyday problems and encouraged Mr. and Mrs. Dawe to role play these situations. For example, we suggested the following:

> Mrs. Dawe becomes hungry at 3:00 p.m. She thinks about the bag of candy in the kitchen that she had intended to give her grandchildren. How can she deal with this situation?
>
> Mr. Dawe comments that the green beans taste bland when they are cooked without bacon or pork. How can Mrs. Dawe respond?

Through this approach, learning activities became problem centered, and the patient and her family were encouraged to develop problem-solving skills.

Appendix A: Checklist for Assessing Patient-Education Materials

This checklist is designed to be used by health professionals when they review instructional materials for use in patient education. The checklist can be used with any type of instructional material (*e.g.*, print, films). Some items may not be applicable; however, each item has been included because it is considered to be desirable. The checklist is fairly exhaustive and may be shortened for use in a particular setting.

Title _____

Author_____ Publication date_____

Specified intended audience:

Age span:_____ to_____ years

Language or ethnic background _____

Socioeconomic group _____

I. Accuracy

A. Accuracy of factual information

1. Are facts, diagrams, pictures, and other visual representations accurate and presented objectively, without major distortions (sometimes due to oversimplification)?

     2. Is subject matter up to date? (Are there statements in the material that are no longer true or about which there is currently debate?)

II. Content
  A. Breadth or scope of coverage
     1. Does the subject matter or content presented address major area(s) of difficulty experienced by many patients with the specific medical problems (*e.g.*, need for factual information, need for attitude development, or need for physical skills development)?
     2. Is there content (subject matter or product endorsements/ advertising) included that is inappropriate for the intended audience?
  B. Balance of coverage
    Is the subject matter balanced in terms of the emphasis on various major areas?
  C. Inclusion of appropriate important "grey areas," "areas of uncertainty," or "areas of current debate" in the literature

III. Educational Methods
  A. Organization of content
     1. Is there an organizational structure or logic that is apparent to the patient?
     2. Are major content areas "set off" so that material can be put into perspective?
     3. Is the organizational structure obvious enough so that sections can be readily identified (for emphasis by patient educator or review by patient)?
  B. Contribution of organization of content to efficient learning
     1. Are concepts or terms introduced in an appropriate sequence?
     2. Does material start with simple concepts, then move to the more complex?
     3. Are elementary concepts introduced that are requisite for more advanced ones?
     4. Is there a summary?
  C. Educational objectives or goals and methods for assessing learner achievement (see 1 *or* 2 below)
     1. If objectives or goals *are* explicitly stated and included in the educational material
       a. Are objectives stated so that patients will understand them? (They should not "scare" the patient away, but rather should orient the patient.)
       b. Is it likely that patients will reach the objectives by study of the material? (Is there logical congruence between the objectives and the content?)
       c. Are learner-assessment methods congruent with the stated objectives? (Do test items or evaluation procedures reflect the objectives?)

2. If objectives or goals *are not* explicitly stated or are not present
   a. Are the implicit objectives easily inferred from the instructional materials? (*Implicit objectives* are learning outcomes that the author of the instructional material considers important and expects students to achieve. These are inferred from information such as content, selected author's emphasis, repetition of ideas, and intended level of generalization.)
   b. Are learner-assessment methods congruent with the implicit objectives?
      i. Is it possible for patients to do well on the evaluation instrument?
      ii. Are significant learning outcomes that are likely to occur reflected on the evaluation instrument? (Include anticipated as well as unanticipated and desirable as well as undesirable outcomes.)
D. Appropriateness of objectives (implicit or explicit)
   1. Do the objectives address areas that are generally of concern *to most physicians* who treat patients with this problem?
   2. Do the objectives address areas that are generally of concern *to most patients* with the particular problem?

IV. Communication
A. Appropriateness of the reading level for the stated audience
   1. Are other key audience characteristics specified?
   2. Whenever possible, are sentences short and simple, containing only commonly used terms, and is medical jargon avoided?
B. Availability of appropriate places for the patient to practice and obtain feedback about mastery of the facts, concepts, or principles taught? Are there appropriate places for the patient to practice and obtain feedback about instances in which the application of principles or methods is *not* appropriate (overgeneralization)?
C. Concreteness of the communication
   1. Is abstract communication avoided?
D. Adequate technical quality of the material
   1. Is the print size adequate?
   2. Are spacing and layout attractive?
   3. Are pictures attractive?
   4. Are diagrams simple and clear?
E. Availability of material for the patient to take home
   1. Does the material include key information or ideas?
   2. Does the material include a step-by-step explanation of any task the patient is to perform?

V. Faculty Guidebook
A. Inclusion in the instructional material of a guidebook to help members of the health-care team work together in their use of the material
   1. Does the guidebook contain
      a. Behavioral objectives for the program?

    b. A clear description of the instructional methods that are recommended? (This includes "how-to" information)

    c. A method for charting patient-education problems and attainment of objectives?

    d. A description of "pitfalls" or "problems to be avoided" when using the program (*e.g.*, common misunderstandings that occur with the materials)?

    e. Suggested methods for assessing attainment of the objectives?

VI. Evaluation
  A. Provision of data by the materials developer that proves that the materials are indeed effective (Testimonials do not count here)
    The evaluation report should contain a clear summary of the findings of the evaluation-research study and a description of how these results were obtained. It should also include information about the following:
    1. Antecedents—any conditions existing prior to teaching and learning that may relate to outcomes
      a. What are the characteristics of the individuals in the study (*e.g.*, social class, aptitude, prior experience, kind and phase of illness)?
      b. What is the setting (*e.g.*, rural vs urban, general vs subspecialty practice)?
    2. Transactions—succession of engagements that compose the process of education. Was the instructional process described as it actually happened? Did all the participants experience the instruction (*e.g.*, watch the film, read the printed material)? How much time did they spend engaged in study?
    3. Outcomes—results of the educational process. Consider participants' achievement, attitudes, health, and use of the health-care system as well as the effects on the providers and the system.
  B. Likeliness that patients will misunderstand, become confused by the materials, or misapply the principles learned from the material

VII. Authorship and Sponsorship
  A. Evidence that physicians who are knowledgeable about the area have been involved in the development and review of the materials
  B. Approval of the materials by the appropriate professional group

VIII. Cost-effectiveness/Practicality
  A. Excessive cost of the material
  B. Possibility that the same objectives can be reached by other methods
  C. Practicality of the methods
    Comments _____

_____

_____

_____

_____

Overall Evaluation			Very	
Poor	Fair	Good	Good	Excellent
1	2	3	4	5

(From The Society of Teachers of Family Medicine: Patient Education, A Handbook for Teachers. Kansas City, Society of Teachers of Family Medicine, 1979)

Appendix B: Sources for General Patient-Education Information

Section A: Professional Organizations

Organization	Available Materials
*American Academy of Family Physicians 1740 W. 92nd Street Kansas City, Missouri 64114	Pamphlets and catalogs on cancer
American Academy of Ophthalmology P.O. Box 7424 San Francisco, California 94120	Materials relating to ophthalmology
American Academy of Otolaryngology 15 2nd Street, S.W. Rochester, Minnesota 59901	Materials relating to otolaryngology
American Academy of Pediatrics 1801 Hinman Avenue Evanston, Illinois 60204	Publications on child health (mostly for professional audiences); some information sheets for patients
American Association for Health, Physical Education, and Recreation 1201 16th Street, N.W. Washington, D.C. 20036	Pamphlets, films, slides, catalogs, and other materials on nutrition and weight control
American Association of Ophthalmology 1100 17th Street, N.W. Room 304 Washington, D.C. 20036	Materials relating to ophthalmology

American Association of Poison
Control Centers
4800 Sandpoint Way
Seattle, Washington 98105

Slide presentations for adults;
filmstrip and study guides for
children, slide presentation for
health fairs and clinics; book on
poisons for ages 5–10

American Association of Sex
Educators, Counselors, and
Therapists
Suite 304
5010 Wisconsin Avenue, N.W.
Washington, D.C. 20016

Pamphlets on sex education

American Bakers Association
Public Relations Department
Suite 560
1700 Pennsylvania Avenue N.W.
Washington, D.C. 20056

Pamphlets on nutrition and weight
control

American Chiropractic Association
2200 Grand Avenue
Des Moines, Iowa 50312

Films, slide presentations,
pamphlets, booklets, texts, posters,
displays, and kits on a variety of
health topics

American College of Cardiology
9111 Old Georgetown Road
Bethesda, Maryland 20014

Professional materials only

American College of Obstetrics and
Gynecology
One East Wacker Drive
Chicago, Illinois 60601

Pamphlets and catalogs on cancer,
obstetrics and gynecology

*American Dental Association
211 East Chicago Avenue
Chicago, Illinois 60611

Pamphlets, posters, films,
presentations, flipcharts, and
exhibits on dental health

American Dietetic Association
430 North Michigan Avenue
Chicago, Illinois 60611

Most publications for professional
use; materials for the public on
special diets, vegetarianism, weight
control, allergy; single copies are free

American Home Economics
Association
2010 Massachusetts Avenue, N.W.
Washington, D.C. 20036

Pamphlets and catalogs on nutrition
and weight control

American Hospital Association
840 North Lake Shore Drive
Chicago, Illinois 60611

Numerous publications for the
professional regarding patient
education; numerous patient
publications

American Medical Association
535 North Dearborn Street
Chicago, Illinois 60610

Pamphlets on specific diseases and
on such topics as drug abuse,
alcoholism, physical fitness, mental
health, nutrition; posters and
teaching kits on some topics, books
on health topics

American Nurses' Association
2420 Pershing Road
Kansas City, Missouri 64108

Publications for nurses about
patient education

American Occupational Therapy
Association
6000 Executive Boulevard
Suite 200
Rockville, Maryland 20852

Pamphlets and posters on
occupational therapy and
rehabilitation

American Optometric Association
243 N. Lindbergh Street
St. Louis, Missouri 63141

Pamphlets and posters on eyesight

American Osteopathic Association
212 East Ohio Street
Chicago, Illinois 60611

Printed materials on venereal disease,
poisoning, first aid, immunization,
cancer, and nutrition; single copies
are free

American Physical Therapy
Association
1156 15th Street, N.W.
Washington, D.C. 20005

Pamphlets on rehabilitation

American Podiatry Association
20 Chevy Chase Circle, N.W.
Washington, D.C. 20005

Films and publications on general
foot care and on foot care for the
diabetic

American Psychiatric Association
1700 18th Street, N.W.
Washington, D.C. 20009

Publications on mental health

American Public Health
Association
1015 18th Street, N.W.
Washington, D.C. 20036

Patient-education information for
health workers; general information

Association of American Medical Colleges One Dupont Circle, N.W. Suite 200 Washington, D.C. 20036	General information
National Council on the Aging 1828 L Street, N.W. Suite 504 Washington, D.C. 20036	Professional materials related to starting programs for the elderly
National League for Nursing 10 Columbus Circle New York, New York 10019	Publications on patient-education topics and issues
National Retired Teachers Association/American Association of Retired Persons 1909 K Street, N.W. Washington, D.C. 20049	Total programs on chronic diseases, including films and printed materials; some programs are single sessions on one specific disease
Society for Nutrition Education 2140 Shattuck Avenue Suite 1110 Berkeley, California 94704	Materials on food additives, food and health misinformation, pregnancy and nutrition; special diets and weight control information are available through a search-service format

Section B: Hospitals, Medical Schools, and Educational Centers

Organization	*Available Materials*
Albert Steiner Memorial Lung Clinic St. Joseph's Infirmary 56665 Peachtree Dunwoody Atlanta, Georgia 30342	Pamphlets on respiratory diseases
Brookhaven Memorial Hospital 101 Brookhaven Hospital Road Patchogue, New York 11772	Videotaped materials
Bureau of Audio Visual Instruction The University of Wisconsin 1327 University Avenue Madison, Wisconsin 53706	Films or slides and catalogs relating to obstetrics and gynecology
The Children's Hospital 700 Children's Drive Columbus, Ohio 43205	Pamphlets on diabetes

*Children's Hospital of Los Angeles
4650 Sunset Boulevard
Los Angeles, California 90054

Films or slides on hypertension

Diabetes Education Center
4959 Excelsior Boulevard
Minneapolis, Minnesota 55416

Pamphlets, films, slides, catalogs, books, and other materials on nutrition and weight control in diabetes

Educational Television Department
Auburn University
Auburn, Alabama 36830

Pamphlets, films, slides, and other materials on hypertension

Fairview General Hospital
c/o The Greater Cleveland Hospital
Association
18101 Lorraine Road
Cleveland, Ohio 44111

Videotaped materials

Indiana University School of
Medicine
Medical Educational Resources
Program
1100 West Michigan Street
Indianapolis, Indiana 46223

Videotaped materials

Kaiser Permanente Health Center
Audiovisual Workshop
280 W. McCarther Boulevard
Oakland, California 94611

Films, slides, and catalogs relating to arthritis and obstetrics/gynecology

Martland Hospital
Health Education Project
College of Medicine and Dentistry
of New Jersey
100 Bergen Street
Newark, New Jersey 07102

Videotaped materials

Mercy Medical Center
Patient Education Division
Mercy Drive
Dubuque, Iowa 52001

Films or slides on diabetes

University of Illinois Medical
Center
Public Information Office
1737 West Polk Street
Chicago, Illinois 60612

Videotaped materials

University of Kansas College of Health Sciences and Hospital 39th and Rainbow Streets Kansas City, Kansas 66103	Videotaped materials
University of North Carolina at Chapel Hill Institute of Nutrition Allied Health Sciences Building 311 Pittsboro Street, 256H Chapel Hill, North Carolina 27514	Pamphlets and other materials on nutrition and weight control
University of Toronto Division of Instructional Media Services 8 Taddlecreek Road Toronto, Ontario, Canada M5S 1A8	Videotaped materials

Section C: Voluntary and Nonprofit Organizations

Organization	*Available Materials*
*Al-Anon (Family Group Head- Quarters, Inc.) 200 Park Avenue South Room 1602 New York, New York 10003	Books, pamphlets, cartoon booklets, and monthly publications on life with an alcoholic; some materials in Braille and on tape
*Alcoholics Anonymous World Services, Inc. 468 Park Avenue South New York, New York 10017	Publications, books, and pamphlets for patients, their families, friends, and employers
Allergy Foundation of America 19 West 44th Street Suite 702 New York, New York 10036	Pamphlets on respiratory diseases
American Association for Maternal and Infant Health P.O. Box 965 Los Alto, California 94022	Pamphlets, catalogs, and other materials relating to obstetrics/ gynecology
American Cancer Society 777 3rd Avenue New York, New York 10017	Pamphlets, films, posters, displays, and booklets on cancer
American Council on Alcohol Problems 119 Constitution Avenue, N.E. Washington, D.C. 20002	Pamphlets on alcoholism

American Diabetes Association, Inc. 600 5th Avenue New York, New York 10020	Printed matter for the patient and physician; bimonthly magazines, reprints of magazine articles, programmed instruction booklet on diabetes, cookbook
*American Foundation for the Blind, Inc. 15 West 16th Street New York, New York 10011	Pamphlets, films, posters, and flyers on Braille, dog guides, and rehabilitation employment; most are free
American Health Foundation 320 East 43rd Street New York, New York 10017	General information
*American Heart Association 7320 Greenville Avenue Dallas, Texas 75231	Films, slides, filmstrips, tapes, diagrams, posters, exhibits, models, books, and pamphlets on stroke, arteriosclerosis, smoking, rubella, diet, and other heart-related risks
American Lung Association 1740 Broadway New York, New York 10019	Films, leaflets, and booklets on specific lung diseases, smoking, and air pollution
American Red Cross 18th and E Streets, N.W. Washington, D.C. 20096	Materials provided in health and safety courses; some first-aid materials and instructional films available separately
American Social Health Association 260 Sheridan Avenue Palo Alto, California 94306	Materials on veneral disease and drug abuse
American Society for Psycho-prophylaxis in Obstetrics 1411 K Street, N.W. Suite 200 Washington, D.C. 20005	Books, pamphlets, and audiovisual aids on childbirth preparation
The Arthritis Foundation 3400 Peachtree Road, N.E. Suite 1101 Atlanta, Georgia 30326	Pamphlets and catalogs on arthritis, nutrition, and weight control
Association for Hearing and Speech Action 814 Thayer Avenue Silver Spring, Maryland 20910	Pamphlets on hearing and speech

Better Vision Institute 230 Park Avenue New York, New York 10017	Pamphlets, catalogs, and other materials on eye care and blindness
California Literacy, Inc. 248 East Main Street Aloama, California 91801	Pamphlets and catalogs about nutrition and weight control
Child Study Association of America 9 East 89th Street New York, New York 10028	Pamphlets about parenting
Consumers Union of United States 256 Washington Street Mount Vernon, New York 10550	*The Medical Show,* a guide to home health care; *Health Guide for Travelers;* reprints on dental care, breast cancer, use of drugs during pregnancy, marijuana use, and so forth
Council of Guilds for Infant Survival 1629 K Street, N.W. Washington, D.C. 20006	Pamphlets on parenting
Cystic Fibrosis Foundation 6000 Executive Boulevard Suite 309 Rockville, Maryland 20852	Films, pamphlets, brochures, newsletters, and posters on cystic fibrosis; list of medical centers specializing in CF; information on lung and digestive diseases also available
Epilepsy Foundation of America 1828 L Street, N.W. Washington, D.C. 20036	Pamphlets, films, and audio tapes on epilepsy
Food and Agriculture Organizations of the United Nations North American Regional Office 1776 F Street, N.W. Washington, D.C. 20437	Pamphlets on nutrition and weight control
La Leche League International, Inc. 9616 Minneapolis Avenue Franklin Park, Illinois 60131	Pamphlets and books on prenatal care, childbirth, the practical and psychological aspects of breast-feeding, child care, and family nutrition; pamphlets are free

*Maternity Center Association 48 East 92nd Street New York, New York 10028	Leaflets, books, teaching aids, and reprints on pregnancy, maternity care, childbearing, parenthood, parent education, and nurse–midwifery; slides, charts, bibliographies, and resource lists on nutrition, drugs, and other family-life concerns; films and film catalogs also available
Mental Health Materials Center 419 Park Avenue South New York, New York 10016	Materials concerning mental health and family-life education
MRS Associates, Inc. 535 Lexington Avenue New York, New York 10022	Pamphlets and catalogs relating to obstetrics/gynecology
Muscular Dystrophy Association 810 7th Avenue New York, New York 10019	Pamphlets on muscular dystrophy
National Academy of Sciences National Research Council Food and Nutrition Board 2101 Constitution Avenue, N.W. Washington, D.C. 20418	Pamphlets, catalogs, and other materials on nutrition and weight control
*National Association for Mental Health 1800 North Kent Street Arlington, Virginia 22209	Publications on mental illness and good mental-health practices; also, catalogs on films and prenatal materials
National Association for Retarded Citizens 2709 Avenue East Arlington, Texas 76011	Pamphlets and catalogs on parenting
National Association of the Deaf 814 Thayer Avenue Silver Spring, Maryland 20910	Pamphlets on hearing and hearing loss
National Council on Alcoholism 733 3rd Avenue New York, New York 10017	Pamphlets on alcoholism
The Nutrition Foundation, Inc. 888 17th Street, N.W. Washington, D.C. 20006	Pamphlets, films, slides, catalogs, and other materials on nutrition and weight control

*National Easter Seal Society for Crippled Children and Adults
2023 West Ogden Avenue
Chicago, Illinois 60612

Leaflets, pamphlets, newsletters, and bibliographies on parenting, rehabilitation for cerebral palsy, speech disorders, stroke, learning disabilities, and orthopedic conditions

*National Foundation—March of Dimes
1275 Mamaroneck Avenue
White Plains, New York 10605

Materials and programs on birth defects and prenatal care; pamphlets and audiovisual materials on rubella, Cooley's anemia, Tay-Sachs disease, venereal disease, alcoholism, and genetic counseling

National Hemophilia Foundation
25 West 39th Street
New York, New York 10018

Pamphlets on hemophilia

National Interagency Council on Smoking and Health
291 Broadway, Room 1005
New York, New York 10007

Pamphlets on smoking

National Kidney Foundation
2 Park Avenue
New York, New York 10016

Brochures on kidney disease and organ-donor programs; most are free

National Multiple Sclerosis Society
205 East 42nd Street
New York, New York 10017

Pamphlets and teaching aids about multiple sclerosis for patients and professionals

National Safety Council
444 North Michigan Avenue
Chicago, Illinois 60611

Films, filmstrips, slide sets, pamphlets, calendars, decals, and manuals on all areas of safety, first aid, poisons, child safety, sports safety, traffic safety, and so forth.

National Society for Medical Research
1000 Vermont Avenue
Washington, D.C. 20005

Pamphlets on heart disease

National Society for the Prevention of Blindness, Inc.
79 Madison Avenue
New York, New York 10016

Publications and audiovisual aids on eye care and prevention of blindness; single copies are free

Nutrition Foundation
489 5th Avenue
New York, New York 10017

Pamphlets on nutrition

Parkinson's Disease Foundation
640 West 168th Street
New York, New York 10032

Pamphlets on Parkinson's disease

*Planned Parenthood Federation of
America, Inc.
810 7th Avenue
New York, New York 10019

Printed materials, slides, and
novelties on family planning, specific
birth-control methods, contraceptive
use, childbirth, and human
reproduction

The Public Television Library
475 L'Enfant Plaza, S.W.
Washington, D.C. 20024

Videotaped materials

Sex Information and Education
Council of United States
84 5th Avenue, Suite 407
Hempstead, New York 10011

Pamphlets on parenting, sex
education, family planning, sexual
problems of the handicapped, sex
and aging, and obstetrics/gynecology

Sister Kenny Institute
Chicago Avenue at 27th Street
Minneapolis, Minnesota 55407

Pamphlets, films, slides, catalogs,
and other materials on ostomy

Society for Public Health
Education, Inc.
693 Sutter Street, 4th Floor
San Francisco, California 94102

Professional journal, *Health
Education Monographs,* containing
articles and studies on theory and
practice of health education

United Cerebral Palsy Associations,
Inc.
66 East 34th Street
New York, New York 10016

Publications on cerebral palsy, baby
care, nutrition, early identification of
cerebral palsy; films, slides, and
cassettes

United Ostomy Association
111 Wilshire Boulevard
Los Angeles, California 90017

Pamphlets and catalogs on ostomy

United Way
801 N. Fairfax Street
Alexandria, Virginia 22314

General information

Section D: Commercial Organizations and Companies

D-1: Pharmaceutical Companies

Organization

Available Materials

Asthma Information
Cooper Laboratories, Inc.
110 East Hanover Avenue
Cedar Knolls, New Jersey 07927

Pamphlets on respiratory diseases

Ayerst Laboratories Division of American Home Products Corp. 685 3rd Avenue New York, New York 10017	Pamphlets relating to obstetrics/ gynecology
Bristol Laboratories Division of Bristol-Myers Co. Thompson Road, P.O. Box 657 Syracuse, New York 13201	Pamphlets on hypertension
CIBA-GEIGY Corporation 556 Morris Avenue Summit, New Jersey 07901	Pamphlets, films, slides, and catalogs on hypertension
Davol, Inc. 100 Sockanosset Crossroads Cranston, Rhode Island 02920	Pamphlets, catalogs, and other materials on ostomy
Dorsey Laboratories Division of Sandoz, Inc. P.O. Box 83288 Lincoln, Nebraska 68501	Materials on respiratory diseases
Eli Lilly and Company 307 E. McCarty St. P.O. Box 618 Indianapolis, Indiana 46285	Pamphlets and catalogs on diabetes
Mead Johnson Pharmaceutical Division Division of Mead Johnson & Company 2404 W. Pennsylvania Street Evansville, Indiana 47721	Pamphlets and other materials on parenting, obstetrics/gynecology, respiratory diseases, nutrition, and weight control
Merck Sharp & Dohme Division of Merck & Co., Inc. West Point, Pennsylvania 19486	Pamphlets and catalogs on nutrition and weight control
Ormont Drug and Chemical Co., Inc. 520 S. Dean Street Englewood, New Jersey 07631	Videotaped materials
Ortho Pharmaceutical Corporation Route 202 Raritan, New Jersey 08869	Pamphlets and catalogs on obstetrics/gynecology
Pennwalt Pharmaceutical Division Pennwalt Corporation P.O. Box 1212 Rochester, New York 14603	Pamphlets on nutrition and weight control

Pfizer Laboratories Division
Pfizer Inc.
235 East 42nd Street
New York, New York 10017

Pamphlets and catalogs on diabetes

Riker Laboratories, Inc.
Subsidiary of 3M Company
19901 Nordhoff Street
Northridge, California 91324

Pamphlets and other materials on
respiratory diseases

Roche Laboratories
Division of Hoffman-LaRoche Inc.
Roche Park, 340 Kingslend Street
Nutley, New Jersey 07110

Pamphlets on nutrition and weight
control

Ross Laboratories
Div. Abbott Laboratories
Creative Services and Information
Department
625 North Cleveland Avenue
Columbus, Ohio 43216

Pamphlets, films, slides, and catalogs
on obstetrics/gynecology, eye care,
nutrition, weight control, and
parenting

Searle Laboratories
Division of G.D. Searle & Company
Box 5110
Chicago, Illinois 60680

Pamphlets on obstetrics/gynecology
(available to physicians only),
hypertension, and family planning

Smith Kline and French Laboratories
Division of Smith Kline Corporation
1500 Spring Garden Street
Philadelphia, Pennsylvania 19101

Pamphlets on hypertension

E. R. Squibb & Sons, Inc.
General Offices
P.O. Box 4000
Princeton, New Jersey 08540

Pamphlets on diabetes and ostomy,
catalogs on diabetes, other materials on
ostomy

Syntex Laboratories
1344 Elmwood Avenue
Wilmette, Illinois 60091

Pamphlets on nutrition and weight
control

United States Pharmacopeial
Convention, Inc.
Publication Department
12601 Twinbrook Parkway
Rockville, Maryland 20852

Patient information on drugs and
drug therapy; *Advice for the Patient,*
vol. II (1983) may be used by health
professionals in patient-education
planning and adapted for teaching
programs

The Upjohn Company
7171 Portage Road
Kalamazoo, Michigan 49001

Pamphlets, films, and slides on
diabetes, nutrition, weight control,
and preventive health

Warner/Chilcott Laboratories Div. Parke-Davis 201 Tabor Road Morris Plains, New Jersey 07950	Pamphlets and catalogs on heart disease
Winthrop Laboratories 90 Park Avenue New York, New York 10016	Pamphlets on parenting
Wyeth Laboratories Division of American Home Products Corporation P.O. Box 8299 Philadelphia, Pennsylvania 19101	Pamphlets and catalogs on obstetrics/gynecology and parenting

D-2: Sources of Audiovisual Materials

Abbott Film Service Scientificom Distribution Center 14th Street and Sarian N. Chicago, Illinois 60064	Films, slides, and catalogs on hypertension
Alfred Higgens Productions, Inc. 9100 Sunset Boulevard Los Angeles, California 90069	Videotaped materials
*Ames Company Division of Miles Laboratories, Inc. 1127 Myrtle Street Elkhart, Indiana 46514	Pamphlets, films, slides, and other materials on diabetes
Becton-Dickinson & Company Ruther Ford, New Jersey 07070	"Getting Started" program (diabetes care); pamphlets, films, slides, and other materials on diabetes
Best Foods—Consumer Service Department A Division of CPC International, Inc. International Plaza Englewood Cliffs, New Jersey 07632	Pamphlets, films, slides, catalogs, and other materials on nutrition and weight control
Bluestone Video Makers 4018 22nd Street San Francisco, California 94110	Videotaped materials
BNA Communications, Inc. 9401 Decoverly Hall Road Rockville, Maryland 20850	Videotaped materials

Churchill Films 662 N. Robertson Boulevard Los Angeles, California 90069	Films, slides and catalogs relating to obstetrics/gynecology
Core Communications in Health, Inc. 1916-38 Park Avenue New York, New York 10037	Pamphlets, films, slides, and catalogs on heart disease, hypertension, kidney disease, ostomy, parenting, respiratory disease, stroke, arthritis, diabetes, obstetrics/gynecology, and cancer; publishes *CORE Communications in Health*, a major patient-education newsletter
Education for Health, Inc. 205 Deerwood Lane Minneapolis, Minnesota	Pamphlets, films, slides, catalogs, and other materials on hypertension, and pamphlets on diabetes
Family Communications, Inc. 4802 5th Avenue Pittsburgh, Pennsylvania 15213	Videotaped materials
Film-Com Audience Planners 108 W. Grand Chicago, Illinois 60610	Films, slides, and catalogs on eye care and blindness
Health Films Library P.O. Box 309, One W. Wilson Street Madison, Wisconsin 53701	Films, slides and catalogs on cancer
Hospital Audio Visual Education 606 Halstead Avenue Mamaroneck, New York 10543	Videotaped materials
Johnson & Johnson Health Care Division 501 George Street New Brunswick, New Jersey 05903	Pamphlets, films, slides, and other materials on parenting
Lawren Productions, Inc. P.O. Box 1452 Burlingame, California 94010	Films, slides, and catalogs on hypertension
Learning Resources Facility Institute of Rehabilitation Medicine 400 East 34th Street New York, New York 10016	Films and slides on arthritis
Lee Creative Communications, Inc. P.O. Box 1367, 5 South St. Regis Drive Rochester, New York 14618	Films and slides on arthritis

J. B. Lippincott Company
East Washington Square
Philadelphia, Pennsylvania 19105

Videotapes, filmstrips, and pamphlets
for patient instruction

Medcom, Inc.
1633 Broadway
New York, New York 10019

Videotaped materials

*Medfact, Inc.
1112 Andrew, N.E.
Massilon, Ohio 44645

Pamphlets, films, slides, and catalogs
on parenting, respiratory diseases,
stroke, diabetes, eye care, heart
disease, hypertension, and obstetrics/
gynecology

Metropolitan Life Insurance
Health and Welfare Division
One Madison Avenue
New York, New York 10010

Pamphlets, films, and slides on
parenting; pamphlets and catalogs on
hypertension

*Professional Research, Inc.
12960 Coral Tree Place
Los Angeles, California 90066

Pamphlets, films, slides, and catalogs
on stroke, eye care, heart disease,
hypertension, and obstetrics/
gynecology

Public Affairs Committee
Film Library
381 Park Avenue South
New York, New York 10016

Films and slides on diabetes

Pyramid Films
Box 1048, 2801 Colorado Avenue
Santa Monica, California 90406

Videotaped materials

Richard Milner
Milner, Fenwick
2125 Greenspring Drive
Timonium, Maryland 21093

Films, slides, catalogs, and other
materials on hypertension

Single Concept Films
Two Terrain Drive
Rochester, New York 14618

Pamphlets, catalogs, films, and slides
on heart disease, hypertension,
parenting, respiratory diseases, and
stroke

Teach'Em, Inc.
625 N. Michigan Avenue
Chicago, Illinois 60611

Videotaped materials

Train-Aide
1015 Grandview Avenue
Glendale, California 91201

Pamphlets, films, slides, catalogs,
and other materials on diabetes,
respiratory diseases, and heart
disease; pamphlets, catalogs, and
other materials on ostomy

The Trainex Corporation
P.O. Box 116
12601 Industry Street
Garden Grove, California 92641

Films, slides, and catalogs on diabetes; pamphlets and catalogs on parenting; pamphlets, films, slides, catalogs, and other materials on respiratory diseases and heart disease; pamphlets, films, slides, and catalogs on hypertension; pamphlets and catalogs on ostomy

Vidcom
4470 Chamblee-Dunwoody Road
Atlanta, Georgia 30338

Pamphlets, films, slides, catalogs, and other materials on respiratory disease

Video Communication, Inc.
Suite 904, Watergate Office Building
2600 Virginia Avenue, N.W.
Washington, D.C. 20037

Films, slides, and catalogs on hypertension

Vitamin Information Bureau, Inc.
383 Madison Avenue
New York, New York 10017

Pamphlets, films, slides, catalogs, and other materials on nutrition and weight control

W. B. Saunders Company
W. Washington Square
P.O. Box 416
Philadelphia, Pennsylvania 19105

Films and slides on arthritis

Wells National Services
Corporation
3 Park Avenue
New York, New York 10016

Videotaped materials

D-3: Sources for Printed Materials Only

American Dry Milk Institute
130 N. Franklin Street
Chicago, Illinois 60606

Pamphlets on nutrition and weight control

American Egg Board
1460 Renaissance Drive
Park Ridge, Illinois 60068

Pamphlets on nutrition and weight control

American Institute of Baking
Consumer Service Department
1213 Baker's Way
Manhattan, Kansas 66502

Pamphlets on nutrition and weight control

American Meat Institute
Department of Public Relations
1600 Wilson Boulevard
Suite 1200
Arlington, Virginia 22209

Pamphlets and catalogs on nutrition and weight control

Appleton-Century-Crofts Education Division Meredith Corporation 750 3rd Avenue New York, New York 10017	Pamphlets on nutrition and weight control
Armour Food Company Consumer Services Department Greyhound Towers Phoenix, Arizona 85077	Pamphlets on nutrition and weight control
Beecham-Massengill Division of Beecham, Inc. 501 5th Street Bristol, Tennessee 37620	Pamphlets relating to obstetrics/gynecology
Blue Cross Association 840 N. Lake Shore Drive Chicago, Illinois 60611	Pamphlets and catalogs relating to parenting, nutrition, weight control, and obstetrics/gynecology
Boehringer Ingleheim 90 East Ridge Ridgefield, Connecticut 06877	Pamphlets, catalogs, and other materials on hypertension
The Borden Company Marketing Services 180 E. Broad Street Columbus, Ohio 43215	Pamphlets on nutrition and weight control
California Prune Advisory Board 103 World Trade Center San Francisco, California 94111	Pamphlets on nutrition and weight control
California Tree Fruit Agreement 701 Fulton Avenue Sacramento, California 95825	Pamphlets on nutrition and weight control
Campbell Soup Company Food Service Products Division Campbell Place Camden, New Jersey 08101	Pamphlets, catalogs, and other materials on nutrition and weight control
Carnation Company Medical Marketing Department 5045 Wilshire Boulevard Los Angeles, California 90036	Pamphlets and catalogs on nutrition and weight control
Cereal Institute 1111 Plaza Drive Schaumburg, Illinois 60195	Pamphlets, catalogs, and other materials on nutrition and weight control

Channing L. Bete Company, Inc. 45 Federal Street Greenfield, Massachusetts 01301	Booklets (containing cartoons) and catalogs on arthritis, cancer, heart disease, parenting, drug abuse, obstetrics/gynecology, and a wide variety of other topics
Chicago Dietetic Supply, Inc. 405 E. Shawmut La Grange, Illinois 60525	Pamphlets on nutrition and weight control
Corn Products Company (Best Foods) International Plaza Englewood Cliffs, New Jersey 07632	Pamphlets on nutrition and weight control
Del Monte Kitchens Del Monte Corporation P.O. Box 3575 San Francisco, California 94119	Pamphlets on nutrition and weight control
The Equitable Life Assurance Society of the United States 1285 6th Avenue New York, New York 10019	Pamphlets on nutrition and weight control
Fleischman's Margarine 625 Madison Avenue New York, New York 10022	Pamphlets on heart disease, nutrition, and weight control
Food Council of America 1750 Pennsylvania Avenue, N.W. Washington, D.C. 20005	Pamphlets on nutrition and weight control
General Foods Corporation Consumer Service Department 250 North Street White Plains, New York 10625	Pamphlets on nutrition and weight control
Gerber Products Company 445 State Street Freemont, Michigan 49412	Pamphlets on parenting, nutrition, and weight control
Good Food 1864 E. Washington Pasadena, California 91103	Pamphlets on nutrition and weight control
Good Housekeeping Bulletin Service 959 8th Avenue New York, New York 10019	Pamphlets on nutrition and weight control

Green Giant Company Home Services Department Hazeltine Gates Chaska, Minnesota 55318	Pamphlets on nutrition and weight control
Harshe-Rothman and Druck, Inc. California Avocado Advisory Board 3345 Wilshire Boulevard Los Angeles, California 90010	Pamphlets on nutrition and weight control
Health Insurance Institute 1850 K Street, N.W. Washington, D.C. 20006	General health pamphlets
H. J. Heinz Consumer Relations 1062 Progress Street Pittsburgh, Pennsylvania 15212	Pamphlets on nutrition and weight control
Holister, Inc. 211 East Chicago Drive Chicago, Illinois 60611	Pamphlets and other materials on ostomy
International Apple Institute Public Relations 2430 Pennsylvania Avenue, N.W. Washington, D.C. 20037	Pamphlets on nutrition and weight control
John F. Greer Company 530 East 12th Street Oakland, California 94606	Pamphlets and catalogs on ostomy
Kellogg Company Department of Home Economic Services 235 Proter Street Battle Creek, Michigan 49016	Pamphlets on nutrition and weight control
Kimberly-Clark Corporation Life Cycle Center Box 2001 Neenah, Wisconsin 54956	Pamphlets on obstetrics/gynecology
Knox Gelatin, Inc. Subsidiary of Thomas J. Lipton Englewood Cliffs, New Jersey 07632	Pamphlets on nutrition and weight control
Kraft Foods 500 Peshtigo Court Chicago, Illinois 60690	Pamphlets on nutrition and weight control

Lamb Educational Center 200 Clayton Street Denver, Colorado 80206	Pamphlets and other materials on nutrition and weight control
Libby, McNeil, and Libby 200 S. Michigan Avenue Chicago, Illinois 60604	Pamphlets on nutrition and weight control
Media Medica, Inc. East Hanover, New Jersey 07936	Pamphlets and catalogs on heart disease and stroke
Nabisco 425 Park Avenue New York, New York 10022	Pamphlets on nutrition and weight control
National Dairy Council 6300 North River Road Rosemont, Illinois 60018	Pamphlets and other materials on parenting, heart disease, nutrition, and weight control
National Food Processors Consumer Services 1123 20th Street, N.W. Washington, D.C. 20036	Pamphlets on nutrition and weight control
National Livestock and Meat Board 444 N. Michigan Avenue Chicago, Illinois 60611	Pamphlets and catalogs on nutrition and weight control
New Readers Press 1320 Jamesville Avenue Syracuse, New York 13210	Pamphlets on obstetrics/gynecology
Nutra-Mate Textured Vegetable Protein A. E. Staley Manufacturing Co. Food Service Division 2222 Kensington Court Oak Brook, Illinois 60521	Pamphlets on nutrition and weight control
Pacific Vegetable Oil Corporation Saffola Products Division World Trade Center, Room 130 San Francisco, California 94111	Pamphlets on nutrition and weight control
Perennial Education, Inc. 477 Roger Williams P.O. Box 855 Razinia Highland Park, Illinois 60035	Catalogs and other materials relating to obstetrics/gynecology

Pet Incorporated Office of Consumer Affairs Pet Plaza 400 S. 4th Street St. Louis, Missouri 63166	Pamphlets on nutrition and weight control
Pharmaceutical Manufacturers Association 1155 15th Street, N.W. Washington, D.C. 20005	Catalog of materials available from member drug companies
Pritchett and Hull 2122 Faulkner, N.E. Atlanta, Georgia 30324	Pamphlets, films, slides, catalogs, and other materials on diabetes, respiratory diseases, and heart disease
Prudential Insurance Company of America P.O. Box 388 Fort Washington, Pennsylvania 19034	Pamphlets and other materials on nutrition and weight control
Public Affairs Pamphlets 381 Park Avenue South New York, New York 10016	Pamphlets and catalogs on obstetrics/gynecology
Quaker Oats Company Consumer Services Merchandise Mart Plaza Chicago, Illinois 60654	Pamphlets on nutrition and weight control
Ralston Purina Company Nutrition Service 835 South 8th Street St. Louis, Missouri 63188	Pamphlets on nutrition and weight control
Research Media, Inc. 14 Story Street Cambridge, Massachusetts 02138	Pamphlets, catalogs, books, and other materials on heart disease
Rice Council P.O. Box 22802 9317 Richmond Avenue Houston, Texas 77027	Pamphlets on nutrition and weight control
Robert J. Brady Company Route 197 Bowie, Maryland 20715	Pamphlets, catalogs, and other materials on diabetes, heart disease, hypertension, kidney disease, ostomy, respiratory diseases, and stroke

A. H. Robbins Company 1407 Cummings Drive Richmond, Virginia 23220	Pamphlets on arthritis
Standard Brands DMS, Inc. 60 E. 42nd Street New York, New York 10017	Pamphlets on nutrition and weight control
Stokely, Van Camp, Inc. Home Economics Department 941 Meridian Indianapolis, Indiana 46206	Pamphlets and other materials on nutrition and weight control
Sunkist Growers, Inc. Consumer Services 14130 Riverside Drive Sherman Oaks, California 91423	Pamphlets and other materials on nutrition and weight control
Swift and Company Public Relations Department 115 W. Jackson Boulevard Chicago, Illinois 60604	Pamphlets on nutrition and weight control
United Fresh Fruit and Vegetable Association 727 N. Washington Street Alexandria, Virginia 22314	Pamphlets and catalogs on nutrition and weight control
Wheat Flour Institute Home Economics Department 1776 F Street N.W. Washington, D.C. 20006	Pamphlets, films, and slides on nutrition and weight control

Section E: Governmental Sources

E-1: Federal

Organization

Department of Agriculture

Available materials

Consumer and Foods Economic Institute Room 325A, Federal Building Hyattsville, Maryland 20782	Pamphlets on nutrition and weight control
Department of Agriculture Office of Information Washington, D.C. 20250	Pamphlets on nutrition and farm and home safety

| The Food and Nutrition Information and Educational Materials Center National Agricultural Library Beltsville, Maryland 20705 | Pamphlets on nutrition and weight control |

Office of Consumer Affairs

| 621 Reporters Building 300 7th Avenue, S.W. Washington, D.C. 20201 | General health pamphlets |

Department of Health, Education and Welfare

| Centers for Disease Control Bureau of Health Education 1600 Clifton Road, N.E. Atlanta, Georgia 30333 | Pamphlets on accident prevention and disease control |

| Administration for Children, Youth, and Families P.O. Box 1182 Washington, D.C. 20013 | Pamphlets, films, slides, and other materials on nutrition and weight control |

| Food and Drug Administration Parklawn Building 5600 Fishers Lane Rockville, Maryland 20852 | Pamphlets on safety and accident prevention |

| Division of Long Term Care Health Standards and Quality Bureau Dogwood East Building 1849 Gwynn Oak Avenue Baltimore, Maryland 21207 | Pamphlets on nutrition and weight control |

| National Clearinghouse for Alcohol Information P.O. Box 2345 Rockville, Maryland | Large variety of pamphlets, booklets, and other printed materials on alcohol, drinking, alcohol abuse, and alcoholism |

| National Clearinghouse for Drug Abuse Information 5600 Fishers Lane Room 10A-J3 Rockville, Maryland 20857 | Materials about drug abuse and drug addiction |

| National Clearinghouse for Mental Health Information 22400 Rockville Pike Rockville, Maryland 20857 | Large variety of printed materials about many aspects of mental health; includes materials for the physician, the patient, and the public |

National Institute on Alcohol Abuse and Alcoholism
5600 Fishers Lane
Rockville, Maryland 20857

Pamphlets on alcoholism

National Office on Smoking and Health
5600 Fishers Lane
Parklawn Building, Room 1-58
Rockville, Maryland 20857

Pamphlets on smoking

Nutrition Section
Office of Clinical Services
Bureau of Community Health Services
5600 Fishers Lane
Rockville, Maryland 20857

Pamphlets on nutrition and weight control

National Institutes of Health

National Institute of Allergy and Infectious Diseases
Building 31, Room 7A03
9000 Rockville Pike
Bethesda, Maryland 20205

Pamphlets on allergy and infectious diseases

National Institute of Arthritis and Metabolic Diseases
Building 31, Room 9A52
9000 Rockville Pike
Bethesda, Maryland 20205

Pamphlets on arthritis and metabolic diseases

National Cancer Institute
Office of Cancer Communications
Building 31, Room 10A-29
Bethesda, Maryland 20205

Pamphlets and catalogs on cancer; related materials

National Institute of Child Health and Human Development
Building 31, Room 2A03
9000 Rockville Pike
Bethesda, Maryland 20205

Pamphlets on child health, growth, and development

Diabetes and Arthritis Program
Building 10, Room 9N-222
Bethesda, Maryland 20205

Pamphlets on diabetes and arthritis

National Institute of Dental Research
Building 31, Room 2C34
9000 Rockville Pike
Bethesda, Maryland 20205

Pamphlets on dental health

National Eye Institute Building 31, Room 6A03 9000 Rockville Pike Bethesda, Maryland 20205	Pamphlets on eyesight
National Institute of General Medical Sciences 9000 Rockville Pike Bethesda, Maryland 20205	General information
National Heart, Lung, and Blood Institute Building 31, Room 4A21 Bethesda, Maryland 20205	Pamphlets, catalogs, and other materials on hypertension, heart disease, stroke, and so forth
National High Blood Pressure Education Program Information Center 120/80 National Institutes of Health Bethesda, Maryland 20014	Pamphlets, booklets, posters, films, and other materials on hypertension
National Institute of Neurological Diseases and Stroke 9000 Rockville Pike Bethesda, Maryland 20014	Pamphlets on stroke

Public Health Service

Allergy Research and Introduction Building 31, Room 7A32 9000 Rockville Pike Bethesda, Maryland 20205	Pamphlets and other materials on respiratory diseases
Public Health Service 200 Independence Avenue Washington, D.C. 20201	Pamphlets and catalogs on diabetes, foot care, eye care, blindness, nutrition, and weight control

Department of Labor

Occupational Safety and Health Administration 3rd Street and Constitution Avenue, N.W. Washington, D.C. 20210	Pamphlets on occupational safety

E-2: State

The exact titles of the following state governmental agencies will vary from state to state. Addresses may be found in local telephone directories.

Commission on Alcoholism and Drug Abuse
Commission on Children and Youth

Departments of
  Education
  Environmental Health
  Health and Social Services
  Hospitals and Institutions
  Motor Vehicles
  Vocational Rehabilitation
Nursing Board
Pharmacy Board
Universities and Colleges

E-3: County

The exact titles of the following types of county governmental agencies will vary from county to county. Addresses may be found in local telephone directories.
  Agriculture Department—Extension Agent
  Health Department
  Hospital/Medical Center
  Housing Authority
  Maternity and Infant Care Project
  Mental Health/Mental Retardation Center
  Safety Department

E-4: City

The exact titles of the following types of city governmental agencies will vary from city to city. Addresses may be found in local telephone directories.
  Environmental Health
  Fire Department; Fire Prevention Bureau
  Housing and Urban Development
  Library and Information Service
  Mayor's Office—Community Services Division
  Police Department—Public Information Officer; School Safety Division

(Adapted from The Society of Teachers of Family Medicine: *Patient Education, A Handbook for Teachers.* Kansas City, Society of Teachers of Family Medicine, 1979)
*Some materials are available in Spanish.

References

1. Brunner LS, Suddarth DS: The Lippincott Manual of Nursing Practice, 3rd ed. Philadelphia, JB Lippincott, 1982
2. Kreigh HZ, Perko JE: Psychiatric and Mental Health Nursing: Commitment to Care and Concern, pp 74–77. Reston, VA, Reston Publishing, 1979
3. Hospitals 'warm' to self-help groups as linkage benefits gain recognition. Hospitals 56, No. 5:33, 1982
4. Brown JW, Lewis RN, Harcleroad FF: AV Instruction: Technology, Media and Methods, 4th ed. New York, McGraw-Hill, 1973

5. National Cancer Institute: Readability Testing in Cancer Communications. NIH
   Publication No. 81-1689. Bethesda, Cancer Information Clearinghouse, 1981
6. Frye E: A readability formula that saves time. J Reading 11:514, 1968
7. Bensinger C: The Video Guide. Santa Barbara, Video-Info Publications, 1979

Bibliography

Books

American Hospital Association: Implementing Patient Education in the Hospital.
Publication No. 1488. Chicago, American Hospital Association, 1979
American Hospital Association: Media Handbook: A Guide to Selecting, Producing, and
Using Media for Patient Education Programs, Publication No. 1258. Chicago,
American Hospital Association, 1978
American Hospital Association: Staff Manual for Teaching Patients about Chronic
Obstructive Pulmonary Diseases. Publication No. 1317. Chicago, American
Hospital Association, 1979
American Society of Hospital Pharmacists: Medication Teaching Manual: A Guide for
Patient Counselling. Publication No. 1258. Chicago, American Hospital Associa-
tion, 1978
Anderson RH: Selecting and Developing Media for Instruction. New York, Van Norstrand
Reinhold, 1976
Blevins DR: The Diabetic and Nursing Care. New York, McGraw-Hill, 1979
Bower FL, Bevis EO: Fundamentals of Nursing Practice: Concepts, Roles and Functions. St
Louis, CV Mosby, 1979
DeCecco JP: The Psychology of Learning and Instruction: Educational Psychology.
Englewood Cliffs, NJ, Prentice-Hall, 1968
Espenshade JE: Staff Manual for Teaching Patients about Diabetes Mellitus. Publication
No. 1318. Chicago, American Hospital Association, 1979
Gagne RM: The Conditions of Learning, 3rd ed. New York, Holt, Rinehart and Winston,
1977
Kron T: The Management of Patient Care. Philadelphia, WB Saunders, 1981
Lamonica EL: The Nursing Process: A Humanistic Approach. Menlo Park, CA, Addison-
Wesley Publishing Co, 1979
National Task Force on Training Family Physicians in Patient Education: Patient
Education: A Handbook for Teachers. Kansas City, Society of Teachers of Family
Medicine, 1979
Wallace R, Heiss ML, Bautch JC: Staff Manual for Teaching Patients about Rheumatoid
Arthritis. Publication No. 1320. Chicago, American Hospital Association, 1979
Yura H, Walsh MB: The Nursing Process: Assessing, Planning, Implementing and
Evaluating. New York, Appleton-Century Crofts, 1978

Journals

Barlow DJ, Bruhn JG: Role-plays on television: A new teaching technique. Nurs Outlook
21, No. 4:242–244, 1973
Levin LS: Forces and issues in the revival of interests in self-care: Impetus for redirection in
health. Health Educ Monogr 5:115–20, 1977
Parsell S, Tangliareni EM: Cancer patients can help each other. Am J Nurs 74:650–657,1974
Witt GA: Six media guidelines for memorable training. Training 19, No. 2: 56–57, 1982
Tarver J, Turner AJ: Teaching behavior modification to patient's families. Am J Nurs
74:282-283, 1974

Chapter 9
Evaluation

Evaluation is an essential component of the nursing process, yet it is one that is often neglected and misunderstood. Why is it that we frequently cannot find time to evaluate patient education, or that we fail to document learning? Why does the word *evaluation* cause us to feel uneasy and uncertain?

To evaluate is "to determine the significance, or worth of by careful appraisal or study."* All to often, nurses and patients alike feel threatened by the thought of evaluation. We worry about being personally devalued or judged unworthy. We recall our humiliation when, as children, we failed in a test or a spelling bee, and we do not want to feel that way again. We fear that if we fail to achieve what others expect of us we will lose love, support, assistance, esteem, and credibility.

The actual intent of evaluation is not to place a value or worth on patients or nurses. Its purposes are to measure the degree to which goals have been met and to redirect patient care. Evaluation of patient education involves collecting specific and descriptive data related to behaviors targeted as patient-learning objectives. Through evaluation, the nurse and the patient determine the value of the nursing interventions in helping the patient to carry out desired behaviors.

In addition to misunderstanding the meaning of evaluation, many nurses underestimate its importance in patient education. In the past, we thought about patient teaching as simply giving information. It had not been thought of as a valid nursing intervention for response to specific client needs or problems. As we become aware that the nursing process directs the delivery of patient education, just

*By permission. From Webster's New Collegiate Dictionary © 1979 by G. & C. Merriam Company, publishers of the Merriam-Webster® Dictionaries.

as it directs other nursing interventions, we recognize that evaluation is a component of the nursing process, deserving of our attention (Fig. 9-1).

This chapter is intended to offer a better understanding of evaluation, to address methods of data collection, and to discuss how to use the information gained in evaluation to reinforce learning and to plan future learning opportunities for patients. The examples offered in this chapter specifically focus on patient education of individual patients and their families. Chapter 3 addressed the evaluation of formal teaching programs.

Scope of Evaluation

Evaluation is closely related to assessment. Both involve formulating criteria or questions, gathering and categorizing data, and writing a summary statement. These findings are used in patient-care planning. *Assessment* usually refers to building a data base that includes nursing diagnoses and outlines the patient's needs or problems. *Evaluation* refers to the *follow-up assessment* that is continuously conducted as nursing interventions are carried out. Therefore, evaluation takes place throughout the learning activities and is used to assess the patient's progress toward meeting learning objectives. Understanding of the information and skills introduced in Chapter 6 is important in preparing for evaluation. We encourage the reader to review that chapter about the assessment process.

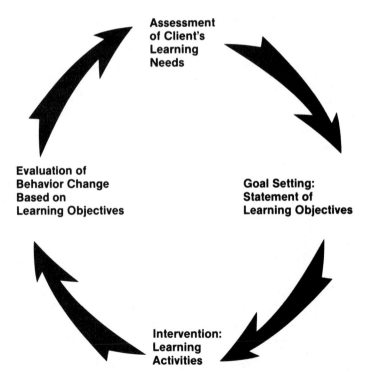

Assessment of Client's Learning Needs

Goal Setting: Statement of Learning Objectives

Intervention: Learning Activities

Evaluation of Behavior Change Based on Learning Objectives

Fig. 9-1. Evaluation: Part of a continuous process in patient education.

Evaluation is conducted using the behavioral objectives discussed in Chapter 7. If the patient objectives are clearly defined, evaluation is straight-forward. Measurement is based on the stated behaviors. The patient and his family should be active participants in evaluating learning. Through self-evaluation, based on his own learning objectives, a patient can define what is expected of him, he can plan and participate in learning activities, and he can seek feedback to direct his performance. Evaluation becomes a learning experience that can increase the patient's self-esteem as he recognizes his own accomplishments and gains positive feedback and support from others.

Evaluation is also a learning opportunity for the teacher. The feedback she receives from the patient's progress or lack of progress helps her to modify her approach and to consider alternate teaching strategies. These may include providing the learner with more review, clarifying learning objectives, and changing teaching/learning methods and media.

Evaluation is thus a continuous process conducted by the teacher and learner throughout patient education. Using the evaluation process, both parties benefit from feedback that reinforces successes and readdresses problems. There are certain times when evaluation is more formally conducted, and includes the use of written documentation as well as oral feedback. This documentation usually takes place at the ends of nursing shifts, after classes or skills training, and prior to the patient's discharge from the hospital or office. Just as the assessment process involves asking questions in order to gather specific information, so does the evaluation process. The evaluation process should include the following steps:

1. Measuring the extent to which the patient has met his learning objectives
2. Indicating when there is a need to clarify, correct, or review information
3. Noting objectives that are unclear
4. Pointing out shortcomings in the patient-teaching interventions, specifically addressing content, format, activities, and media

In patient education it is the teacher's responsibility to initiate the evaluation, summarize the findings, document findings in the medical record, give constructive feedback to the patient and his family, plan future experiences to reinforce learning, and design learning opportunities to foster behaviors that were not initially accomplished.

She must prepare herself by knowing what questions to ask and by having a good understanding of each component of the patient-education process. In addition to first measuring behavior, the nurse looks critically at nursing care and identifies problems that have prevented learning.

Thora Kron suggests that nurses formulate a series of questions to provide direction in the evaluation of patient care.[1] We find this suggestion especially practical and productive when used in the evaluation of the patient-education process. We have constructed a checklist with our questions (Fig. 9-2). We have included references to the text to encourage readers to review principles introduced in other chapters.

Questions

✓ Did the objectives clearly state observable patient behaviors?‡

✓ Were the objectives realistic for the client?†‡

✓ Was the original assessment complete?†

✓ Did the client perceive the identified problem as important? Did he want to change?*†‡

✓ Did new problems pose obstacles to behavioral change?†

✓ Did the client participate in goal setting?*‡

✓ Were the interventions tailored to meet the objectives?§

✓ Was behavioral change measured and documented accurately?//

✓ Is there a skill deficiency? Should there be changes in the nursing interventions?§//

* See Chapter 4
† See Chapter 6
‡ See Chapter 7
§ See Chapter 8
// See Chapter 9

Fig. 9-2. *Nurse's checklist for evaluation of patient education.*

Measuring Behavioral Change

Applying Learning Objectives

Learning objectives describe the behaviors the patient will perform to show that he has mastered knowledge, attitudes, and skills. They are tailored to the patient's individual goals.

Recall that a learning objective has three components: performance, conditions, and criteria. *Performance* states what the learner will do and uses an action verb that describes a measurable activity. In choosing the action verb, the teacher asks herself: "Can I measure this behavior?" The verb is carefully selected so that the learner and the teacher both have a clear understanding of how the learner will demonstrate his competence. *Conditions* state special activities to be included in the learner's performance. Sterile technique used in insulin administration is an example of a condition. *Criteria* state how well or how long the behavior must be performed to show mastery. To summarize, the three characteristics of a learning objective are that it is specific, that it is measurable, and that it is attainable.

To evaluate patient education, the teacher uses performance, conditions, and criteria to measure the patient's progress. The measurements should be collected accurately and should reflect qualitative and quantitative data.

In Chapter 7, the following learning objective was offered as an example: *The patient will draw up and administer 22 units of U100 NPH Insulin using sterile technique at 7:00 a.m. on three consecutive days.*

Qualitative data might include the following statement: "The patient was able to perform sterile technique in preparing the injection, but could not accurately measure the units of insulin." Quantitative data might include this statement: "The patient was able to perform sterile technique correctly only once. In the other two efforts, he contaminated the needle by placing it on the table uncapped." Specific data helps the nurse and the patient to focus on problem areas and to acknowledge progress which is made toward meeting the objective.

Methods of Measurement

There are several ways to gather information to evaluate learning. The nurse should remember that adults learn best with immediate application of knowledge, attitudes, and skills. Evaluation becomes a learning experience when it is prompt and when it is an exercise shared with the learner. The feedback reinforces positive behaviors and guides the correction of misunderstandings and performance problems. Because evaluation is a problem-solving process, the learner gains skill in managing problems by working with the teacher.

There are seven methods commonly used by nurses to evaluate patient learning.

Direct Observation

Watching the patient perform a skill or having him role play a situation offers two valuable opportunities. First, accurate, descriptive data can be collected. Second, the learner receives immediate feedback and guidance. We encourage nurses to use direct observation whenever possible, rather than to rely on reports and assumptions. Patients should be encouraged to demonstrate self-care activities and should be given professional guidance to reinforce learning. Examples of opportunities for direct observation are when the patient changes dressings, administers medication, performs breast self-exam, or selects foods according to a prescribed diet plan.

Patient Records

We must often rely on patients to keep records of their performance. While teaching begins in the company of health-care professionals, much of the actual learning takes place in the home when the patient and his family assume total responsibility. Although reinforcement of positive behavior is essential to the continuance of learning, it is not easily provided when opportunities for observation are lacking. Asking the patient to keep specific records and to present them to the nurse at a later time reinforces the patient's responsibility, reinforces positive behaviors, helps the patient to evaluate his own progress, and provides the nurse with data for her evaluation. This method has worked well in evaluating cooperation with medical regimens, diet modification, stress management, and treatments carried out at home. Whenever it is possible to supplement patient records with direct observation by the nurse, this should be done to increase objectivity.

Reports

Patient and family reports are used as sources of data, although their objectivity is often questioned. Reports can be accompanied with measurements such as pill counts, weight, and blood tests. Reporting should be solicited from the patient and his family through carefully constructed questions. For example, the nurse will get more specific and descriptive data by asking, "What medications did you take today and at what times did you take them?" than she would by asking, "Are you taking your medication as you were instructed?" Patients can be taught to be good reporters if they are given specific directions about collecting and recording significant information and if they are told how they are expected to contribute to the evaluation process.

Tests

Oral and written tests can be used prior to learning activities and repeated at intervals following instruction. This method is very effective in measuring the patient's progress toward meeting cognitive objectives and it offers objective data about his ability to retain what he has learned. Tests require the patient to be an active participant in defining his learning needs and in recognizing positive change. Tests are often used to teach and evaluate daily-management decisions made by patients and their families dealing with chronic illness. As with the tests discussed in Chapter 8, tests used for evaluation should present problems in a sequence, from simple to complex, and the tool should be appropriate for the patient's literacy level.

Interviews and Questionnaires with Patients and Their Families

Patients and their families may be interviewed or given written questionnaires to assess their degrees of confidence in new knowledge and skills. They may evaluate their own progress, define their learning needs, and offer suggestions for future training. We have used questionnaires of this nature in the evaluation of prenatal classes, newborn-care instruction, and stress-management classes. Again, we emphasize the importance of asking specific questions that do not require long, general responses, and of phrasing the questions so that the learner can understand them. Questionnaires are inappropriate for illiterate patients and family members.

Interviews and Questionnaires With Staff

Staff members contributing to the patient's care can offer important information about his progress. Although one nurse coordinates his care, many health professionals, including those from other disciplines, gather evaluative data. They should be asked to contribute these important measurements. This can be done efficiently with brief, carefully worded questions used in interviews and surveys. The questions should focus on specific, measurable behaviors. Data are also found in their notes in the medical record.

Research Using Statistical Comparison

This method of evaluation takes a broader look at the patient's course before and after the learning of new behaviors. Information is collected about absences from work or school, hospitalizations, episodes of acute complications, and daily management. Research data are usually gathered to measure the long-term value of patient-education interventions. In addition, they may be used to substantiate requests for third-party reimbursement of patient teaching.

Assessment of Learning

Data from a combination of evaluation sources should be assimilated and the results should be summarized. This procedure is very similar to that of the categorization of information and the writing of a summary statement in assessment.

The first question to be answered is "To what extent were the learning objectives accomplished?" The answer to this initial question guides us in asking further questions:

"If the behavior was successfully performed, how can it be reinforced?"

"If the behavioral objective was *not* met, was the patient able to perform the behavior in the past?"

"If he was able to perform it in the past, why has he failed to perform it now?"

Evaluation does not simply provide us with one "Yes" or "No" answer. Instead, it becomes another starting point in the continuous nursing process. We gather data and offer feedback about the learning experience to the patient, his family, the health-care team, and the institution. We also look to others for return feedback about the quality of our nursing interventions. Feedback is a learning tool that can be very powerful in guiding behavior when it is used positively. Tips on giving feedback are offered later in this chapter.

Assessment of Learning Needs and Performance Problems

In Chapter 7, we introduced a flow diagram to illustrate the use of behavioral objectives in the learning process (Fig. 7-2). This figure guides the nurse in following up the evaluation.

If the desired behavior is accomplished, the nurse provides opportunities for reinforcing the positive behavior. Clinic visits, home visits, telephone calls, and community resources offer such opportunities. The patient and his family can demonstrate the knowledge and skills they have retained and ask for the review or guidance that they need. The health-care team should encourage clients to take advantage of these learning resources.

When learning behaviors are not accomplished, or are only partially accomplished, the patient educator must reassess and readdress barriers to behavioral change. Mager provides a model for problem solving to determine client-learning needs (Fig. 9-3).[2] We must reconsider whether or not the particular behavior is important and necessary. If so, we ask if a skill deficiency is present. If the patient has never been able to perform the skill, the teacher should provide additional training. If the skill will be used infrequently, feedback and practice should be arranged. For example, insulin injection is often learned with some initial difficulty, but the skill is used so often that it is retained and reinforced. Breast self-examination is performed less often, so this technique and the importance of its performance may need more reinforcement.

If the patient has demonstrated the ability to perform the skill but has not continued to perform it, four additional questions direct the teacher's problem solving. Mager suggests that if performing the skill somehow punishes the patient, we should identify the source of punishment and remove it. *Why does the patient feel punished?* For example, patients who are on special diets often complain that they are not able to combine socializing with friends and cooperating with their diet plans. Locating other sources of support, such as support groups of dieters, may remove the feeling of being "different" or "punished."

Does the patient see the performance as unrewarding? If so, the teacher can arrange positive consequences by offering additional support and more frequent follow-up visits and reporting mechanisms, so that the patient will see his improvement more clearly.

Does the patient feel that it doesn't matter whether he performs the behavior? If this is the case, as with hypertensive patients who fail to take their medications regularly, more frequent blood-pressure checks can reinforce the patient's awareness of the seriousness of omitting the medication.

Are there obstacles that prevent the patient from performing the behavior? If so, the teacher will want to look at these and try to help the patient deal with them. For example, the snack machine at work, which contains only candy and chips, may be less of a temptation if the patient takes a more nutritious snack with him to work in the morning. If a millworker feels self-conscious about wearing a protective mask on the job because "nobody else wears one," the company manager

WHEN CLIENTS FAIL TO MEET LEARNING OBJECTIVES: IS THERE A SKILL DEFICIENCY?

Yes	No
1. Has the client ever demonstrated the ability to perform the skill? If not, *formal training* is required.	1. Is the performance of the skill punishing? If so, *remove punishment*.
2. Is the skill used often? If not, *arrange practice*. If so, *arrange feedback*.	2. Is nonperformance rewarding? If so, *arrange a positive consequence*.
	3. Does the client feel that it doesn't matter if he performs the behavior? If so, *arrange a consequence*.
	4. Are there obstacles to performing the behavior? If so, *remove obstacles*.

Fig. 9-3. *Assessment of performance problems. (Content adapted from Mager RF, Pipe P: Analyzing Performance Problems. Belmont CA, Fearon-Pitman Publishers, 1970.)*

and employee-health nurse may be able to insist that all employees wear the recommended masks. Chapter 4 offers additional discussion about dealing with barriers to behavioral change.

The nurse must become a "detective" to help patients overcome stumbling blocks in the learning process. This requires the skills of making acute observations, using active listening, and approaching individual situations creatively.

Review of Learning Objectives

The continuous cycle of teaching and learning brings us back to formulating objectives. The nurse, the patient, and the patient's family must once again discuss their mutual goals: where does the patient want to be in terms of his behaviors, and what can the nurse offer to assist him in carrying out these new behaviors? Just as negotiation and the formulation of a learning contract were emphasized in Chapter 7, they are also priorities in evaluation. The original learning contract should be modified according to the oral agreement between the nurse and the patient.

Evaluation of Interventions

The nurse should take a critical view of the teaching/learning interventions that were designed to help the patient achieve his goals and gain knowledge, attitudes, and skills. The following questions help in determining which interventions have been effective and in what areas changes might be made to improve nursing care.

Format. Was the patient taught by self-study, individual instruction, or group instruction? Was the format compatible with the learning objectives and with the patient's condition and learning style?

Content. Did the patient receive the necessary facts and training to learn the desired behaviors?

Teaching/Learning Activities. Was the patient given an opportunity to actively participate, ask questions, and practice? Were the patient's past experiences used as a resource for learning? Were the patient's social roles and developmental tasks acknowledged? Was learning practical and problem centered? Was there an opportunity for immediate application by the learner? Were the learning methods and media appropriate for the types of learning objectives?

Media. Were the media able to deliver the message in a manner that the patient and his family could understand?

Patient-Family Satisfaction. Do the patient and his family have suggestions for improving the patient-education experience? Which activities did they find most helpful and which seemed least helpful? Did they feel supported in the learning environment? Were their concerns addressed? Did they feel confident of the staff's preparation to teach? Was the content understandable and practical?

Time, Cost, and Resources Involved. Were resources of staff and facilities adequate for teaching? If not, which unmet staff needs posed barriers to patient learning?

Recommendations of the Staff. Do nurses and other members of the health-care team have suggestions? How do they assess the quality of the patient-learning experience? Were the contributions of staff members in teaching the patient and his family coordinated? Did they feel prepared to teach? If not, what training should be offered to the staff?

Feedback

Feedback is a communication process that involves a sharing of perceptions. The patient and his family can be supported and guided in learning when they are given constructive feedback. They can be directed toward meeting their goals. Nurses often comment that they wish patients, families, and staff would give them more positive feedback about the nursing care they provide. Health-care institutions ask for feedback from the public about how they are meeting community health-care needs.

Feedback is seen as a valuable commodity. People generally refer to two types of feedback: *positive* and *negative. Positive feedback* is complimentary of a person's behavior. *Negative feedback* communicates displeasure or disappointment with a person's behavior. Most people describe *positive feedback* as being of great importance to them. It means more when it comes from someone we respect, from someone who values us, and from someone who understands our situation. Feedback is provided in the home, the workplace, and also in health-care settings. In patient learning, patients and their family members expect to receive feedback from nurses and other team members.

There are guidelines that can be offered to increase the likelihood that the feedback offered by professionals to clients will be constructive and helpful. Rather than focus on positive *vs* negative feedback, we consider how we can use the evaluation process to offer a maximum number of opportunities for useful feedback. First, we describe the characteristics of constructive feedback. Second, we offer tips for conveying the message to the patient and his family so that it is understood. Third, suggestions are provided for the nurse to solicit feedback about her performance from others.

Characteristics of Constructive Feedback

1. It is descriptive rather than judgmental. It offers objective data and suggestions for improvement.

2. It is specific rather than general. It does not include absolute words such as *always* or *never*. It is concerned with the here and now.

3. It is focused on the person's *behavior* rather than on the person *himself.*

4. It is given at the earliest opportunity after the behavior is performed. It is timely.

5. It takes into account the needs of the learner. It is given to help, not to hurt.

6. It is directed toward a behavior about which the learner can do something. The person will only become frustrated and discouraged when he is unable to control a situation.

7. It involves sharing information and offering guided choices rather than giving advice such as "You should . . . "

8. It takes into account the amount of information that the learner can handle. It does not overload the person.

Tips for Giving and Soliciting Feedback

1. Ask whether feedback is wanted. It is most useful when it is solicited rather than imposed.

2. Be prepared to listen.

3. Give positive feedback first. Reinforce positive behaviors, then discuss weaknesses.

4. Don't argue or push. Present alternatives.

5. Check to be sure that your feedback is interpreted correctly.

6. When requesting feedback from others, tell them what kinds of specific information you want. Offer them structured questions but encourage them to use open-ended responses.

7. When you want feedback from others, be open to it. Observe patients' expressions or comments. Listen for the intended message.

Written Documentation

Written documentation of the evaluation of learning is important for communication among team members, for quality assurance, for problem identification, and for problem solving.

The Learning Contract

This tool, which was first used to formalize goal setting between the patient and the nurse, assigns a specific time for learning to be evaluated and for the contract to be renegotiated. This written record is not usually a permanent part of the chart, but it can be placed in the chart to increase team collaboration and communication. Learning contracts emphasize the patient's role in the evaluation of behavioral change.

Medical Record

Patient education should always be documented in the progress-notes section of the medical record. Because patient education is a problem-solving process, documentation includes a clear statement of needs or problems, significant data contributing to these nursing diagnoses, and the plan for nursing care. The evaluations of the outcomes of care are essential ingredients in the care plan.

In Chapter 1, we heard comments from health professionals. Many of them addressed documentation concerns or problems. Although many of them stated that progress notes were important to communication and planning, they worried that their contributions to the medical record were ignored.

Dr. Lawrence Weed offered us the problem oriented record (POR) as a systematic tool for communication and problem solving. All team members (physicians, nurses, physical therapists, dietitians, pharmacists, and social workers) contribute to one problem list that focuses on *patient* problems rather than on *provider* problems. Each problem is assigned a number. Team members write narrative and discharge notes using the *SOAP* format to address the identified problems. This method increases awareness of the contributions of others and encourages the members to function as a team. There are no divisions of nurses' notes, physicians' notes, and so forth. All health-care professionals document information on the patient's progress notes. The patient is clearly the center of the team and the focus of care.[1]

We recommend this method, and in our own experiences in patient education it has increased communication and collaboration. It helps team members to know what has been taught by others and facilitates reinforcement of learned behaviors.

The POR highlights the use of the nursing process, which is based on problem solving. Narrative notes begin by naming the problem, and they then offer subjective and objective data, the assessment, and the plan.

#_____: Problem

S: Subjective data—what the patient reports

O: Objective data—what is observed through the senses and diagnostic tests

A: Assessment—the nursing diagnosis based on categorization and interpretation of data

P: Plan—includes diagnostic, therapeutic, and patient education interventions and reflects immediate and future actions and the evaluation of these actions

---

The reader will find sample *SOAP* notes, based on our case study of Mrs. Dawe, in Figures 9-4*A* and 9-4*B*. It is noteworthy that patient education is not named as a problem. It is designated in the plan as a nursing intervention that is offered along with treatments and therapy. The assessment includes the educational diagnosis, which is a definition of the patient's learning needs.

Report

Summaries or reports written at the time of discharge or transfer communicate to other health-care providers the patient's needs for reinforcement and continued learning. This documentation is very important because learning is a process that occurs over time. It is often begun in the hospital, but must be resumed in the clinic or home. Nurses are encouraged to use written as well as telephoned consultations in planning to meet the patient's learning needs. Calling to mind experiences with patients who have newly diagnosed diabetes, for example, reminds us that much of their learning takes place after they leave the sheltered hospital environment and that most of them need continuous patient teaching to become responsible and capable in managing their daily care.

Case Study: Mrs. Dawe At our first follow-up visit with Mrs. Dawe, we measured behavioral change using her learning objectives and her learning contract. The nursing-care-plan sheet was updated to include the evaluation of behavioral changes (Fig. 9-5). The care plan was

3/31/82 HOME VISIT

Nursing Note

3/31/82 HOME VISIT

1. OBESITY

   S: "I want help with my weight problem. I know I'm too heavy and it's making my diabetes difficult to manage. My diet is too limited. I just can't follow it."

   O: 5'8" tall, weight 280 pounds at last visit. 120 pounds above prescribed weight. Unable to follow 800-calorie ADA diet. Gets little exercise except for housework.

   P: Negotiate weight-loss goals. Change diet plan to 1200-calorie ADA diet. Outline menus with Mrs. Dawe and make referral to the dietitian to build variety into her diet plan. Discuss importance of weight loss in management of diabetes. Refer to Diabetic Luncheon. Schedule clinic visit for one week from now.

2. HYPERTENSION

   S: "I know I need to cut down on salt and lose weight to get my pressure down."

   O: Blood pressure 220/190 today. Reports taking hydrochlorothiazide, 100 mg daily.

   A: Blood pressure poorly controlled. Diet recall reveals salt used in cooking and at the table, with canned foods frequently included.

   P: Continue medication as ordered. Patient to keep written records. Follow weight-reduction diet as ordered in No. 1. Omit salt in cooking and avoid canned foods. Mrs. Dawe is in agreement with the plan. We discussed high-sodium foods to be avoided. Return to clinic in one week for blood-pressure check.

   Sally H. Rankin

   Sally Rankin, RN

Fig. 9-4A. *Nursing entries in the Problem-Oriented Record (POR).*

modified as the teaching/learning process continued. Sample entries are included from the POR progress notes (Fig. 9-4*A* and *B*).

Summary

Patients often find changing very difficult in spite of good intentions, new knowledge and skills, and behavior-modification strategies. The case of Mrs. Dawe illustrates this situation. Obstacles to change are often less tangible than, for example, exposure to party foods or pressure from family and peers. They are closely related to self-esteem—the patient's view of himself as a whole person. The feedback and counseling offered to patients in the health-care setting may help them to place greater values on themselves and their health. This often takes time to develop and many patients have difficulty accepting their own responsibilities in daily-health management.

The provider–patient relationship offers an opportunity to help the patient grow in assuming his role as a member of the health-care team. It is important to communicate confidence in the patient's ability to choose responsibly. It is also important to offer encouragement and guidance for change. Evaluation is a tool used to strengthen the provider–patient relationship and to continue patient-centered care through the nursing process.

4/7/82 CLINIC VISIT

Nursing Note

1. OBESITY

   S: "I followed my diet the first two days but cheated after that. I just couldn't pass up deserts when I thought about having them. I didn't keep records of what I ate because I was embarrased. I really do want to lose weight and wish you would help me to do it."

   O: Weight 280 pounds (unchanged from last visit). The two days of recorded meals did follow diet plan.

   A: Poor cooperation with diet plan. Understands exchanges and is able to select menus. Understands importance of weight control but does not perform necessary behavior modifications.

   P: Review goals. Stress Mrs. Dawe's responsibility. Offer assistance for problem solving and role playing. Reinforce two days of positive behavior. Return visit in one week.

2. HYPERTENSION

   S: Reports taking 100 mg hydrochlorothiazide each morning. Reports omitting salt in cooking.

   O: Blood pressure 188/96 today.

   A: Blood pressure lower. Good cooperation with reducing sodium intake. Knows name and dosage of medication. Identifies high-sodium foods to avoid.

   P: Reinforce progress. Continue weekly blood-pressure checks.

Karen Duffy, RN

Karen Duffy, RN

Fig. 9-4B. *Nursing entries in the Problem-Oriented Record (POR).*

Patient and Health-Team Assessment	Factors Affecting Behavioral Change for Health Promotion	Educational Diagnosis
1. OBESITY Recent weight gain due to the following: a. Inability to follow 800-calorie ADA diet b. Inability to follow exercise program	1. OBESITY + knowledge about health problem + patient cooks + patient makes decisions − self-concept − environment (sweets around house) − feels hungry − feels diet is too restrictive	1. OBESITY Negotiation and behavior modification related to diabetic diet needed
2. SHORTNESS OF BREATH 2° obesity	2. SHORTNESS OF BREATH + interferes with role of caring for others, grandchildren + decreasing mobility and independence; patient wants to be independent − obesity − increasing dependence on husband − inability to follow diet	2. SHORTNESS OF BREATH Negotiation and behavior modification necessary to increase exercise
3. HYPERTENSION	3. HYPERTENSION + knowledge about health problems − poor cooperation with diet, exercise − husband likes food cooked with salt	3. HYPERTENSION Has learning needs related to management of hypertension. Negotiation of plan for medication, diet, weight reduction
4. DIABETES Poor control Hyperglycemia Retinopathies	4. Diabetes + family history + symptoms bothersome + knowledge about disease/management − self-concept, role conflict (care-giver vs. patient − husband not impressed with seriousness of problem	4. DIABETES Self-care attitudes and commitment should be explored. Plan for behaviors to be negotiated with patient/family

(continued)

Goals to Promote Knowledge, Attitudes and Skills

1. GOAL:
   To lose ten pounds by 6/1/82
   OBJECTIVES:
   C—Outline food exchanges for breakfast, lunch, and dinner using a 1200-calorie ADA diet plan.
   C—Describe how one-half cup of ice cream is worked into the weekly meal plan.
   P—Record in notebook all foods eaten during the week.
   A—State why weight control is especially important in the management of diabetes.

2. GOAL:
   To achieve systolic blood pressure below 160 points and diastolic blood pressure below 90 points by 6/1/82
   OBJECTIVES:
   C—State name, dose, and frequency of antihypertensive medication.
   P—Record in notebook when antihypertensive medication is taken each day.
   P—Omit salt in cooking.
   C—Name ten high-sodium foods that should be avoided.
   P—Eliminate canned food from the diet during the week. Substitute fresh fruits and vegetables, recording them in notebook.

Teaching/Learning Formats and Activities

Individual and small-group lecture, discussion, demonstration, return demonstration, and role playing with nurse, using 1200-calorie ADA diet booklet and patient notebook.
Referral to dietitian.

Discussion with husband and nurse.
Referral to Diabetic Luncheon at the county hospital.

Individual teaching with husband.
Lecture, quiz, and demonstration.

Discussion and simulation.
Label reading in the home.
Role playing of shopping for groceries.

Evaluation of Behavioral Changes

Goal 1

Mrs. Dawe correctly outlined food exchanges for breakfast, lunch, and dinner using her 1200-calorie ADA diet plan. She

Reassessment and Modification

Weight today had not changed from her last clinic visit. We reviewed her goals and learning objectives. Mrs. Dawe stated made up three sample menus for each meal. She included one-half cup of ice cream in one of these meals and substituted exchanges accurately. She returned to the clinic for her first weekly visit with two days of food intake recorded in her notebook. Both days she had followed her diet plan. She reported that on the last five days she "cheated" on her diet and ate several desserts, failing to record what she ate. She stated that she felt guilty not following the diet and proceeded to explain why controlling her weight was important in the management of her diabetes.

Goal 2

Mrs. Dawe reported that she was taking hydrochlorothiazide, 100 mg, once a day (in the morning). She did record taking the medication in her notebook. She reported that she omitted salt in cooking during the week and that she did not use any canned foods except for water-packed fruits. She recalled ten high-sodium foods when asked to do so.

that she was still interested in losing weight and wanted a nurse's help in doing so.
We reinforced Mrs. Dawe's knowledge about her diet and her understanding of the importance of weight control in diabetic management. We stressed that she would have to take responsibility for changing her habits but that we would help her to work out strategies to confront problems. She stated that she would like to resume her diet plan today and see us next week. We agreed and reinforced her two days of success with her plan.

Blood pressure was 188/96 today.
Mrs. Dawe reported that it was less difficult than she thought to avoid high-sodium foods and that Mr. Dawe had encouraged her to do so. In fact, when she was about to use canned tomato sauce in cooking, it was Mr. Dawe who reminded her of its high sodium content. We commended Mr. and Mrs. Dawe on their positive behaviors and showed them how the blood-pressure measurement also highlighted their success.

Key:
+ = Positive factors affecting behavioral change
− = Negative factors affecting behavioral change
C = Cognitive learning objective
A = Affective learning objective
P = Psychomotor learning objective

Fig. 9-5. *Mrs. Dawe's nursing-care plan for patient education.*

References

1. Kron T: The Management of Patient Care, pp 199–207. Philadelphia, WB Saunders, 1981
2. Mager RF, Pipe P: Analyzing Performance Problems. Belmont, CA, Fearon-Pitman Publishers, 1970

Bibliography

Books

Berne E: Games People Play. New York, Grove Press, 1964

Blevins DR: The Diabetic and Nursing Care. New York, McGraw-Hill, 1979

Bower FL, Bevis EO: Fundamentals of Nursing Practice: Concepts, Roles and Functions. St Louis, CV Mosby, 1979

Douglass LM, Bevis EO: Nursing Leadership in Action. St Louis, CV Mosby, 1974

Feeley EM, Shine MS, Sloboda SB: Fundamentals of Nursing Care. New York, McGraw-Hill, 1980

Gage NL, Berliner DC: Educational Psychology. Chicago, Rand McNally, 1975

Hanson PG: Giving feedback: An interpersonal skill. In Jones JE, Pfeiffer JW (eds): The 1975 Annual Handbook for Group Facilitators. San Diego, University Associates Publishers, 1975

Jones JE, Kurtz RJ: Confrontation: Types, conditions and outcomes. In Jones JE, Pfeiffer JW (eds): The 1973 Annual Handbook for Group Facilitators. San Diego, University Associates Publishers, 1973

Lamonica EL: The Nursing Process: A Humanistic Approach. Menlo Park, Addison-Wesley, 1979

Mager RF: Preparing Instructional Objectives. Belmont, CA, Fearon-Pitman Publishers, 1975

Yura H, Walsh MB: The Nursing Process: Assessing, Planning, Implementing and Evaluating. New York, Appleton-Century Crofts, 1978

Journals

Shaw LM: The patient as an adult learner. AORN J 33, No. 2:233–239, 1981

Tarnow KG: Working with adult learners. Nurs Educ 4, No. 5:34–40, 1979

Woody M, Mallison M: The problem-oriented system. Am J Nurs 73, No. 7:1168–1177, 1973

Chapter 10

Continuity and Transition in Patient Education: Cardiac Rehabilitation in Acute and Outpatient Settings

Diane Shea Pravikoff

Differences Among Critical-Care, Intermediate-Care, and Outpatient Settings

The educational needs of patients differ according to the care setting. The patient in the acute-care setting (whether critical care or intermediate care) is different from the patient in an ambulatory-outpatient setting such as a clinic, health center, or physician's office. The teaching goals must be different as well. The goals in the acute-care setting, particularly in critical care, are basically therapeutic. In this setting we need to reduce anxiety, to inform the patient about procedures and equipment, and to teach necessary skills to meet basic survival needs.

In the intermediate-care setting we have both therapeutic and preventive goals. We want the patient to understand, for example, the therapeutic reasons for coughing and deep breathing, wearing support stockings and ambulating frequently and progressively. We also want him to understand the use of his medications, his exercise regimen, or the importance of following a particular diet. We want him to understand his own level of risk of future illness and hospitalization and to know what he can do to modify these risks. We help him to understand how to overcome obstacles and setbacks during recovery, how to handle visitors after his discharge, and how to cope with depression. In the outpatient setting, although we still have some therapeutic goals (*e.g.*, maintenance of medication and diet regimen) we are primarily concerned with prevention and management.

Psychological, Physiological, and Environmental Considerations

In order to accomplish our therapeutic, preventive, or management goals we have to consider the psychological, physiological, and environmental aspects of different settings. Some inhibit education; others may facilitate it. In the critical-care setting, anxiety may be a major inhibitor. Medications may interfere with understanding. In this setting inhibitors outweigh facilitators and this is the reason for the limited amount of teaching we can do in this environment. Pain, dyspnea, restlessness, and sensory overload are other inhibitors. Telemetric equipment, ventilators, intravenous monitoring devices, noise, and constant activity are other inhibitory factors of which we need to be aware in the assessment of these patients.

In the intermediate-care setting, anxiety is still present but it is better controlled. The patient has, at least, survived and improved enough to be transferred. We are, however, still coping with such inhibitors as medications, which may dull the patient's consciousness or even make him sleep through the teaching session. Environmental inhibitors, including ventilators, IV lines, and monitoring equipment have been mostly, if not completely eliminated. One of our greatest facilitators in this setting is motivation. The patient is generally anxious to learn what has happened to him, as well as what he can do to help himself. There is more staff time available for teaching because the patient's condition has been stabilized, allowing the staff to be less task oriented. Family involvement is a potential facilitator, as mentioned in Chapter 7.

In the outpatient rehabilitation setting, the patient is less anxious and physically stronger. We have found that patients in this setting often have a tendency to minimize what has happened to them. Coronary-artery-bypass patients may be aware of their condition longer because they have scars that are difficult to ignore. However, they too have to be reminded that a problem still exists because they may feel that surgery has been a cure. Although denial can be useful, it can also be a harmful defense mechanism. It may have initially caused a patient to delay in seeking medical care, but it may be helpful later in lifting spirits and preventing depression and extreme anxiety. Still later, during hospitalization and in long-term care, denial is an inhibitor to learning and prevention. It is difficult to teach a person with high blood pressure or a high cholesterol level when there is no physiological feedback to reinforce the need for a change in life-style or dietary habits. The environmental factor is not an inhibitor in the case of outpatient education because the setting is typically one in which the patient feels comfortable. In the rehabilitation setting it is convenient for the family to be present and included in the teaching.

Cardiac Rehabilitation and Patient Education

Cardiac rehabilitation is an area that is obviously suitable for patient education. Cardiac rehabilitation begins when the patient is in either the acute-care or the outpatient setting, depending on his particular disease process. For example, a patient who has suffered an acute myocardial infarction (MI) or who has undergone coronary-artery bypass-graft surgery is initially seen in the acute-care setting and then progresses to outpatient status. Patients who are being managed medically may be seen almost entirely in the outpatient setting. Our approach is one of modifying all possible risk factors for any patients with evidence of atherosclerotic heart disease, including patients with MI or coronary bypass surgery. It makes no sense, for example, to treat the bypass patient as if he has undergone a cure for the disease process. Unless he does something to change his life-style, the disease may continue to progress. We certainly do not guarantee the patient that our program will ensure that he will have no more difficulty, but we do tell him that he will at least be able to do something constructive for himself and, in that way, take some control.

We have a broad educational program in which we combine many methods of instruction and various team members. We are fortunate to have two excellent closed-circuit television channels devoted to patient education. Each program has been carefully selected by the patient-education coordinator and specialists—both physicians and nurses—in each field. In the case of cardiac rehabilitation, there are programs discussing all aspects of the disease process, recovery, angiography, surgery, and risk-factor modification. These are high-quality productions that help to reinforce information that is presented in books, pamphlets, or diagrams. The programs are included as part of the process of achieving educational goals and participation.

Presentation of Information

Timing of the presentation to the patient is important. In the work we have done with MI patients, we have found that attempting to discuss *in detail* the disease process while the patient is still in the coronary care unit (usually three days) is generally useless. The patient is still asking questions such as, "Why me?" "Will I live?" and "What happened?" He does not necessarily want to know *everything* about atherosclerosis at this point, nor would he be able to comprehend it all. This patient should be educated on the basis of immediate needs. He needs to know what is happening to him at the particular moment. Time should be spent discussing the environment, blood tests, monitors and oxygen equipment, and activity or lack of it. We should also be dealing with the patient's feelings of denial, anger, frustration, and fear. If the patient asks questions about the disease process, these questions should be answered. All responses should be made with awareness of ongoing assessment of the patient's level of understanding, and answers should be kept short and to the point. One fundamental rule is that the answers at this time should be simple and limited in scope. We can always go into more detail after we are sure that we have a base on which to build.

Inclusion of Family

Including the family in the patient education is very important. Illness is generally a family problem and all members need to have the information they seek. The major difficulty we have dealt with in this area is a lack of availability of family members. During the crisis period we have no difficulty locating them, but the crisis period is not the ideal time for in-depth teaching of the patient's family. When the crisis is over the patient's spouse returns to work and his children to school or work, so that they are often not available for daytime classes.

Because daily evening classes are not a possibility in our situation, we have to compromise by having a monthly evening session in which various aspects of atherosclerosis are discussed by experts in their fields. Each of these sessions is attended by 100 to 200 people, most of whom are former patients or their family members.

We also recommended strongly the institution's educational television programs to the patients and their families. Literature from sources such as the American Heart Association is distributed to the patients as part of the cardiac kit. This kit is offered to the patient when he begins the cardiac teaching classes upon transfer to the progressive-care unit. Participation in these classes is by physician's order. However, the order is a formality and it usually determines only the actual day the patient will start classes, rather than whether the patient will attend at all. We are fortunate in maintaining the cooperation and enthusiam of the physicians. In cardiac rehabilitation we have not encountered the "ignorance-is-bliss" attitude, which is unfortunately prevalent in some other areas.

Content and Format of Classes

The classes were established to discuss and reinforce basic information about heart disease. There is a sequence of five classes; each is limited, with some leeway for discussion and questions, to thirty minutes. The first class covers the process of atherosclerosis and MI. A slide-tape presentation that is shown gives an overview, from symptoms of heart disease to recovery. Discussions of sexual activity and exercise programs are included in this segment. A nurse clinician is present to handle discussion. One of the clearest examples we use is a corroded and obstructed pipe from a house built in 1927; this graphically demonstrates what can happen to the arterial vasculature.

The second session is conducted by a registered dietitian, who helps the patient understand the principles of his diet, usually emphasizing low-fat or low-salt use. Patients and their family members participate actively in this session, with a stimulating question-and-answer format. The dietitian is also available for individual or family consultation at no charge to the patient. Patients will frequently request another meeting with the dietitian following discharge because putting the diet into practice often brings up new problems and questions.

The third session is held by a physical therapist, who describes a good cardiovascular conditioning program. We try to stress exercises that our patients are able to do and safe means of accomplishing them. All of the classes need to be directed toward the particular population that uses the facility. Ours is a population of older patients who have little desire, for example, to be joggers. Frequently we encounter patients who claim that playing golf two or three times a week is adequate exercise, even when they use a golf cart. Our response is to tell these patients that we know of no one who is able to hit the ball hard enough that 30 minutes of walking is required to retrieve it! We then remind them that they need 30 minutes of brisk walking for cardiovascular fitness.

The fourth class includes an overall description, presented in a readily recallable fashion, of risk factors. It combines much of the information already presented and elaborates further on diet and exercise. We also discuss sexual activity again and we delve into the subject of depression that may follow a coronary event. A volunteer who assists us in this presentation is someone who once smoked three packs of cigarettes a day, had been hypertensive, hyperlipidemic, overweight, and lazy, and then had a cardiac arrest and open heart surgery. The patients can identify with him; he has been where they are. This gives him a credibility that we do not have. He is able to show the patients that change is possible and that they too can enjoy full and active lives. I heartily recommend volunteer assistance of this type in patient education.

The fifth, and final, class is concerned with the emotional aspects of both the illness and discharge from the hospital. This is a group class for families to discuss the patient's reaction to the illness, his family's reaction to the illness, and ways to promote the best possible adaptation for all. It was originated as a result of a patient's request: "I didn't know what to say to my 17-year-old son, who stood over me as we waited for the paramedics to arrive while I could see the fear in his face." It is basically a class that stresses the importance of communication between patients and their families during the acute phase as well as the recovery phase. We ask questions to encourage discussion, such as the following inquiry to patients: "Do you think your family will try to 'put you on a shelf' and overprotect you?" or to the family: "Do you think your spouse will try to show how healthy he or she now is and do things that are too strenuous?" We also discuss the possibility of the patient's using the illness to control family members. One 70-year-old woman who participated in our outpatient program informed us that she would no longer allow her husband to accompany her to the sessions because if he saw how well she was doing she would have to resume the vacuuming and cleaning that he was now doing for her. An 80-year-old aortocoronary-bypass patient had had the surgery because he had been incapacitated by angina and unable to work in the garden he loved. He was recovering very well but was unhappy and frustrated because his family had told him that he would have to give up gardening because they did not want him to work that hard. Communication is obviously crucial.

We should also consider and discuss the fears of the family about taking the patient home. Staff members will have just spent seven to ten days hovering over the patient, monitoring every activity, and being ready to respond if any problem occurred. Suddenly the patient is being turned over to the spouse to take home, where there are no monitors, emergency medications, or crash carts. The family will naturally be a little nervous and apprehensive.

The area of medications is very important in our educational efforts and we try to inform the patient that all medications have the potential of producing side-effects. We recommend that, rather than simply discontinuing the medication abruptly when the patient feels it is causing a side-effect, he should telephone the physician and discuss the problem. We also recommend that the patient carry a list of his medications and current doses with him for quick reference in all situations. Antihypertensive medications are a particular problem in two ways: the disease itself produces so few symptoms that the patient wonders why he should take medication, and the medication produces multiple side-effects. One patient told me that he only took his medication when he felt as if the top of his head were going to "blow off." At such times his blood pressure was as high as 240/140.

Evaluation of Patient Education in the Cardiac-Rehabilitation Setting

In addition to direct observation of changes in behavior, pre- and post-tests are another useful method of evaluation in the acute-care setting. We have used these on a spot-check basis and we find them helpful in evaluating our teaching competence, as well as helping the patient to see what he has accomplished or needs to accomplish.

Our patient-education coordinator conducted a nonrandomized study of our patient television programming to determine whether patients were aware of its existence and whether it had produced any changes in their behavior. Approximately 40% of her sample of 600 returned the questionnaire saying that they had viewed the available programs, 23% of the respondents had watched some of the programs related to their hospital stay. Of these, 18% said they had actually made life-style changes as a result. The changes ranged from discontinuing smoking to beginning to exercise. We believe that this form of instruction offers many benefits in terms of flexibility and time management.

Evaluation is vital to any patient-education program and, although we believe our program is comprehensive, we know there is always room for change and improvement. For example, one of our patients had a severe myocardial infarction followed by coronary-bypass surgery. He attended the series of classes twice, as did his wife. The couple also received instruction from our cardiovascular clinician (prior to the surgery), the surgeon, the cardiologist, their family doctor, and me. They saw each of us on an individual basis. The patient recovered from the surgery. Although somewhat disabled because of the severity of the disease, he participated in our outpatient program for six weeks and then transferred to the long-term program. During this period he saw films and heard discussions. One evening, about 14 months after we had originally met him, he experienced chest pains, which the cardiologist diagnosed as angina. At the physician's request we discussed nitroglycerin administration. We had a long talk about the timing of taking his medication, how much he should take, and when he should call the physician. His wife was present throughout this discussion. The next day I received a call at work from his wife, who told me how much they appreciated the time I had spent the evening before but that they had failed to ask one specific question: "What is angina?" This is one of the most fundamental pieces of information we can present, but it had somehow never been incorporated into that particular patient's working knowledge of the disease.

It was at that point that I changed my approach in establishing goals and objectives for the classes we offer. Prior to that time I had used a form that simply listed the information presented—in effect, it was an attendance record. We are now working with a form (see Appendix A at the back of this chapter) that is more complete and serves our purposes better. It also makes us accountable for what we are doing. The form is individualized and can be used repeatedly for all participants. It is kept with the physician's progress notes. It not only helps to justify the need for a cardiac-rehabilitation nurse, but it is also an aid, when a patient is readmitted, in determining what the patient had been told in the past and what he has apparently understood. Documentation of the education we are doing has often been a problem in the acute-care setting. Although very detailed, a form such as this makes record keeping fairly easy and it can be placed on the chart at the time of admission. It is a combination of assessment (*i.e.,* the risk-factor evaluation), and documentation of attendance and participation in the class. I record details such as whether the patient seemed to sleep through the majority of the class. This way I know what I have to emphasize the next time the patient attends the class.

Patient education also provides some humorous experiences. When I first decided that I was going to include a discussion of sexual activity in one of our classes, I tried to assess the group of patients first to see if they might still be interested in sex or if they were "too old." I had a group of men one day, the youngest of whom was 75. I decided this group was too old and finished my discussion on risk factors, asking for comments or questions. One 83-year-old gentlemen put me properly in my place by saying, "You have told us all the boring stuff. Now what about sex?" I have not omitted that topic from the discussion since.

Case Study: Mr. Connelly

Mr. Connelly is a 58-year-old policeman who suffered excruciating jaw pain while in pursuit of a robbery suspect. When he slowed his pace the jaw pain decreased, and when he stopped to rest it disappeared completely. He visited his dentist, thinking a dental problem was the source of his pain. The dentist, fortunately, found nothing wrong with his teeth and recognized this as a possible case of variant angina pectoris. The patient was referred to a cardiologist, but hesitated to make an appointment because "nothing could possibly be wrong with my heart." Following three more episodes, each more severe and lasting slightly longer, Mr. Connelly made and kept an appointment with the cardiologist, who ordered a treadmill test. The results of the treadmill test indicated possible myocardial tissue ischemia. Mr. Connelly was hospitalized and right and left heart catheterizations were performed. The angiograms revealed a right coronary artery that was completely obstructed near its origin, a left main artery stenosis of about 50%, a completely obstructed left anterior descending artery, and a circumflex artery that was virtually untouched by disease.

Because is appeared that still-viable remaining muscle was endangered, the patient underwent triple-vessel coronary-artery bypass-graft surgery. His preoperative instruction was limited more to the procedure and the equipment involved than to the process of the disease. Education about atherosclerosis and risk-factor modification began on his return to the Definitive Observation Unit (DOU) three days following surgery. He attended all five classes and participated quietly although he was somewhat sleepy initially. His particular areas of concern were what his activity level would be following discharge and what he could do to prevent the recurrence of disabling angina. He was not concerned about returning to work because of an excellent retirement program. He had realistic ideas about staying active and productive and was relieved to have an opportunity to eliminate job stress from his life because he felt that it was a major contributor to his disease. The modifiable risk factors identified were hypertension (160/100), cigarette smoking (2 or more packs a day), elevated serum cholesterol (318 mg/dl), and lack of a regular exercise program.

Mr. Connelly handled the emotional impact of heart surgery well and, although he became depressed at times during the immediate postoperative period as well as during the postdischarge period, he recovered from these episodes quickly. He wanted to be active and has continued to be so. Our education continued in the outpatient cardiac-rehabilitation program, which he currently visits on a monthly basis at his own request.

Summary

We have discussed various components of a patient-education program in the acute-care setting. We have touched on problems that must be confronted, rewards and challenges of the program, and some philosophy. The remaining challenge that we face is to maintain our enthusiasm in the face of patients' disappearing for treatments or tests at the time of class, of the realization that often everything else seems to come before patient teaching, and of the small number of tangible results we are able to demonstrate. We must believe that what we are doing is essential— not simply because it is mandated by regulation, but for the overall well-being of our patients, now and in the future—and that we are helping to give our patients the tools to manage their future.

We have included a case study involving a patient with heart disease. A nursing-care plan, using the format presented in Chapters 6, 7, 8, and 9, is presented to illustrate the appropriate patient education during the cardiac-rehabilitation phase (Fig 10-1).

Fig. 10-1. Nursing-care plan for a patient with atherosclerotic heart disease.

Patient and Health-Team Assessment	Factors Affecting Behavioral Change for Health Promotion	Educational Diagnosis
1. HYPERTENSION Essential 160/100	1. HYPERTENSION + knowledge about health problems + will not be returning to same job + BP well controlled while hospitalized − poor dietary habits with salt and "junk food" − long hours away from home − dislike of medications − asymptomatic − likes to add salt before tasting food	1. HYPERTENSION Has learning needs related to management of hypertension (HTN). Negotiation of plan for medication, exercise, diet, stress reduction.
2. CIGARETTE SMOKING 2 or more packs a day (70-pack year history)	2. CIGARETTE SMOKING + knowledge of effects of nicotine on cardiovascular system + hospitalization required cessation of smoking + views emphysema as frightening. − stress of job − physiological/psychological dependence − wife continues to smoke	2. CIGARETTE SMOKING Has learning needs related to discontinuation of smoking. Negotiation and behavior modification necessary for stress reduction.
3. ELEVATED CHOLESTEROL 318 mg/dl	3. ELEVATED CHOLESTEROL + knowledge − poor dietary habits − lack of uniformity in research − dislikes poultry, fish − self-concept as "meat-and-potatoes man" − patient and wife enjoy eating out as major social activity − weight 210 pounds, height six feet	3. ELEVATED CHOLESTEROL Has learning needs related to low cholesterol diet. Negotiation of plan for diet

(continued)

Patient and Health-Team Assessment	Factors Affecting Behavioral Change for Health Promotion	Educational Diagnosis
4. INACTIVITY	4. INACTIVITY + knowledge + enjoyed exercise in younger years + not returning to work + wife also wants to exercise	4. INACTIVITY Has learning needs related to good cardiovascular exercise program

Goals to Promote Knowledge, Attitudes, and Skills	Teaching/Learning Formats and Activities
1. GOAL: To maintain BP below 140/90 OBJECTIVES: To take medication daily and keep list of medications on his person To restrict salt intake by using salt substitute recommended by physician To use fresh fruits and vegetables whenever possible; eliminate processed and packaged foods	Educate as to importance of medications (C; 1:1); inform physician if side-effects occur. Help patient make chart detailing times and dosages of medications (P; 1:1) Have patient attend group classes with dietitian regarding low-sodium meals (C; G, L)
2. GOAL: To maintain discontinuation of cigarette smoking OBJECTIVES: To continue use of sugar-free gum to assuage cigarette craving To avoid situations where cigarette smoking occurs To record instances when desire for cigarette was strong	Reinforce information presented regarding problems related to smoking (C; 1:1) Encourage spouse to limit smoking around patient (A; 1:1) Encourage attendance at health-education classes on smoking (C; A; G, L)
3. GOAL: To maintain cholesterol level at 200 mg/dl OBJECTIVES: To record diet for two weeks To outline low-cholesterol, low-triglyceride diet according to	Educate patient and wife regarding source of high-cholesterol, high-triglyceride foods (C; 1:1) Give pamphlets from AHA: *Dine to Your Heart's Content* (C) Suggest AHA cookbook (C)

American Heart Association (AHA) guidelines

To find restaurant menus that fit low-cholesterol diet.

4. GOAL:

to maintain 30–45 minutes of aerobic exercise 3–4 days a week

OBJECTIVES:

To record distance, time, and pulse rate

To list warning signs of over-exertion

Educate patient and wife regarding principles of aerobic exercise (C; 1:1, G)

Expose patient and wife to various types of aerobic exercise.
Suggest organized programs (P; G)

Suggest that heart rate and blood pressure be maintained under monitored parameters during exercise (C; 1:1)

Evaluation of Behavioral Changes

1. BP has averaged 120/70 during monthly visits over two-year time period

2. Patient has not smoked since surgery. Wife does not smoke in patient's presence.

3. Cholesterol level varies from 200–250 mg/dl. Weight has decreased to 170–180 pounds.

4. Patient has gradually increased workload to appropriate heart-rate and blood-pressure responses. He has maintained this exercise level over two years.

Reassessment and Modification

1. Continue monitoring blood pressure.

2. Refer wife to smoking clinic.

3. Reassess level of knowledge regarding cholesterol and tri-glycerides. Reinforce teaching related to correct diet.

4. None.

Key:
C = Cognitive
P = Psychomotor
A = Affective
L = Lecture
1:1 = One to one
G = Group

Appendix A: Program Evaluation Form

Glendale Adventist Medical Center

PATIENT/FAMILY EDUCATION

DIAGNOSIS:

DATE INITIATED _____

Educational Goals	Dead-lines	Date of Teaching Patient/ Family	Comments/ Evaluation
Patient will be able to do the following:			
1. Explain the purpose of CCU/DOU a. Supervision by skilled personnel b. Special equipment c. Controlled environment to stress activities Met ___(Date)___			
2. Understand the principles of progressive activity/ambulation Met _____			
3. Define atherosclerosis as a disease of the blood supply; the role of the coronary arteries			
4. Define angina or chest pain and give the possible causes and treatment Met _____			
5. Define MI and identify possible symptoms Met _____			
GAMC-TV Ch. 8 "Post Coronary Care" Ch. 6 "The Heart: Counterattack"			
6. Form a list of controllable risk factors and identify them for self			
___Age ___Family Hx ___Stress ___Sex ___Blood Fats ___DM ___B/P ___Smoking ___Obesity ___Inactivity			
GAMC-TV Ch. 6 "Let's Call it Quits" Ch. 8 "High Blood Pressure"			
7. Explain reasons for limited diet and list four appropriate and four inappropriate foods: _____ _____ _____ _____ _____ _____ _____ _____			
GAMC-TV Ch. 6 "Eat Right to Heart's Delight"			
8. Explain the benefits and principles of cardiovascular exercise Met _____			
GAMC-TV Ch. 6 "Coping with Life On The Run" Ch. 8 "Be Fit and Live"			
9. Verbalize the importance of CPR training Met _____			
GAMC-TV Ch. 6 "CPR Quiz"			

(continued)

Educational Goals	Dead-lines	Date of Teaching Patient/ Family	Comments/ Evaluation
10. Identify several symptoms requiring emergency assistance			
11. Be aware of potential emotional swings following MI or CAB Met _____			
12. Recognize sexual activity as a normal form of exercise Met _____			

(Used with permission of Glendale Adventist Medical Center)

Diane Shea Pravikoff, R.N.
Cardiac Rehab Coordinator

Bibliography

Books

Czerwinski BS: Manual of Patient Education for Cardiopulmonary Dysfunction. St Louis, CV Mosby, 1980

Knowles M: Informal Adult Education. New York, Association Press, 1961

Narrow B: Patient Teaching in Nursing Practice. New York, John Wiley & Sons, 1979

Storlie F: Patient Teaching in Critical Care. New York, Appleton-Century-Crofts, 1975

Journals

Clark M: The utilization of theoretical concepts in patient education. Nurs Adm Q 4, No. 3:55–60, 1980

Devney AM: Rehabilitation of the cardiac patient: Bridging the gap between inhospital and outpatient care. Am J Nurs 80, No. 3:446–449, 1980

Falkiewicz JT: Are group classes helpful for teaching cardiac patients? Am J Nurs 80, No. 3:444, 1980

Hart LK, Frantz RA: Characteristics of postoperative patient education programs for open-heart surgery patients in the United States. Heart Lung 6, No. 1:137–142, 1977

Chapter 11
Health Promotion in the Community

Educating communities or groups of people is more difficult than educating one person or family. The boundaries of communities are amorphous and not always clearly defined. When a needs assessment (see Chap. 3) indicates that community education is desirable, the implementation process must proceed in a very careful and organized fashion. Methods of evaluation must be included in the program design and the economic realities of undertaking such a program should be considered.

This chapter discusses two community health-education projects: prenatal classes and a cardiopulmonary resuscitation (CPR) program. One of the projects, the prenatal classes, has been mentioned previously. We are including the prenatal classes as an example of community education because they were open to all pregnant members of the community, not just to clinic patients. The prenatal clients also met the definition of a *group* because they were a group of people with common goals interacting independently. Neither the prenatal nor the CPR clients, however, were groups until the interventions began. Instead they met the definition of *community:* they were a specific population living in a defined area having shared institutions, values, and problems.

We present guidelines for establishing such community health-education and health-promotion classes. We include the philosophies of the programs, the objectives established for classes, the evaluation methodologies, and appendices that include outlines and appropriate materials to use. Before we embark on discussion of the specifics about each set of classes, we mention the problems encountered when health education is attempted at the community level.

Observations

Just as the client exists not in a void but rather as the sum of family, socioeconomic, educational, and cultural influences, so must the community be considered in relation to many interfacing systems. A community health-education program cannot be created as if the community existed in a vacuum. Social, economic, organizational, and environmental influences must instead be considered.[1] Each community is unique. For example, a community venereal-disease education program for teenagers in Beverly Hills should differ considerably from one planned for a small Appalachian community in West Virginia.

Just as a needs assessment is required for the patient, so may an assessment of the community's health-education needs be performed. Any type of health-education or health-promotion program should be requested by the community. Because it generally requires greater time and financial expenditure to plan and implement programs for a community than for one patient, and because the community as a whole, directly or indirectly, will probably pay for all or part of the program, it is essential that the community recognize and express a need for the services. Needs of communities can be ascertained in various ways. An effective manner of gathering data pertaining to health-education needs is to first approach medical personnel involved in the delivery of community health care. Public health departments are one obvious place to collect these data. Next, formal and informal community leaders should be polled about their perceptions of health-education needs. Congruence between these two needs lists must then be determined. One of the greatest causes of past failures in community health education has been the imposition of programs, perceived as needed by health-care professionals, on a population that neither perceives the same need nor desires the program.

The school-age population, unlike the adult population, cannot adequately express its health-education needs. This group is a prime target for prevention programs. The "Know Your Body" program in New York City was implemented in the schools to decrease risk factors leading to atherosclerosis, stroke, and nutrition- and tobacco-related cancers. The health-care professionals who evaluated the program found that educational interventions were ineffective with the children, but behavior-modification techniques did produce desired changes.[2] Therefore, an implication for health-education programs with children is that behavior-modification techniques, such as rewards for not assuming smoking behaviors, are more useful than educational programs for effecting attitude changes.

Another factor that must be considered in planning community health-education programs is the credibility of those teaching the material. One study found that an inner-city community preferred and better responded to health education offered by a nurse who was a member of the community than that offered by outside health-care professionals.[3] Another community health-education project involved indigenous community leaders to act as lay health educators. The leaders were trained to facilitate health-knowledge acquisition and to recognize health problems that needed professional attention.[4] Such programs are especially successful in minority communities that have developed distrust of outside professionals, who they perceive as trying to impose their ideas on communities that they do not know or understand.

Credibility in highly educated and sophisticated communities must be maintained by employing health professionals at similar educational and socioeconomic levels to those of the population being served. For example, a community hospital in a prosperous Southern California community always uses physicians to present health-education seminars to the public because the community would not be responsive to less highly trained professionals.

Another factor is financing of community education programs. In the case of the prenatal classes, charges for clinic patients were covered by the obstetrical package fee; nonclinic patients were charged $25 for five classes. The CPR classes were taught by community volunteer paramedics. The only charge to participants was the cost of photocopying the self-study booklets.

Our experience has been that a community is willing to pay for the service when it wishes to participate in health education. When we are considering a group such as schoolchildren, however, monies usually come from foundation grants or federal- or state-government funds. Obviously the state of the national economy is very important to the funding of such programs. During recessions we see very little federal funding of what is viewed as unessential. A good example of the economy's effects on health-care delivery is the issue of nationalized health care. During the middle-to-late 1970s, many of us believed that nationalized health care was soon to become a reality. The advent of a new administration in the 1980s, however, repealed that expectation. Certainly, community health education must become more self-supporting and also look to the generosity of the private sector if it is to continue.

Another factor in the success or failure of community health education involves its general appeal. To succeed, community health education must be timely, well presented, and able to attract the attention of many people. The advertising profession has accumulated a vast store of knowledge that enables businesses to sell their products. Unfortunately we usually do not employ advertising research to sell health education. All too often, community health-education projects are the brainchildren of single-well-meaning health-care professionals who determine a need and decide to fill it.

Research on the usefulness of television's ability to affect health education is embryonic. Most such research however, indicates that although television does not produce behavioral changes it will arouse interest and inform people of health matters.[5] One specific evaluation indicated that a series of programs on alcoholism, broadcast on a public-television network, heightened public awareness of alcoholism but did not stimulate corrective action.[6] Due to this finding, and to obvious cost reasons, the use of television in health education must be carefully considered.

Godfrey Hochbaum, a well-known health-education specialist, suggests that we promote healthful practices by showing them to be pleasant and easy, rather than by trying to scare people into healthy behaviors.[7] We cannot force health education onto a community any more than we can force a person to practice contraception. However, by using advertising technology and by promoting the positive aspects of health practices, we may enjoy more success in future community health education.

Strategies

Strategies of community organization can be applied to the promotion of health awareness in the community setting. Community organization is a methodology enabling communities to develop their own human and economic resources. The techniques of community organization are taught in many schools of social work and have been effectively applied by such individuals as Saul Alinsky.[8,9] Three community-organization techniques useful in promoting community health awareness are *community development, social action,* and *social planning.*[10]

Community development is an effective community-organization technique that uses a self-help approach to problem solving. The application of community-development techniques is most successful when the community is homogeneous and has well-defined issues and problems. The role of the health educator is to enable the community to recognize its need for health education and then to aid in securing necessary funds. Lobbying can be done at the local level for state and federal money, which is disbursed through local agencies empowered to make funding decisions.

The CPR community-education project that we present in this chapter is a good example of community development. In this instance, a community of 900 families living in a well-demarcated, middle-class housing development recognized the need for training community members in CPR and basic lifesaving techniques. This community was located in a rural area, approximately eight miles from the nearest hospital. Local volunteers had previously taken Emergency Medical Technician (EMT) training and the community had financed its own ambulances. The community nevertheless recognized the need for proficiency in CPR and basic lifesaving techniques for all of its members, so that they would not have as great a risk of dying before being transported to the hospital.

The concept of *social action* involves underprivileged populations that make demands for needed services and changes. While community development assumes that consensus exists in attempts to attain desired goals, social action often pits one social class against another.[10] Protests against the building of nuclear-power plants are an example of one segment of the community's attempts to direct public opinion against economic forces in the community. These protesters believe that nuclear-energy plants can negatively affect their health or the health of their children. Social action requires strong indigenous community leadership and followers who are willing to actively put themselves on the line to obtain needed health education and services. One of the problems with the application of social action in the promotion of health education is that, in many cases, the community's beliefs related to perception of illness do not match the actual illness present.[3] When this situation prevails, the underserved portions of the community cannot identify which health services they need, and they do not know where or how to lobby to get their needs met.

Social planning is the method used by planning and welfare agencies when they plan and implement health and education programs they deem necessary. Unfortunately, there is little indigenous community participation when this type of community organization is used. Social planning can be a rational approach to solving the problem of an overabundance of poorly planned health-care services. Health Systems Agencies (HSA) were instituted as a form of social planning to address this problem, and they have consumer membership on their boards. However, the consumer board members, consistent with the history of consumer membership, had inadequate numbers to make themselves heard or tended to be co-opted by more vociferous members who had vested interests in maintaining the *status quo*. One successful example of social planning, occurring in the 1960s and 1970s, was the advent of free clinics. These clinics were organized and maintained by members of the health-care establishment in response to consumers' demonstrated need for free health care offered in a nonjudgmental setting. Social planning, like community development and social action, has been a useful strategy to implement health education and services at the community level.

We now discuss two community health-education projects with which we are familiar. Both of these projects could be implemented in any community. Appendices at the end of the chapter have an actual "how-to" discussion of implementation. Our readers are welcome to use the ideas in planning their own programs.

Prenatal Community Education

Our prenatal classes have been mentioned in other chapters of this book. They were originally developed as part of a clinical practicum in graduate school. The classes evolved in response to an informal needs assessment that was conducted at the outpatient clinic of a university's family-medicine residency-training program. Faculty, residents, and nurses designated prenatal classes as the outstanding patient-education need for clinic patients. When the Family Practice Clinic assumed the leadership of the prenatal classes, the following philosophy about the delivery of prenatal education was developed:

> There is a strong agreement within the Family Practice Clinic that education is an essential ingredient in the health care we deliver to our prenatal patients. Although there have been many attempts to provide this education in the past, it was not until recently that a commitment was made to offer prenatal classes to all of our patients on a regular basis.
>
> We believe that prenatal classes should be attended as early as possible in pregnancy. There are numerous advantages to the patient, her family, the physician, and the nurse:
>
> 1. The mother's participation in her own care is essential, especially in the areas of nutrition and care of her body. The classes give both parents the information they need to work in partnership with the physician and nurse.
>
> 2. Classes dealing with the labor-and-delivery process give expectant parents an opportunity to verbalize anxieties or fears about childbirth.

3. Expectant parents enter a supportive relationship with other expectant parents.

4. Relaxation and breathing techniques are learned. This may make both routine obstetric examinations and the labor and delivery better experiences.

5. Expectant mothers and fathers are encouraged to communicate their feelings effectively with one another and to consider ways to keep the communication lines open during stressful events surrounding the birth of their child.

6. Parents gain knowledge about newborn care and helpful suggestions for dealing with the new baby's siblings and other family members.

The prenatal-care curriculum offers a blend of general childbirth education and Lamaze techniques. We do not promote any one specific approach to the birth experience or child care. Our aim is to provide expectant parents with information that enables them to consider their own needs and wishes. We stress the importance of openness and flexibility in planning for labor and delivery and in considering each couple's special circumstances.

We believe that expectant parents learn from us and from each other. As health-care providers, we also learn a great deal from our patients in an informal group in which all members are supported and encouraged to share their thoughts and feelings with one another.

A commitment to patient education is demonstrated by our willingness to become team members in health care with our patients. It is a statement of our respect for patients as consumers. Finally, offering an attractive prenatal-care package is an important step toward enrolling new families in the practice.

Development of the philosophy continued the Family Practice Clinic's history of interest in the consumer. The philosophy was viewed as an attempt to specify and to advocate the rights of the prenatal client and her support system. Evolution of the philosophy preceded the establishment of behavioral objectives and methods of evaluating participants' satisfaction.

Care was taken to ensure continuity of the prenatal classes regardless of changes in clinic staff and residents. To this end guidelines and standards were developed to help each prenatal-class coordinator handle the logistics of the classes as well as to allay anxiety she might have about the program. The guidelines can be found in Appendix A at the end of this chapter.

Following the development of guidelines, objectives were written for each class. Outlines for each class were also written; objectives and outlines are contained in Appendix B. Included with the outlines is a listing of the audiovisual and printed materials used with each class.

During the first class meeting a learning-needs assessment was filled out by each client and her significant other. The learning-needs assessment data were then fitted into the general schema of classes. In this way the prenatal clients were able to set their own agenda (*i.e.,* the class was taught to meet their needs, not the health-care professionals' needs). Data from the learning-needs assessment was transferred to the client's chart, with her knowledge, so that during routine office visits the physician could discuss her stated concerns. The learning-needs assessment form is found in Appendix C.

Classes were enlivened by group discussions and demonstrations. During the first class we enlisted the assistance of a couple who had attended the previous set of classes and were willing to bring their infant to a new series of classes. The expectant parents always had many questions for the parent visitors, and seeing the outcome of the prenatal period—a healthy baby—focused the class for everyone. We also separated the participants into smaller groups of five or six to discuss such topics as sexual activity during pregnancy and to play educational games related to nutrition. During the fourth class, which discussed the care of the newborn, a family nurse practitioner or a family medicine resident demonstrated physical assessment of a neonate. The couples were invariably amazed to see the newborn's range of behaviors. We felt this class helped them better envision their forthcoming infant and also helped them to lay the foundation for infant-stimulation practices. During the class on contraception we obtained samples of all the different contraceptive devices and passed them around the room. The demonstration segments of the classes helped to break the tedium that can occur with the lecture format and also allowed the participants an opportunity to become acquainted with one another.

At the end of the last class each participant was asked to complete the evaluation form found in Appendix D. Evaluations were useful in planning future classes and in giving specific teachers feedback on their performance in the classes.

In Chapter 3 we referred to another evaluation format, called a confidence survey. It was used during the first class series to obtain information related to the participants' growth in confidence levels during the five class meetings. One of the purposes of any type of prenatal education is to instill confidence in the couple so that they will be able to manage self-care practices related to pregnancy, as well as care of the neonate. Confidence levels on 19 different items were determined on a pre- and post-test basis (*i.e.,* at the beginning of the class series and after the last class). When the data were tabulated, they showed that all clients had increased their confidence levels or remained the same on every item, except for three items on which two patients had decreased their confidence level. If the prenatal patient-education project were applied to the model presented in Chapter 3 it would appear as in Figure 11-1. Any increase in confidence level as measured by this instrument was accepted as an indication that the intervention had created a positive change. Using a control group that had not attended the classes would have been one method of verifying that the experimental prenatal patients had indeed increased their confidence levels as a result of the classes. Below is the confidence-level survey that was used (Fig. 11-2).

Confidence levels as an evaluation methodology are only one outcome that can be considered when determining the efficacy of the intervention. When prenatal

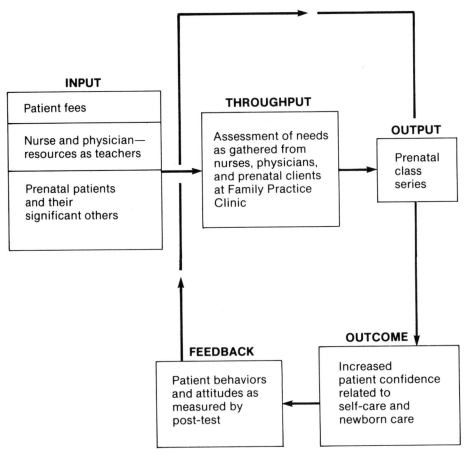

Fig. 11-1. *Systems evaluation of prenatal community education program.*

patient education is evaluated, we can focus upon different outcomes. We have presented one outcome and one instrument through which to obtain feedback. Another obvious outcome is knowledge acquisition, which could also be measured by pre- and post-test. The outcome that is evaluated by the questionnaire in Appendix D is patient satisfaction. All patient-education programs, whether individual, group, or community oriented, must be evaluated in terms of outcomes. As stated previously, cooperation/compliance is not the only outcome worth evaluating and, as in the case of prenatal education, compliance may be very difficult to determine. The purpose of prenatal education is to maximize the desired outcomes of a healthy mother and infant and the promotion of family bonding. Since there are many variables that affect whether the infant and mother will be healthy, it is wise to evaluate the specific intervention (prenatal classes) in terms of the clients' response to them.

We have used the prenatal classes as an example of a successful teaching program for one group in the community. The next community-teaching program we discuss did not consist of a group bound together by the common tie of

Fig. 11-2. *Prenatal Questionnaire.*

INSTRUCTIONS:

We are interested in knowing how confident you feel about your knowledge associated with pregnancy, labor, and delivery. Please answer these questions carefully by circling the response that refers to your confidence level.

A sample question will help you understand how to fill out the questionnaire.

I know how to fill out this questionnaire.

VC   C   ?   I   VI

VC—I feel very confident and secure in my knowledge of this material.
  C—I feel confident that I can deal adequately with this material.
  ?—I have no particular feelings about this material; I do not know what this material means.
  I—I feel insecure, knowing that I would have a difficult time dealing with this material.
VI—I feel very insecure, knowing that I definitely could not deal with this material at this time.

1. I know which foods a pregnant woman should eat and why.

    VC   C   ?   I   VI

2. I understand the changes in my breasts.

    VC   C   ?   I   VI

3. I know about the effects of alcohol on my body.

    VC   C   ?   I   VI

4. I know how many pounds I can gain during my pregnancy.

    VC   C   ?   I   VI

5. I understand restrictions placed on me because of my job.

    VC   C   ?   I   VI

6. I know how to do a pelvic tilt.

    VC   C   ?   I   VI

7. I understand the reasons for frequent urination during pregnancy.

    VC   C   ?   I   VI

8. I know the danger signs to watch for during pregnancy.

    VC   C   ?   I   VI

9. I understand the fear–tension–pain cycle.

    VC   C   ?   I   VI

10. I know how to do breathing exercises to be used during labor.

    VC   C   ?   I   VI

11. I know what to expect from a newborn baby.

    VC   C   ?   I   VI

(continued)

12. I understand the differences between bottle feeding and breast feeding for the mother and baby.

        VC   C   ?   I   VI

13. I know how to give a baby bath.

        VC   C   ?   I   VI

14. I know what kind of contraception to use while nursing.

        VC   C   ?   I   VI

15. I know what kinds of anesthetics are available during labor.

        VC   C   ?   I   VI

16. I know at least three signs of beginning labor.

        VC   C   ?   I   VI

17. I know how to get my body into shape following delivery.

        VC   C   ?   I   VI

18. I understand the various forms of birth control and the ones best suited for me.

        VC   C   ?   I   VI

19. I know the types of equipment and clothing necessary for myself and my baby.

        VC   C   ?   I   VI

pregnancy. Instead, this group was united primarily by a desire to learn how to assist drowning, accident, and cardiac victims while awaiting the arrival of paramedics.

*Cardiopulmonary-Resuscitation and Basic-Lifesaving Classes**

As mentioned earlier in this chapter, the community program to teach CPR and basic-lifesaving techniques was developed and taught by members of a community that recognized the need for wider citizen participation in emergency situations. The fact that the community was homogeneous and had its own schools, churches, and voluntary organizations made the technique of community development very successful. The community had a long history of giving financial and volunteer support to the maintenance of its own rescue squad. Community members and trained Emergency Medical Technicians (EMTs) were extremely proud of their vehicles and highly trained volunteers.

    The justification for the program was the perceived importance of citizen participation in critical situations that warrant bystander intervention. Besides skills to aid in situations involving cardiac and respiratory arrest, seven other basic skills were identified as necessary lifesaving techniques. A written justification for the program was supported by studies, conducted in Baltimore County and Seattle, indicating that mortality outcomes were improved when there was intervention by a trained bystander.[11,12] Old fears of lacerated livers and broken ribs induced by

*This section was written with the collaboration of Kathy Finch, R.N., B.S.N., Duke University Medical Center, Durham, NC.

nonprofessionals practicing CPR are not warranted and volunteers do, indeed, accomplish more good than harm.[13]

A philosophy was therefore developed emphasizing the importance of prevention, detection, early diagnosis and treatment, education of health personnel and the public, and research and evaluation. This component of emergency services was viewed as an adjunct to the already existing paramedic services provided by the EMTs. The purpose of the training program was to teach the average citizen basic skills that could be performed on an acutely ill or injured victim until more highly trained help could arrive.

The following objectives were developed for the program:

1. To teach the public how to recognize a life-threatening situation
2. To teach the public how to intervene in a life-threatening situation and to perform lifesaving procedures
3. To teach the public how to alert EMTs and paramedics
4. To orient the public to the statewide Emergency Medical Service (EMS) system.

Classes lasted three hours each, with two sessions required. The first class consisted of seven basic lifesaving skills and the second class covered CPR. The seven basic skills that were identified as crucial to the bystander's attempts to intervene follow:

1. Entering the system, including dialing the 911 emergency number, giving appropriate information to the emergency operator, and so forth
2. Opening and maintenance of an airway
3. Techniques of the Heimlich maneuver
4. CPR using one-man-rescue technique
5. Control of bleeding and hemorrhage
6. Care of the person in shock
7. Handling acute poisoning emergencies

CPR was taught using the self-instructional booklets developed by the American Red Cross, for which the students paid a minimal fee. The basic-lifesaving skills were developed by the coordinator of the program, a registered nurse. The lifesaving skills followed guidelines suggested by the American Red Cross. If students wished to purchase the lifesaving-skills manual they were able to do so at cost. A local manufacturing company had been approached and had expressed interest in underwriting the cost of printing the booklet.

Innovative approaches were used in teaching the classes. Students read their self-study booklets and then moved around the room in pairs from station to station. Class size was restricted to ten adults. Two instructors were always present to help the students practice their skills and to certify them as competent. Students also practiced together and critiqued one another's skill performance. Reinforcement of skills was provided by watching and critiquing another student's performance and by obtaining "hands-on" practice. Students were encouraged to visualize between classes what the skills included and also to visualize a contingency plan (*i.e.*, "What do I do if . . . "). The purpose of the visualization of skills and the frequent opportunities for practice was to make the most necessary skills automatic. The ability to respond automatically in life-threatening situations is of primary importance.

An advantage of the self-instructional approach was that variations in instructor ability to teach were minimized and use of volunteers was maximized. All instructors were volunteer members of the community rescue squad and certified EMTs. They were also certified American Heart Association and American Red Cross instructors.

There were minimal charges for the classes because of volunteer participation. Overhead costs for building usage were absorbed by the rescue squad because the classes were taught in the squad house.

The potential for research and evaluation of this program of community health promotion and preventive maintenance is apparent. Because the community had well-defined boundaries and had been demographically described, it would have been relatively simple to compare morbidity and mortality data of this community with those of another community, of corresponding size and characteristics, without a training program. Remember, however, that there are a number of variables, such as rural *vs* urban nature, level of education, mean age, and socioeconomic background, that must be controlled in such a study.

The success of this program was related to the following considerations:
1. The need for the program was recognized by the community
2. The community had a history of voluntarily supporting emergency medical services
3. The program was developed and taught by indigenous community members
4. The community was homogenous in nature, with common goals shared by all
5. The cost to participate in the program was minimal

Appendix A: General Guidelines for Prenatal Classes

1. There must be one person teaching each series of classes to allow for continuity.
2. Resident and nursing-student participation is encouraged.
3. Teachers should use the behavioral objectives previously developed.
4. With advance notice, secretaries can duplicate handouts. Teachers may wish to make their own.
5. Materials suggested in class outlines are free of charge from HEW and the March of Dimes.
6. Pertinent information about patients and their concerns should be communicated to the providers orally or documented in the chart.
7. Posters at the front of the family practice clinic are good publicity. Fliers with a phone number for patients to call to register for classes are also helpful.
8. Billing is handled by the business office.
9. All patients should sign an attendance sheet at *each* class.
10. Evaluation of classes should be made after the last class.

Appendix B: Objectives, Outlines, and Guidelines for Prenatal Classes

Objectives for Class I: Nutrition During Pregnancy

At the close of Class I, each participant will be able to do the following:

A. Answer the following questions correctly:
  1. How much weight do you plan to gain during your pregnancy?
  2. Now that you are pregnant, how many more calories do you think you need: 2 times normal, 3 times normal, only 300 calories more, only 100 calories more?
  3. Which of the following foods do pregnant women especially need: dairy products, sweets, fatty foods, fresh vegetables, protein foods?
  4. Which of the following items might be dangerous to eat or use while you are pregnant: alcoholic beverages, salt, sugar, nicotine, caffeine?
  5. In which of the following situations would a pregnant woman be wise to lose weight: if the woman were overweight before pregnancy, if the woman is diabetic and overweight, if the woman suddenly gains ten pounds that are primarily fluid?
B. List three advantages of breast-feeding.
C. State three advantages of exercise during pregnancy.
D. Choose one type of exercise and describe where and how often it will be done.

Materials*

  Nutrition and Pregnancy pamphlet—March of Dimes
  Be Good to Your Baby Before It's Born pamphlet—March of Dimes

Teaching Aids

  Flipchart and markers
  Food-group posters

Class I Outline

A. Needs Assessment
B. Introduction
  1. Key staff people
  2. Restrooms
  3. Group exercise†
C. Nutrition (pre- and postnatal)
D. Exercise
  1. Discussion of fitness, exercise
  2. Care of the back, body mechanics
  3. General body awareness

*Obtain through The National Foundation/March of Dimes, Box 2000, White Plains, NY 10602 or from a local March of Dimes agency.
†Each person takes about five minutes to get to know the person next to her (not the person with whom she came). At the end of this time, each person will introduce the other to the group. Staff members should scatter themselves throughout the group.

Prenatal Nutrition Guidelines

- Eat a balanced diet, drawing from the four food groups
- Gain between 24 and 30 pounds at the appropriate rate
- Take your folate and iron supplements daily
- Avoid weight-reduction diets
- Avoid salt restriction
- Do not use diuretics (fluid pills)
- Use iodized salt *ad lib*
- Consider breast-feeding your baby

Table 11B-1. **Prenatal Exercise Plan**

Class Session	Topics
I	Fitness, personal exercise plan Musculoskeletal system changes Body mechanics General body awareness
II	Kegel exercise Slow, deep-chest breathing Pelvic rock—knees
III	Verbal cues, positioning Bent leg lifts Pelvic rock—back Shallow breathing
IV	Panting Nonverbal cues, comfort measures Pushing
V	Review of breathing techniques Mock labor and delivery

Objectives for Class II: Physiologic and Psychological Changes of Pregnancy

By the close of Class II, each participant will be able to do the following:

A. Identify on a diagram:
1. Spine
2. Rectum
3. Amniotic fluid
4. Uterus
5. Amniotic sac (bag of waters)
6. Cervix
7. Pubic bone
8. Vagina (birth canal)

B. Describe breast changes and care of the breasts during pregnancy

C. Describe recommendations for the following during pregnancy:
1. Rest and sleep
2. Smoking and alcohol
3. Dental care
4. Travel and work
D. Name two common discomforts of pregnancy and recommended treatments
E. State why the doctor should be consulted before *any* medication is taken during pregnancy
F. Identify three warning signs for which the doctor should be notified immediately
G. Describe the Kegel exercise for toning pelvic musculature, demonstrate the pelvic rock for controlling low-back pain, demonstrate slow, deep-chest breathing used during the initial stage of labor

Materials

      Prenatal Exercises booklet—Family Practice Center (agency-created booklet)
      How Your Baby Grows sheet—Lederle Laboratories*

Teaching Aids

      Blackboard, flipchart
      Diagram of pregnant anatomy

Class II Outline

A. Review of needs assessment
B. Outline of class, introduction of staff
C. Class content: physiologic and psychological changes during pregnancy
D. Exercises, breathing techniques
1. Kegel exercises
2. Pelvic rock
3. Deep breathing

Objectives for Class III: Labor and Delivery

At the close of this class, each participant will be able to do the following:
A. Describe the work of the uterus in labor
B. Describe the changes of the cervix in labor
C. Describe three signs of labor
D. Demonstrate the timing of contractions
E. Describe how and when to contact the doctor when there has been a sign of labor
F. Describe three stages of labor

*Obtain through Lederle Laboratories, Public Affairs Department, Middletown Road, Pearl River, NY 10965.

G. Consider own plans for labor and delivery (*e.g.*, birthing room, rooming-in arrangements, early discharge)
H. Describe some variables that make cesarean section necessary

Materials
    "Prenatal Exercises" booklet—Family Practice Center

Teaching Aids
    Film: *The Miracle of Birth* (40 minutes) from Brigham Young University, Salt Lake City, Utah
    Birth Atlas flipchart from: Maternity Center Association, 48 East 92nd Street, New York, NY 10028

Class III Outline

A. Introduction of staff and guests
B. Class content
   1. Informal group discussion
   2. Elicit feelings about pregnancy, fears, dreams, fantasies from both partners
C. Exercises, breathing
   1. Verbal cues, positioning
   2. Bent-leg lifts
   3. Pelvic rock
   4. Shallow breathing

Labor and Delivery Topics to Cover

- OB tour
- Birthing room
- False labor—Braxton Hicks sign
- Things to take to the hospital
- Stop eating when labor begins—why?
- Early labor—clinic procedure
- Length of labor
- Stages of labor, transition
- Emotions
- IVs
- Pitocin
- Fetal monitoring
- Analgesia
- "Prep"
- Stirrups
- Urge to push
- Forceps
- Episiotomy
- Umbilical cord, clamping
- Placenta
- Checking over baby

- Silver nitrate drops
- C-section

Objectives for Class IV: The Newborn

At the close of this class, each participant/couple will be able to do the following:

   A. Describe why fatigue is a problem that most new parents face
   B. Discuss two ways new parents can minimize unnecessary fatigue
   C. Consider what "helpers" might be staying with them when they come home from the hospital and describe what they can do to help
   D. Describe three infant-care problems for which the doctor should be notified
   E. Describe three needs for which babies depend on their parents
   F. Describe two issues that new parents often confront as a couple

Materials

   Resources for New Parents (list of local community resources)
   La Leche League leaders and support group

Teaching Aids

   New parents/babies in practice

Class IV Outline

A. Introduce staff and guests
B. Class content
   1. Encourage participants to share what they already know about baby care
   2. Ask participants to anticipate their concerns in taking care of baby and describe them to group
C. Exercises, breathing
   1. Nonverbal cues
   2. Panting
   3. Pushing

The Newborn Topics to Consider

- Communication between couple
- Flexibility in schedule
- Fatigue
- Will there be family members or help at home?
- If so, what can they do to help?
- Advice of parents or others
- The "blues"
- Siblings
- What do you need for the baby?
- Bath
- Sleeping (baby)
- Breast-feeding problems
- Skin changes in baby

- How do you know if the baby is sick?
- Physiological jaundice of neonate
- Intimacy
- Suggested reading

Baby Needs
    Changing
    Safety/protection
    Comforting
    Bathing

Parent–Couple Issues
    Fatigue
    Sharing
    Sex/intimacy
    Parents

Baby Problems
    Diarrhea
    Constipation
    Fever
    Fussiness
    Crying

Objectives for Class V: The Postpartum Period

At the end of this class, each participant will be able to do the following:

A. Identify two common postpartum discomforts and describe how to initiate relief measures
B. Identify two symptoms or problems for which the doctor should be notified
C. State how and where (anatomically) conception occurs
D. Consider a method of contraception that is acceptable to them
E. Demonstrate the following in a mock labor and delivery
    1. Deep-chest breathing
    2. Shallow breathing
    3. Panting
    4. Pushing

Materials
    Contraception pamphlet—Department of Health and Human Resources—Government Printing Office, DHEW Publication #HSA 76-16024, Rockville, MD 20852
    Prenatal Exercises booklet—Family Practice Center
    Getting Back into Shape—Ayerst Laboratories, 685 Third Avenue, New York, NY 10017

Teaching Aids
    Poster or diagram of female reproductive anatomy
    Contraceptive teaching kit
    Flipchart

Class V Outline
A. Introduction of staff
B. Class content
C. Exercises, breathing, mock labor and delivery
D. Evaluation of classes

Appendix C: Learning-Needs Assessment

Please fill out one form per family and return it to the staff by the end of class.
1. How many previous pregnancies have you had? _____
2. What is your expected date of delivery? _____
3. Will someone attend classes with you? _____ If so, what is his relationship to you? _____
4. Have you had any previous prenatal education? _____ If so, please describe: _____
    _____
5. What do you want to learn in these classes? _____
    _____
    _____
    _____
    _____
    _____
    _____
6. Your name: _____
7. Your doctor's name: _____

Appendix D: Evaluation of Prenatal Classes

Please help us to evaluate the prenatal classes you have just attended at the Family Medicine Center so we can improve them in the future.
1. My favorite class was _____
    I liked this class because _____
    _____
2. My least-favorite class was _____
    It could have been improved by _____
    _____
3. I wish more time had been spent on _____
    _____
4. I wish less time had been spent on _____
    _____
5. Can you think of more effective ways of presenting the material? _____
    _____
6. Do you have any comments about the film *The Miracle of Birth?* _____
    _____

7. How do you feel about the exercises that were taught? _____
   _____

8. Other comments _____
   _____

References

1. Green LW: To educate or not to educate: is that the question. Am J Public Health 70, No. 6:625–627, 1980
2. Williams CL, Arnold CB: Teaching children self-care for chronic disease prevention, obesity reduction, and smoking prevention. Patient Counselling and Health Education, 2, No. 2:92–98, 1980
3. Dyson BC, Dyson EU: The health team in primal community: A new context for community medicine. Patient Couns and Health Educ 1, No. 3:122–127, 1979
4. Salber EJ: The lay advisor as a community health resource. J Health Polit Policy Law 3, No. 4:469–478, 1979
5. Richman LA, Urban D: Health education through television: some theoretical applications. Int J Health Educ 21:46–52, 1978
6. Dickman FB, Keil TJ: Public television and public health: The case of alcoholism. J Stud Alcohol 38, No. 3:584, 1977
7. Hochbaum GM: An alternate approach to health education. Health Values 3, No. 4:197–201, 1979
8. Alinsky S: Rules for Radicals. New York, Random House, 1971
9. Alinsky S: Reveille for Radicals. New York, Vintage, 1969
10. Green LW, Kreuter MW, Deeds SG et al: Health Education, Planning: A Diagnostic Approach pp 103–105. Palo Alto, Mayfield Publishing, 1980
11. Eisenberg MS, Bergner L, Hallstrom A: Paramedic programs and out-of-hospital cardiac arrest: I. Factors associated with successful resuscitation. Am J Public Health 69, No. 1:30–38, 1979
12. Cobb LA, Alvarez H, Kopass MK: A rapid response system for out-of-hospital cardiac emergencies. Med Clin North Am 60, No. 2:283–290, 1976
13. Copley DP, Mantle MJ, Rogers WJ et al: Improved outcome for prehospital cardiopulmonary collapse with resuscitation by bystanders. Circulation 5, No. 6:901–905, 1977

Bibliography

Books

Beatty SR (ed): Continuity of Care: The Hospital and the Community. New York, Grune and Stratton, 1980
Freeman RB, Heinrich J: Community Health Nursing Practice. Philadelphia, WB Saunders, 1981
Jarvis LL (ed): Community Health Nursing: Keeping the Public Healthy. Philadelphia, FA Davis, 1981
Reinhardt AM, Quinn MD: Current Practice in Family-Centered Community Nursing. St Louis, CV Mosby, 1977
Smith ED: Maternity Care: A Guide for Patient Education. New York, Appleton-Century-Crofts, 1981
Spradley BW: Community Health Nursing: Concepts and Practice. Boston, Little, Brown, 1981

Journals

Bryant NH: Consumer health education in New Jersey community hospitals: A medical school initiative. J Community Health 3, No. 3:259–270, 1978

Hughes GH et al: The multiple risk factor intervention trial (MRFIT): V: Intervention on smoking. Prev Med 10:476–500, 1981

Pigg RM: The impact of health advertising on the consumer. Health Values 3, No. 4:206–8, 1979

Pisa Z: Comprehensive cardiovascular control programs in the community. Excerpta Medica ICS (Amsterdam) 470:169–172, 1979

Worden JK, Waller JA, Ashikaga T et al: Respiratory disease in Vermont: A population survey for planning a public education program. Prev Med 9, No. 1:120–134, 1980

Chapter 12

Answers to Questions About Common Problems Encountered in Practice Settings

This chapter is an attempt to answer the questions that may have occurred to our readers during the previous chapters. We try to answer the "yes, but . . . " questions that probably arose after reading our earlier approaches and suggestions. We have found that many texts propose grand and glorious schemata and frameworks while ignoring the daily irritating and confounding problems we encounter in our practice settings. Therefore, we examine such common problems as how to motivate patients and staff involved in patient education and how to get the health team together. Obtaining publicity and choosing teaching materials will be discussed. Delivering patient education to various age groups (pediatric through gerontologic) and in special settings (*e.g.,* to the dying patient and the psychiatric patient) will also be considered.

We begin with a discussion of the differences between *patient teaching* and *patient education.* We have found that these terms are frequently used interchangeably and we feel strongly that they are not synonymous. We present a question-and-answer format to aid in ease of reading.

What is the difference between patient education and patient teaching?

Patient education has been defined as " . . . the process of influencing patient behavior, producing changes in knowledge, attitudes, and skills required to maintain and improve health. The process may begin with the imparting of information, but also includes interpretation and integration of the information in such a manner as to bring about attitudinal or behavioral changes which benefit the person's health status."[1] This definition states that patient education is a process with various components. It considers the patient holistically, with all his needs and concerns, and sets goals with the patient for desired outcomes. The process of patient education also includes an evaluation of the patient's learning, its usefulness to him, and the ease with which he has integrated it into his self-care practices. On the other hand, *patient teaching* refers to only one component of the patient education process—the actual imparting of information to the patient.

Patient education *vs* patient teaching is a process-*vs*-content issue. The content of the actual teaching is very important and, obviously, must be accurate but the total process of patient education is much more important than the teaching itself. The transfer of knowledge that takes place with patient teaching does not ensure behavioral change. There are many research projects that give ample evidence of this.[2,3,4] As stated earlier, we believe that it is our ethical obligation to supply the patient with information related to his problem. We cannot assume, however, that because we fulfill our responsibility the patient will make the desired behavioral changes. If we use the process of patient education, instead of merely impart the content, we can hope that the patient may cooperate more with his regimen. (For more information related to the process of patient education see Chap. 6-9).

How can we motivate patients to learn?

Probably the most important factor in motivating patients to respond to patient education with the desired behavioral changes is the recognition of what motivates each individual patient. For one patient, motivation may be assurance that he will be in control of his own life; motivating factors for another patient may be predicated on his desire to please the health-care professionals. Some patients are able to state clearly what motivates them, but other patients may not recognize what works as a motivator. Clues to the individual motivation factors can be obtained from the client's life-style, his family members, his socioeconomic status, and his growth and development data. Health-care professionals must avoid the assumption that their own motivators apply to their patients.

Frequently motivation is divided into *intrinsic* and *extrinsic* factors. *Intrinsic factors* are those factors that are internally integrated into the client's personality and *modus operandi.* They include such things as the patient's anxiety level, his success in past educational settings, and his openness to learning. *Extrinsic factors* include the environment for learning, the pleasure of acquiring new knowledge, and the type of interaction in the learning process. Extrinsic motivation factors are factors we, as patient educators, can control. If we establish a climate of mutual trust and safety, the environment for learning can be a positive motivator. Likewise, by injecting fun and some levity into the learning situation, we can make the pleasure of learning become a positive force.

The type of interaction in the learning process is another extrinsic motivating factor that the educator can control. Transactional analysis provides a vocabulary useful to describe the desired interaction. If our interaction with the learner is structured so that the adult learner is programmed as the child in an adult/child or parent/child situation, the interaction will have negative motivational effects on the learner. The adult learner will profit most from an adult/adult type of interaction. An example of an adult/adult type of interaction would be that of group-learning experiences for ostomy patients in which one patient would share with the group his experiences in coping with his ostomy. Another example of an adult/adult type of interaction includes the patient educator who encourages the client to set his own agenda for learning the management of heart disease. Adult/adult interactions require the client to take responsibility for his own learning, an issue that will be discussed shortly.

One of the most important roles the nurse can play in motivation is that of helping the client to recognize the gap between what his situation is and what he wants it to be. Malcolm Knowles, in his formative text on adult education, describes the gap as a central aspect of motivating patients to learn.[5] For example, a young couple with whom we worked recognized that they did not want to use corporal punishment with their three-year-old daughter but they did not know how else to achieve necessary obedience. Once we were able to help them to recognize this gap, they eagerly asked for, and then applied, other techniques of discipline. Once the patient has recognized the gap, written contracts are an effective means of motivating patients. The formulation of such contracts is covered in Chapter 7.

If motivational techniques do not seem to be working, the nurse should consider reviewing her assessment and then reassessing the patient if necessary. Perhaps something has changed in the patient's own situation and previous motivators are no longer effective. For example, a low-to-moderate level of anxiety is an intrinsic motivator and may be used effectively to motivate the patient with coronary-artery disease to learn about necessary diet, medication, and life-style changes. However, if this same patient has a successful coronary-artery bypass-graft operation, he may believe he is "cured" and out of danger and anxiety may no longer be an effective motivator. At this point the nurse must reassess the patient and determine other motivators.

There are undoubtedly further questions about motivation, the primary one being "How much responsibility to learn does the patient have?" When all factors are considered, it is the patient who must ultimately decide whether he is going to accept our attempts to teach him, whether he accepts selectively, or whether he completely ignores us. Nurses and health-care professionals are not responsible for patients' behavior. We can try our best to enhance the learning situation and use extrinsic motivation factors, but motivation is essentially an inner drive and if this drive and a sense of personal responsibility are not operating in our particular clients there is little we can do to foster them. Ideally, we should be able to teach patients to be their own advocates and to expect patient-education services on inpatient and outpatient basis. Many patients will respond to this approach and, in fact, various books have been written detailing the approach that patients should take when dealing with the medical world.[6,7,8] However, we must be cognizant of the few patients who do refuse to take responsibility for their own learning; once we have made every attempt to provide patient education to them, we must finally release our own sense of responsibility for them.

How can we motivate staff to become involved in patient education?

Some of the issues related to motivation of staff in patient-education settings are discussed in Chapter 3. Other means of motivating staff to provide high-quality patient education follow.

Nurses and other health professionals frequently complain that they do not understand the process of patient education. One- or two-day *workshops* offered to all health professionals are an effective means of imparting teaching/learning principles and securing interest in patient education. The bonus of giving continuing-education units may be influential, especially to those nurses who work in states with mandatory continuing-education requirements. We have offered many of these seminars to nurses and a basic outline of such a workshop can be found at the end of this chapter in Appendix A. We have usually employed case studies and role plays in these seminars to enhance the learning process. Sometimes we ask participants to develop their own teaching programs, applying the content learned in the seminar.

Another aspect that can be problematic is the actual disease-process or health-promotion content that must be conveyed to patients. Many nurses remark that they do not know what to teach. Although we believe that most nurses usually do have the pertinent information stored away, we feel that anxiety can be decreased by *helping the staff to organize* and review the information that patients need. Frequently, staff members become so enthusiastic about teaching after attending such classes that they recognize other areas of need and develop teaching protocols with very little assistance from the patient educator. Such seminars and classes satisfy both intrinsic and extrinsic motivational factors for the staff. Negative intrinsic factors such as anxiety about lack of knowledge are modified and such positive extrinsic factors as gaining continuing education units are resolved.

Nursing rounds oriented toward patient education can be an effective motivating force because they add novelty to the learning situation. In such instances, nurses or other health professionals should be asked to prepare some information about a patient with whom they are familiar. This material may be related to assessment of the client's patient-education needs, to goal setting, to the actual process of teaching skills, or to any number of patient-education tasks. During nursing rounds the nurse performs the chosen tasks with the patient. Following rounds the task is critiqued by the observing staff. Nursing rounds can become an excellent means of learning from others and expanding one's own repertoire of patient-education behaviors.

Support at the administrative level for patient education is necessary if the programs are to maintain validity and credibility. Such support also acts as an extrinsic motivator to staff members because they feel that their efforts are being appreciated at the highest levels. Developing and enhancing administrative support is covered in Chapter 3.

Reward and incentive programs for staff who provide patient education can be a strong motivator. Sometimes the reward is the ability to move from night or evening shifts to day shifts. Another possibility is for a staff nurse who has developed special skills to be advanced up a clinical career ladder to a position that may be called clinical teaching nurse or nurse clinician. Usually such promotions are accompanied by merit pay raises but have no increase in administrative duties. As mentioned in Chapter 3, these promotions keep good nurses at the bedside rather than shift them into administration. Such rewards and incentives also serve to show other staff members that patient-education activities are valued in their institution.

Peer support is another important motivating factor for the staff. Staff members who can convene on a formal or informal basis to discuss their problems and their successes in patient education can add a great impetus to the widespread adoption of patient-education efforts. As a profession, nursing suffers from a lack of internal validation. Too often we feel we are the only ones on the battle lines, and we refuse to allow ourselves to ask for support when we need it. Greater team efforts and support within nursing would improve patient-education efforts and act as a motivator to inexperienced nurses looking for guidance.

We mentioned the benefits that accrue from increased *physician-nurse collegiality* and its resulting improvement in team effort in Chapters 2 and 3. Certainly such collegiality can be seen as a motivator for the staff. Nurses who know that physicians approve of their patient-education efforts will experience confirmation and validation as motivators. Because collegiality is a two-way proposition, it is important that nurses also validate the patient-education efforts of physicians. Collegiality as a motivator can, and should, extend to other health-care-team members. The sense of colleagueship we experienced with dietitians and pharmacists was a very positive aspect of our participation in the diabetic luncheons referred to in Chapters 2 and 3. Another extrinsic motivator is nurses' better sense of their own professional identity in such collegial relationships.

How is the teaching of children and adolescents different from the teaching of adults?

Children are not just small adults and teaching them demands an ingenuity and an approach very different from that of teaching adults. Adolescents' learning needs vary from those of children and from those of adults, and so will be discussed separately.

Teaching/learning principles, when applied to children, should always consider the growth-and-development level as well as the cognitive level of the child. Table 12-1 is based on Piaget's well-known work regarding the development of perceptual and cognitive processes from infancy through adolescence.[9] We purposely chose Piaget instead of Erikson because we feel that an understanding of cognitive processes is of equal importance to an understanding of developmental processes for pediatric patient education. A helpful chart that uses Erikson's developmental stages and applies them to patient education can be found in Donald Bille's *Practical Approaches to Patient Teaching.*[10] Table 12-1 outlines the cognitive and perceptual stages of development and then suggests an approach to pediatric-patient teaching.

Before embarking upon pediatric-patient education, remember that children have shorter attention spans, have greater needs for support and nurturance, and learn even more easily through active participation than do adults. This means that material must be presented in abbreviated format over short periods of time. Staff members must remember to consistently and

Table 12-1. **Cognitive Stages and Approaches to Patient Education with Children**

Cognitive Stage	Approach to Teaching
Ages From Birth to 2 Years—Sensorimotor Development	
Begins as completely undifferentiated from environment	Orient all teaching to parents
Eventually learns to repeat actions that have effects on objects	Make infants feel as secure as possible with familiar objects from home environment
Has rudimentary ability to make associations	Give older infants an opportunity to manipulate objects in their environments, especially if long hospitalization is expected
Ages From 2 to 7 Years—Preoperational Development	
Has cognitive processes that are literal and concrete	Be aware of explanations that the child may interpret literally (*e.g.,* "The doctor is going to make your heart like new" may be interpreted as "He is going to give me a new heart"); allow child to manipulate safe equipment such as stethoscopes, tongue blades, reflex hammers; use very simple drawings of the external anatomy because children have limited knowledge of organs' functions
Lacks ability to generalize	Comparisons to other children are not helpful nor is it meaningful to compare one diagnostic test or procedure to another
Has egocentrism predominating	Belief that he causes events to happen may result in guilty thoughts that he caused his own pain, hospitalization, and so forth; reassure child that no one is to blame for his pain or other problems
Has animistic thinking (thinks that all objects possess life or human characteristics of their own)	Anthropomorphize and name equipment that is especially frightening; explain medications such as antibiotics as "Luke Skywalker destroying Darth Vader's forces," and so forth

Table 12-1. **Cognitive Stages and Approaches
to Patient Education with Children** *(continued)*

Cognitive Stage	Approach to Teaching

Ages From 7 to 12 Years—Concrete Operational Thought Development

Has concrete, but more realistic and objective, cognitive processes	Use drawings and models; children at this age have vague understandings of internal body processes; use needle play, dolls to explain surgical techniques and facilitate learning
Is able to compare objects and experiences because of increased ability to classify along many different dimensions	Relate his care to other children's experiences so he can learn from them; compare procedures to one another to diminish anxiety
Views world from more objective viewpoint and is able to understand another's position	Use films and group activities to add to repertoire of useful behaviors and establish role models
Has knowledge of cause and effect that has progressed to deductive logical reasoning	Use child's interest in science to explain logically what has happened and what will happen to him; explain medications simply and straightforwardly (*e.g.,* "This medicine [insulin] unlocks the door to your body's cells just as a key unlocks the door to your house. By unlocking the door to the cell, the insulin can deliver the food and energy in your blood to the cell.")

(Content adapted from Petrillo M, Sanger S: Emotional Care of Hospitalized Children, pp 38–50. Philadelphia, JB Lippincott, 1980 and Kolb LC: Modern Clinical Psychiatry, 9th ed, pp 90–91. Philadelphia, WB Saunders, 1977)

persistently show affection and offer praise to their young clients during patient-education sessions. By actively involving children in the learning process, we help them to more readily assimilate the information. It is an old adage that the child's play is his work. In his play he integrates new and unfamiliar information. Play, therefore, becomes a primary vehicle through which he learns about his disease or acute problem, about what will happen, and about how to take care of himself to the best of his ability. Play therapy should also be used to help the child to postprocedurally integrate and understand the painful or frightening experience he has undergone. Follow-up to surgery and procedures is just as important as preparation for these events because most children have many unresolved feelings and questions that need expression.

Although our case study will focus on a school-age child, we note that current research is proving the efficacy of early-childhood and infant intervention and stimulation.[11,12] Parents are being instructed in techniques of infant stimulation by community agencies such as community colleges, public-health departments, and YWCAs. Certainly pediatric-staff nurses should use their knowledge of child development to both initiate and reinforce such infant-stimulation techniques with hospitalized infants. Role modeling these techniques is an effective teaching intervention for parents.

The case study that follows will be used to illustrate the appropriate teaching for a ten-year-old boy with newly diagnosed idiopathic recurrent seizures.

Case Study: Eric

Eric experienced his first grand mal seizure during recess at elementary school. He was hospitalized immediately for observation and a diagnostic work-up. Eric's primary-care nurse initiated patient education two days prior to his planned discharge. Remembering that Eric's stage of cognitive development had been characterized by Piaget as "concrete operational thought," she began by teaching him the basic pathophysiology of seizure activity.[9] Eric was not capable of abstract thought processes but he did understand the simple drawings the nurse provided of the brain and her explanation that the seizures were caused by too much electrical activity in the brain. The nurse did not stress the term *electrical activity,* instead, she compared the problem in his brain to an electric toy train that goes so fast that it runs off the track. She completed her analogy by saying that the phenobarbital he was going to take every day would act on his brain as if it were slowing down the speed of the electric train. Eric's nurse remained aware of the fact that at this stage of development in the child's language skills he may not always manage to indicate whether he has fully comprehended her explanation. She therefore used a great deal of repetition and asked Eric many questions.

Children from ages seven to twelve are generally able to handle many of the aspects of their medical regimen. Eric was made responsible for administering his own medication at the prescribed times. He began preparing and taking the phenobarbital himself while he was still hospitalized.

Children of Eric's age are more socially involved with their peers than are younger children and it is important not to disrupt their attempts to join groups and participate in team sports. Eric was told that he could continue riding his bike as long as he wore his bike helmet and was accompanied by another child or an adult. He was also informed that he might continue swimming provided there was always someone with him.

Finally, Eric was taught to begin to recognize the signs of his aura. The nurse defined an *aura* as the peculiar sensations Eric would grow to know as a warning sign of a seizure. After determining that Eric had previously experienced nausea and vomiting with the flu, she told him that an aura was the special warning that takes place before a convulsion, just as there was a certain warning that occurred before vomiting. Eric was told that when he began to recognize his aura, which might be a smell, sound, color, or sensation, he should try to lie down immediately.

All of the teaching was accomplished with both of Eric's parents in attendance. The parents could later act as reinforcers of the information imparted to Eric and could also offer support to him during the sessions. The nurse presented the material to Eric during three half-hour sessions so that he had an adequate amount of time to assimilate the information and ask questions. She also spent time with Eric's parents alone, giving them more detailed information and answering their questions. Eric was discharged from the hospital and he and his parents were encouraged to call the primary-care nurse or Eric's pediatrician if they had questions or experienced any problems.

Adolescents have a different cognitive style from that of the school-age child. Piaget asserts that around the age of 12 children develop "formal operational thought."[9] During adolescence the ability to think abstractly becomes well developed. Cognitive processes are of an adult type and the adolescent develops the ability to reason deductively. Therefore, when considering the cognitive style to employ during patient teaching, we should be aware that the adolescent can be taught in a fashion similar to the way an adult is taught.

The aspect of the adolescent's development that clearly differentiates him from the adult, however, is his social development and the importance of his peer group. Knowledge of the adolescent's psychosocial task, "identity *vs* role confusion" as defined by Erik Erikson, is of primary importance to the nurse working with the adolescent in a patient-education setting.[13] The nurse must remember that, because the adolescent develops his identity in relation to his peers and in opposition to his parents, teaching should take place without the parents present.

Frequently, we assume that adolescents have more knowledge about their own anatomy and physiology than they do. This applies to functions of body organs as well as sexuality. Illustrations are helpful with this age group, although they can be more sophisticated than those used with the school-age population.

Honesty with adolescents is very important. If a change in body image is expected as a result of surgery or during the course of a disease, the adolescent must be adequately prepared because body image is of paramount importance to the adolescent. Because of the desire to be "one of the gang" and to look like everyone else, the adolescent who faces a change in his appearance will need help from health-care professionals in hiding or camouflaging the change.

What do we do about the physician who blocks all our attempts at patient education?

Although we may try our hardest to use our change-agentry skills (see Chap. 2) and may have tried our best to implement a high-quality patient-education program according to the precepts outlined in Chapter 3, we most likely still will be confronted by the physician who absolutely refuses to allow any of his patients access to patient education offered in the agencies in which he practices. It makes no difference to this physician that the programs have been approved by the medical staff, and it is usually impossible to tell what is at the root of his intransigence. Fortunately, such physicians are the exception but they can frustrate the intentions of a conscientious patient educator. If you, as the patient's nurse and advocate, feel that patient education is absolutely necessary for the well-being of the patient, and if you have exhausted every approach including speaking personally with the physician, it may be necessary to have the patient himself request patient teaching and put pressure on his doctor to provide it.

I am documenting all my patient education but no one is reading my notes. What should I do?

This is frequently a problem for the nurse who scrupulously documents all of her patient teaching in the nurses' notes section of the chart. We feel that all documentation related to a patient should be put in the progress notes section of the chart, so that the entire health team has easy access to the data. Our experience has been that charting style and format quickly improved when nurses documented in the progress notes, whether this documentation was solely related to patient education or whether it encompassed all of the old nurses'-notes data. In many institutions all other health-care-team professionals (*e.g.*, dietitians, physical and occupational therapists, and social workers) chart in the progress-notes section; it seems that someone as important to the team and to the patient as the nurse should also chart there.

Historically, nurses' notes have been poorly written and have conveyed very few data. However, as nursing education and nursing's theory base have improved, so has nurses' charting. We believe that problem-oriented charting in the *SOAP* (subjective, objective, assessment, and plan) format forces everyone to chart pertinent, concise data related to the patient's problems. The *SOAP* format also lends itself well to charting of the progress of patient education. The nurse who understands and uses problem-oriented charting correctly, with proper grammar, spelling, and punctuation, will find that her charting is read.

How can I get the health-care team together to coordinate patient education?

Coordinating patient education can be a difficult job when many disciplines are involved. For example, the patient with newly diagnosed diabetes is usually taught by nurses, dietitians and, in some settings, pharmacists. The diabetic's physician is also involved and, if some sort of community referral is needed, social workers will frequently join the team. Trying to figure out who is going to do what, and when things will be done, is similar to trying to run a three-ring circus. A general planning meeting can be useful in saving time for everyone and avoiding replication of efforts. If this meeting is set up around the physician's scheduled time on the unit or in the agency, the process will be facilitated. Mutually derived goals should be written at the planning meeting. Notifying the patient's family of a time to be present for planning is also helpful and, because the focus of the team is the patient, he should also be present. It is also important that the nurse make the patient's family aware of the times when health-team members will be teaching the patient so that they can be present if this is appropriate.

Continuity of care and logical progression of the teaching plan can be accomplished by having all health-care-team members use the same problem list and document their teaching in the progress-notes section of the chart. The team approach, when applied to patient education, is one of the most effective uses of a group-management technique. Communication is rendered coherent and concise, teaching efforts are not replicated, and the entire health team, especially the patient, benefits.

Some patients seem to be receiving more patient-education services than others. What can we do about this inequity?

It is important first to determine why some patients are receiving more patient education and what underlying circumstances exist. For example, if patients of a certain physician are not receiving diabetes education because the physician refuses to allow his patients to participate, then the patients have to put pressure on the physician, as discussed earlier in this chapter. However, if one notes that all the cardiac-disease, diabetic, and ostomy patients are being well educated but that the stroke patients and their families have no services offered, then it becomes necessary to document the need for patient education for the stroke group. In institutions where all patients are assessed a fee for patient education, it behooves the institution to make patient education available to all for whom it is a documented need.

Need can be documented in terms of the numbers of patients hospitalized with certain diseases or health-promotion needs, the number of return visits to the agency related to lack of self-care skills, data on local morbidity and mortality, and data obtained from practitioners and national organizations. Once need has been established, agency administrators should be approached with a plan and a request for start-up funding (see Chap. 3).

When are home visits for patient-education purposes efficacious? Which health-care professionals should make them?

We are strong advocates of home visits for many purposes, not the least of which is patient education. The different data that the discerning health-care professional can gather on a home visit far surpasses what she can assess in the hospital. Socioeconomic and educational status, family dynamics, and availability of home and community resources are just a few of the more obvious facts that are evident during home visits.

In addition to home visits' enabling us to perform a thorough family assessment, they also help most clients to feel more comfortable in patient-teaching situations because they are buttressed by familiar objects and family members. We have had very successful home teaching sessions with young mothers about basic child-health and safety practices, when the mothers were fearful or unwilling to attend teaching sessions in the clinic. Observations from such visits were shared with other members of the team and were often instrumental in making future plans for and with clients.

One of our more unique home-visit situations involved introducing two elderly diabetic women to one another, in the home of one, so that they could help one another with management problems. The more experienced patient effectively demonstrated insulin injection and urine testing to the woman whose diabetes was newly diagnosed. This teaching session was facilitated by the nurse but was managed by the patients.

Home visits are expensive in terms of personnel time and driving costs. We are familiar with one outpatient agency that made very effective use of senior-year nursing students by using them as the liaison between the clinic and patients families. The students conducted effective patient education, followed up problems, and assessed the home situations, all of which were course objectives. In this type of situation it is imperative that communication channels between students and providers be open and that students document their visits. Hospitals can also use students to make home visits following patient discharge; the students can then pass the results of their teaching and other information to the attending physician.

What are some of the sources of patient-education resources in my own institution?

Frequently we are vaguely aware that there are resources available for patient education in our institutions but we are not sure what source to tap to find them. The *hospital librarian* is an excellent resource and we have found that when patient-education materials were not available in the library, the librarian always knew where to direct us. Useful audiovisual media are often kept in the library and, if not, they are at least cataloged so that we know where to find them.

Many patient-education resources can be found at the nursing station or somewhere on the nursing unit. One hospital with which we are familiar has excellent *teaching cards* covering diagnostic tests and medications. These are neatly filed at the nurses' station but are rarely used by staff, who either are unaware of their existence or simply do not take the time to deliver them to patients. *Procedure manuals and journals* frequently found at the nurses' station can be valuable teaching resources.

Resources of importance in planning patient-education activities include checklists *in the chart* such as the discharge-planning checklist, the quality-assurance checklist, and patient-education flow sheets. In a given institution, some or all of these may be found. Occasionally these checklists or flow sheets need revising. They can be very useful adjuncts to patient teaching and, if used properly, they make the process more logical and time conserving.

Other resources are *committees* composed of various health-care professionals who are planning future patient-education programs. Committee members usually have a wealth of knowledge about appropriate resources and are happy to share it. If the committee does not include such professionals as dietitians, pharmacists, social workers, and physical, occupational, and respiratory therapists, do not hesitate to approach such persons; they are valuable resources for nurses seeking help with patient education.

If the hospital is of a moderate to large size, it probably will have a *patient-education coordinator* on the staff. Obviously this person is pivotal in the attempts of a hospital to deliver patient education. In an outpatient setting, such as a public-health department, the equivalent position is held by a health educator. If there is no health educator, then frequently nursing in-service, staff training and development, or educational services departments have someone who (officially or unofficially) has developed a role in patient education.

Can the idea of "networking" be applied to patient education to increase resources for patients?

    Networking is a term currently in vogue that refers to pooling resources to assist a certain cause. For example, a *women's network* is a group for women with common interests such as the fact that they are all university-faculty members. Networking as a family-therapy modality means bringing family, extended family, neighbors, and friends together to help a family resolve a problem and gain needed support.

    When we refer to networking in patient education, we mean either bringing together various community services to serve a patient's educational needs or developing a bank of resources that we can refer to when we need help. Obtaining referral sources and information from Visiting Nurse associations, public-health nurses, and specialty-oriented nurses is one form of networking. Use of a directory of community resources and the Yellow Pages of the phone book is another method of developing a network.

    Another form of networking is sharing the teaching needs of a particular patient with the community nurse who will see the patient upon his discharge from the hospital. All too often there is little continuity of care because no one bothers to contact nurses in outpatient settings. If the patient is readmitted to the hospital then the outpatient-agency nurse can give useful information to the inpatient team involved in the patient's care. Sharing of information can take place on an informal basis over the telephone. Such reciprocity is unnecessary in many situations but we are aware of complex patient circumstances in which a great deal of teaching and continuity of care was needed and in which patients benefited from the extra effort nurses put in to smooth transitions from community to hospital and *vice versa*. Remember, however, that confidential information regarding patients may not be shared without their permission.

How can I obtain teaching aids without spending a great deal of money?

    Patient education has become big business ever since the Joint Commission on the Accreditation of Hospitals mandated that hospitals provide it.[14] Many companies already producing learning materials for health-care professionals have begun marketing films, filmstrips, videotapes, books, and anatomic models. Some of these products are very sophisticated and moderately priced and are able to meet the needs of institutions that are unable to produce their own materials. Other commercial products are expensive and do not meet the needs of most institutions because their content and approach are too general. Audiovisual hardware and software can be very expensive and agencies should carefully consider their needs in this area before purchasing one of the package deals promoted by many of the large companies. Also, research on the effectiveness of such media as closed-circuit television is still not complete and we may discover that the outcomes do not justify the huge outlay of funds necessary to develop in-house, closed-circuit television, patient-education systems.[15]

We have seen agency-developed slide-tape programs, videotape programs, films, brochures, and pamphlets that have met the special needs of the agencies and their patients without being prohibitive in cost. Frequently these are supplemented by commercially printed materials or films. Other sources of free or inexpensive rental audiovisual materials are state health-film libraries and public-library systems.

Other resources for free materials are the pharmaceutical, medical-supply, and infant-formula companies. Sales representatives of these companies are very willing to lend films and distribute free literature. We have found that if a given firm does not have the type of brochure we desire for our clients we can request it and often be supplied with what we needed. For example, the brochures produced by the infant-formula companies tended to be directed toward white, upper-middle-class families and we served primarily lower socioeconomic groups of white and black clients. We requested a change in format and also inclusion of material in favor of breast-feeding, and we later received these new brochures.

The Government Printing Office in Washington, D.C. is also an excellent source of free or low-cost printed materials. They are frequently well illustrated and written very simply so that all clients can understand them.

See the Appendices at the end of Chapter 8 for a comprehensive list of patient-education materials.

My institution plans to buy ready-made teaching materials. How can I best use them?

As mentioned, there are some good ready-made teaching materials that save development time and have the advantage of being pretested for validity and reliability. The most important thing to bear in mind when using these materials is that they must be individualized and tailored for each patient. No teaching materials negate the need for personal instruction. Such materials can supplement the instructor but not replace her. Therefore, the patient educator should personally review the materials with the patient, pointing out areas that do not apply and reinforcing others.

Another crucial aspect of using printed materials, or other materials that rely heavily on the written word, is the patient's literacy level. (Chap. 6 mentions the use of tests for determining literacy level.) We had an unfortunate experience, with a patient who had newly diagnosed diabetes, that poignantly illustrates the importance of assessing literacy level. The patient was instructed by a dietitian and a nurse about diet, insulin injection, and recognition of signs of hypoglycemia and ketoacidosis. He attended our diabetic-teaching luncheon and seemed to be one of our more successfully educated diabetic patients. Three days after discharge he franticallly called his physician to report that he had not eaten anything since his discharge because he could not read and did not know what he should eat. None of us had determined his literacy level but, instead, had simply assumed he could read and understand all the written materials we had given him.

What are some examples of quick and easy ways to teach during a busy day?

We feel that many nurses miss golden opportunities to teach because they believe teaching requires long, uninterrupted periods of time. There are many times during the care of patients, both inpatient and outpatient, when the opportunity can be seized to teach. For example, during a dressing change it is very easy to talk through the procedure with the patient, beginning with the reasons for aseptic technique (explaining why the area is scrubbed with povidone iodine from the inside out). If this same patient will have to perform his own dressing changes at home, this talk relieves some of the burden from discharge teaching. When carrying out routine prenatal checks we can say, "I am measuring the height of your fundus (the top of your uterus) to find out how much the baby has grown since your last visit. Usually the fundal height increases about one centimeter per week." When the prenatal patient's urine is tested we can say, "I am checking your urine for sugar and protein. Sometimes pregnant women have a little sugar in their urine but if you have a lot of sugar, we will want to do some blood tests so that we can make certain you have a healthy baby. We check the protein in your urine because this gives us an idea of your kidney function. During pregnancy more stress is placed on your kidneys. Protein in the urine usually develops with a serious condition called toxemia and we want to watch you carefully to prevent development of toxemia." Anticipatory guidance and reassurance should always accompany such teaching because some of the information may be upsetting to patients.

Taking blood pressures also presents a good opportunity for teaching. All patients, hypertensive or not, should know the significance of the blood pressure measurement and should know what is normal for them. This is also a good opportunity for health-promotion teaching related not only to blood pressure, but also to eating habits, and heart disease.

There are literally hundreds of opportunities for brief teaching. By using these opportunities we promote health and self-care practices and also give our patients one more mechanism to reduce their feelings of powerlessness and dependence on us.

What types of things can be do to promote our agency's image as a provider of patient education?

Because the consumer is beginning to expect more patient-education services from his provider, many hospitals, clinics, and private-practice settings are trying to promote an image as a provider of patient education. Such devices as *filmstrips, videotapes, and slide-tape programs* in waiting rooms help to provide this image and have been used by various agencies.[16,17]

Less expensive means are *posters,* either handmade or provided free by organizations such as the American Dairy Association or the March of Dimes. Posters can also be used to advertise seminars or classes open to the public. Many hospitals are promoting their community images by providing free monthly forums on topics of widespread interest such as respiratory disease, prevention of heart disease, and other common health problems. Frequently posters are prominently displayed in hospital lobbies to inform the public of such events.

The *hospital-admissions brochure* may contain information about patient education so that both the patient and his family are immediately aware of inpatient educational services. Likewise, outpatient offices and clinics can stress their roles in patient education in the brochures that are usually given to new patients.

In hospital and outpatient units and waiting rooms, information relevant to the unit can be displayed. For example, information related to child-safety practices can be exhibited on *bulletin boards and waiting room tables.* One nurse who taught prenatal classes told us that the free literature on birth control was so popular on the maternity ward that she could not restock it fast enough.

Now that many hospitals and outpatient agencies have employed computerized billing it is possible to put a patient-education message *on the monthly bill.* For example, "CPR classes will be held June 1, free of charge for all patients, from noon–2:00 p.m. and 7:00–9:00 p.m." could be programmed to read out on all May bills.

Media coverage of patient-education offerings widely extends the image of the agency into the community and can be obtained for free. Public-service spots are available on radio and television for community services that are offered without charge to all members of the community. Newspapers will also print notices of such events if they meet this criterion. The University of North Carolina has provided short television broadcasts on safety and prevention techniques such as the Heimlich maneuver. These free public-interest teaching spots provided an image of the University of North Carolina's hospital and health-professional schools as being concerned about the public.

Another means of making patient education better known in the community is by *gaining access to schools and groups* such as Parent–Teacher Associations. While employed in a hospital's educational-services department, we conducted classes on labor and delivery in a high school's human-sexuality classes. These classes were a public service to the high school and were meant to increase the hospital's image as a provider of health education. Obviously such image enhancement is helpful to hospitals worried about use of beds.

What are some of the common mistakes made when attempting patient education?
In our own experience with patient education and in our enthusiasm to try out our ideas, we have made a number of mistakes. We have also noted mistakes made by others and will enumerate them all below.

1. *Assessment mistakes.* Frequently we do not validate our data with the client, a case in point being the diabetic who could not read.
Another assessment problem is the failure to reassess the situation and the patient following the passage of time or a change in the experience or life events of the patient.

2. *Refusal to work within the restrictions of the patient's environment.* This mistake is related to assessment and involves the health professional who neglects consideration of such factors as lack of family support, educational level, financial assets of the patient, or cultural or ethnic background. We tend to teach from our own backgrounds and experience and may assume a commonality of background that is not present. For example, in the south is makes more sense to teach the poor rural farmer in need of potassium that greens (*e.g.*, collards, kale, spinach, turnip greens) are a good source rather than recommend bananas, which are more expensive. In the Los Angeles barrio, it is unrealistic to expect a prenatal patient's husband to be a coach to her during labor and delivery because Hispanics traditionally do not sanction the presence of men during birth.

3. *Territoriality or "owning" the patient.* Many of us, not just physicians, fall into this trap when we invest a lot of time and effort in teaching our patients. The patient becomes "our" patient and we are loath to believe that anyone else can continue the process we started. As stated before, no one owns patients and we all need to remember the personal responsibility that the patient has for his own behavior.

4. *Denial or oversight of the patient's right to change his mind.* This is a mistake that frequently occurs when, as above, the health professional has overly invested himself in the patient and his progress. We worked for a long time with an elderly woman who was placed on insulin. We were attempting to teach her self-injection of insulin. We tried many creative approaches because she originally had said she would manage her own injections. However, at some point during this lengthy process she had decided that she did not want to give herself insulin, but rather wanted her husband and daughter to do it. Because we had a need to make her independent, we refused to recognize her dependency needs or the fact that she had, indeed, changed her mind. The situation became very frustrating for all until we finally recognized and respected the interpersonal dynamics of the situation.

5. *Inability to learn from our own mistakes.* Nurses tend to be task-oriented and, as such, we often believe that there is only one way to do things. Such an approach is the antithesis of the flexible, open-minded method that is needed with patient education. When conducting the diabetic luncheons, we discovered through an experience with a 12-year-old girl that the luncheon, with its emphasis on food preparation and prevention of long-term complications, was unsuited to any age group other than adult. Later, parents of children and adolescents were invited but the pediatric patients themselves were seen on a one-to-one basis for teaching.

We have seen many nurses continue to use medical jargon with patients when all indications suggested the patients did not understand the teaching. Such practices are self-defeating for the staff and frustrating for patients.

6. *Failure to negotiate goals.* Long- and short-term goals should be established at the beginning of any patient-education endeavor. It is appropriate for the nurse to have goals in mind but she also must determine her client's goals so that he can enjoy some sense of progress. Any discrepancy in goals should be acknowledged by both the nurse and the client, with the nurse recognizing that the client's goals supercede hers. For example, the chronic obstructive-lung-disease patient may set goals for himself that include administering medications and learning breathing exercises. The nurse may agree upon these goals but also set a goal of cessation of smoking. Obviously if the patient does not share this goal he will be unsupportive of, and inattentive to, her efforts and she will be frustrated.

7. *Lack of awareness of the teaching efforts of other members of the health team.* Replication of effort is a common and time-consuming problem, but it is easily corrected by good documentation. Well-meaning health professionals frequently repeat teaching in an area that has just been taught by someone else. Although repetition can be a useful teaching device, it should be planned instead of haphazard. Usually patients are not assertive enough to speak up and tell their teacher that they have already heard this lecture before and would like to hear about something else.

Careful documentation in the appropriate section of the chart (*e.g.*, progress notes, patient-education flow sheet), will solve this problem as well as legally document patient-education efforts. Also, a good assessment of a patient's areas of knowledge and weakness will prevent this repetition. The planning sessions that we referred to earlier in this chapter will help ameliorate the problem.

8. *Overload of information given to the patient.* In our overzealous attempts to teach patients everything we feel they should know, we run the risk of overloading them with more information than they can absorb. Hospitalized patients have low energy reserves and are not usually amenable to long teaching sessions. Two half-hour sessions are more desirable than one hour-long session. Shorter sessions also allow the patient an opportunity to integrate new information and formulate questions for the next teaching session; this opportunity would be unavailable if everything was taught in one hour-long session.

Even the outpatient, whose physical status may be better than that of the inpatient, benefits from shorter sessions. Shorter sessions are also more workable in terms of staff time.

Signs that a patient has been saturated and cannot handle any more material include inability to answer questions regarding the material, fidgeting, yawning, and staring, glazed eyes. When these signs occur tell the patient to prepare questions for the next session and, if appropriate, leave some pertinent literature.

9. *Poor timing and inattentiveness to patient stress levels.* This problem is related to the previous mistake, and is usually caused by a

focus on the needs of the nurse rather than on the needs of the patient. There are advantageous times for teaching and there are some that are very poor. A patient who has just received upsetting or unexpected news should not be burdened by a nurse who wants to teach. Likewise, the time periods immediately prior to or following diagnostic procedures, surgery, or painful episodes are not propitious for teaching.

Patients, such as a new mother with a Downs'-syndrome child, who are under great stress are not good candidates for teaching. Other patients who are not amenable to teaching are patients in denial. For example, a young woman whose acute leukemia had just been diagnosed was in such a strong state of denial that it was impossible to teach her anything about the planned chemotherapy, the importance of diet, or the prevention of infection. Instead, we focused our teaching on her mother and other family members, telling them that we would work with the patient when she came in for chemotherapy on an outpatient basis.

Sometimes the length of inpatient stay does not allow for adequate teaching, in which case either the patient must return to the hospital or plans must be made for outpatient teaching through the Visiting Nurse Association or public-health-department nursing service. It is important for someone to take charge of the situation so that the patient does not lose the services he needs.

10. *Failure to arrange for feedback and evaluation.* As nursing instructors, we see this mistake made more frequently than any other by students and we suspect that it is also one of the most common errors committed by health professionals. Most of us spend time familiarizing ourselves with the material to be taught and then get so involved in our teaching that we forget to evaluate and gather feedback on the patient's comprehension of what we have taught. Patients tend to want to appease and please the nurse or other health-care professional who is teaching them and usually act as if they understand more than they really do. When we do ask for a return demonstration or verbal feedback we are frequently appalled by how little we have managed to make comprehensible.

Another facet of this problem is our failure to provide time for patients to ask questions. Typically we teach an instructional unit at a rapid pace, quickly ask for questions, and then leave the room satisfied that the patient has understood our teaching because he did not ask any questions. In reality the patient probably either understood so little that he was unable to formulate questions or felt that the nurse did not have time to answer him.

Skill building is an important aspect of the teaching/learning process and must also be considered as an important item when planning time requirements. Any type of skill requiring physical manipulation must be practiced by the patient alone and in the presence of the instructor to ensure its integration into the necessary self-care behaviors. Lack of time for building skills frequently accounts for patients who do not want to be discharged when the physician says it is time. Good communication among members of the health-care team will alleviate this common problem.

All of this discussion emphasizes the importance of completing the total process of patient education: assessment, goal setting, teaching, and evaluating (see Chap. 6–9).

11. *Using materials that have not been reviewed or using media exclusively.* The development and popularity of patient education has been followed by the emergence of sophisticated patient-teaching media. We have used media to great advantage with groups and single patients but we believe in the importance of carefully reviewing the media and evaluating their applicability for the intended audience. This point was delineated clearly to us on one occasion when we made the mistake of showing a film on breast-feeding that we had not previewed. The film had been produced by one of the breast-feeding advocacy groups and not so subtly suggested that adequate mothering and bonding could only be achieved through breast-feeding. We were dealing with a group of women who had received very little family or social-group support for breast-feeding and, unfortunately, the film had the effect of polarizing or frustrating our prenatal patients.

Total reliance on media is obviously an inadequate approach to patient education. Such an approach makes it impossible to individualize patient teaching, to allow the patient to ask questions, or to gather feedback from the patient. Obviously mail campaigns and large mass-media health-education projects use this scheme with the assumption that some information is better than none. There are some data that indicates that this assumption is untrue. For example, mass media are believed to be efficacious in informing the better-educated segments of society, but most of the public believes they are part of a ploy to sell something.[19] In any case, individualized patient education for clients who must learn skills or information for managing self-care practices is essential and cannot be managed by reliance on media.

What is the role of the student nurse in patient education?

We believe that providing for patient education is an integral function of nursing practice. Because nursing students are learning to be practitioners, they should deliver patient education as part of nursing care. Patient education is not something that should be excluded from nursing school curricula in the belief that it will be learned on the job. It is a function basic to all good nursing care and, therefore, must be emphasized in nursing school while the theoretical framework for nursing is being presented. As students progress through the program, the faculty should stress the importance of applying teaching/learning concepts, as well as appropriate content, to patient-education situations in clinical settings. Clinical-evaluation tools should be designed to evaluate student competency in patient education.

Most nursing students are not involved in formulating agency needs assessments or planning large-scale programs while in nursing school, but they should be familiar with the issues involved so that they can buttress their array of skills for future use.

Many times the most creative teaching of patients is completed by students. Nursing students frequently have recent knowledge about patient education and enthusiam for attempting innovative approaches. Staff members can learn a lot from students if they drop their defensive attitudes and approach students with a greater sense of collegiality. Students, in turn, can learn a great deal from the staff by observing the techniques staff members have found useful in teaching patients.

As instructors we have found it useful to accompany students on home visits that have been planned for patient-education purposes. Another means of evaluating students' skills in patient education is for the instructor to arrange for students to conduct discharge teaching, diagnostic-test teaching, or perioperative teaching and to then accompany the students when they instruct the patients. The instructor must first ascertain, however, that the students know the material because an unfamiliarity with the content causes embarrassment for the students and confusion for the patients.

In our desire to encourage varied clinical experiences instructors frequently push students into situations in which they do not feel comfortable. Sexuality is an area with which the younger student, or perhaps even older students or practicing nurses, may feel uneasy in teaching situations. Until students express an ease with material related to human sexuality we believe they should not approach this sensitive area. We remember one nursing student who had professed a desire to teach the prenatal class unit on contraception. When she did so, however, she remained suffused with a deep blush and was obviously ill at ease. Patients greeted her teaching with nervous laughter and we suspect little was learned that evening about contraception.

How can patient-education principles be applied in the psychiatric setting?

Traditionally we conceive of the application of patient education to pediatric and adult medical–surgical settings. This is most likely a remnant of our medical-model approach and not representative of a holistic model of man, in which we consider the total individual. Psychiatric patients have the same basic patient-education needs as have medical–surgical patients (*i.e.*, to function to the best of their ability on the wellness–illness continuum and in a manner consistent with their expressed needs and desires).

Benfer recognizes patient education as one of the functions of the psychiatric nurse on an interdisciplinary health team.[20] The psychiatric nurse should perform the traditional function of teaching necessary information about medications and health. In addition, she should also teach the patient how to relate to the environment of the psychiatric agency, how to use unstructured time, and how to establish necessary structure in daily life.

It is the nurse's responsibility to orient patients to the psychiatric environment, whether inpatient or outpatient. This orientation can be crucial to the patient's adjustment to the therapeutic milieu.

Many psychiatric patients have had problems structuring their time to meet the demands of daily existence. Therefore, the nurse's role in facilitating the patient's ability to order his time in a meaningful manner is pivotal to his ability to function in the community. Lancaster also recognizes this need to help patients structure their time and feels that patients can be taught to develop leisure-time skills through group therapy.[21] Planned recreational activities such as exercise, volleyball, crafts, and cooking classes are other means of helping psychiatric patients gather tools to structure their time. These activities can be taught in inpatient or outpatient settings. We observed senior nursing students teaching a very successful cooking course to clients attending sessions at an outpatient mental-health center.

Inpatient psychiatric clients with long histories of institutionalization have problems adapting to the communities into which they are discharged. On admission these patients already have been recognized as having difficulties with social interaction and problem-solving skills. If reintegration into the community is to be successful, it is imperative that coping skills are taught both prior to and following discharge. Social interaction and problem-solving skills are frequently learned in group-therapy contexts. Other skills, such as the ability to perform the basic activities of daily living, can be taught by nurses in a combination of didactic and practical approaches. In many instances patients must be taught such basic activities as personal hygiene or how to use a stove or they must be oriented to a technology that has overtaken them, such as the use of microwave ovens or automatic bank tellers. Patient teaching with psychiatric patients requires creativity and patience, but the rewards can be great.

What are some of the special aspects and needs related to teaching the gerontologic patient?

Many health professionals, recognizing that the gerontologic patient is different from the younger or middle-aged adult patient, approach him as if he were a child. Although there are some qualities of the two age groups that are held in common, it is both insulting to the patient and demonstrative of the health professional's lack of sensitivity and knowledge to take this approach.

We know that as people grow old, their cognitive efficiency declines. Older people have been found to have increasing difficulty understanding complex sentences, to be less proficient in drawing inferences, and to have more difficulty in determining the point of a story.[22] Institutionalized elderly persons do even more poorly on tests of cognitive ability than do their counterparts living in the community. Despite these sobering facts, many creative programs have been implemented. These emphasize conversation and problem-solving skills. They result in improved cognitive abilities and help to prevent deterioration of existing abilities.

In patient-education situations with the elderly, the following points should be remembered:[23]

1. Presentation of information should proceed at a much slower rate than usual
2. Plenty of time should be allowed for the assimilation and integration of conceptual material

3. Any or all of the following causes may be related to the elderly client's reduced capacity to learn: cerebral changes, psychosocial issues, and change in self-concept with probable loss of self-esteem
4. Group experiences can improve the elderly client's problem-solving ability.
5. Aged clients are very cautious and do not make changes easily

The implications for patient education are that we must take more time in teaching and that we should deliver the educational material in small increments so that the material can be integrated. The health professional should be aware of the cause or causes of the elderly individual's reduced capacity to learn so that she can intervene and perhaps change such modifiable causes as psychosocial losses and low self-esteem. Many skills involving social interaction can be successfully taught in a group setting. Examples would be helping the elderly to acquire assertiveness skills to secure better housing or more neighborhood police protection. In deference to the cautiousness and reluctance to make changes that older people display, the health professional should avoid making changes in the medical regimen whenever possible and should attempt to maintain a constant environment and schedule for the elderly patient.

Are patient-education services appropriate for the terminally ill patient?
One might logically assume that once a patient's illness status has changed from chronic to terminal patient education would no longer be involved. However, as long as a patient has options open to him and choices to make, patient education should be available. Patient teaching is a form of offering hope to our dying clients because it is a way of telling them that they can make choices about their futures.

Examples of patient education for terminally ill clients include delineating the choice between going home and staying in the hospital. If a patient wishes to go home to die, he and his family will have questions about control of pain, ability to manage baths, hygiene, and meals, and the impact on the remainder of the family. Sometimes we can tell the dying patient about the services of his local hospice organization and this may offer the necessary support he needs in making his decision to go home. The dying patient must be given the opportunity to revoke his decisions in the same way as any other patient. The offering of choices allows a sense of control that must be respected until the end.

The emotional-support aspects of patient education, which are always an important thread, become even more paramount with the dying patient. We may decide to teach the patient's family members or friends how to employ reminiscence as a therapeutic treatment modality, allowing the client an opportunity to view his life in retrospect with a sense of unity and completion. Emotional support is also given by the nurse who offers her physical presence and shows family members how they can make the patient more comfortable.

How do I offer patient education to clients of different ethnic backgrounds?
There are almost as many different ethnic, cultural, and religious groups as there are subjects to teach. We will not attempt to specify which approaches

work best with which groups. Madeleine Leininger and Rachel Spector have both written excellent books on the concept of transcultural nursing and we recommend them for a good discussion of the impacts of different cultural values on the delivery of health care.[24,25] We believe that every nurse must attempt to transcend her own value system and not judge her clients from her own vantage point. When applied to delivery of health-education services, this means that what may have been found useful or important in teaching clients from our own ethnic, cultural, or religious background might not apply to people from other backgrounds.

Health-and-illness teaching related to diet, sexuality, contraception, childbirth, childrearing, and medications may have to be completely refocused and redirected. For example, when working with Samoan families in Southern California we found that our concepts of obesity had to be completely revised. Among these people, desirable weights according to Western standards were considered much too low, especially for women, in whom plumpness approaching gargantuan size was valued. Their diets were heavily dependent on starchy foods and their incomes were frequently limited. Diet planning and nutritional teaching, therefore, required a great amount of creativity and revised goals.

Of course, we cannot teach a patient unless we have a working knowledge of the patient's language. In such instances it is preferable either to find another health professional, proficient in the language, or use an interpreter. Trying to instruct a client using sign language is frustrating to both the nurse and the client and is not recommended. Nurses and other health professionals should be aware that there is a growing amount of patient-education literature and audiovisual media available in Spanish.

In which situations should one-to-one teaching be used? When should group teaching be used?

We feel that there are distinct advantages inherent in both one-to-one and group teaching. It is difficult to generalize and say when one is more effective than the other because of the individual characteristics of patients.

We have determined individual patient teaching to be more effective than group teaching (whether with a family group or a large, unrelated group) in the following situations:

1. When the health professional has very little knowledge of the patient and an assessment of the patient for education purposes has not been completed, an individual session is required. Trying to assess individual knowledge in a group situation is difficult and usually impossible because most clients do not want to reveal their knowledge deficits to a group.

2. When family members or friends try to co-opt teaching sessions. Some family members have been noted to use teaching sessions to make the patient feel guilty for not following a medical regimen or to attract attention to themselves and their roles as care-givers.

3. When the information to be taught provokes a great deal of anxiety (such as teaching related to cardiac surgery) or is considered to be in the realm of topics not generally discussed in public (such as sexual function, reproduction, or bowel function), then one-to-one teaching is preferable.

When a patient does seem to be a good prospect for a group learning experience, he should first be assessed individually.

We have found group teaching to be useful both as a very helpful adjunct to one-to-one teaching and also as the primary format for patient education. Group teaching sessions lessen the feelings of alienation and being "different" that many people experience with both acute and chronic conditions. Patients frequently remark after attending group teaching that it was very helpful to hear that others share the same problems and feelings. Groups in which patients are encouraged to formulate their own agenda and conduct the group session seem to be even more successful in terms of compliance than instructor-led groups. Nessman, Carnahan, and Nugent studied a large group of noncompliant hypertensive patients who were divided into an experimental patient-operated group and a control group of traditional one-to-one nurse management. The patient-operated group was supervised by a nurse and a psychologist but the emphasis was on the patients' feelings of control and group self-help; the patients concentrated on learning to take their own blood pressure and choosing an appropriate antihypertensive. At the end of six months both groups demonstrated reductions in diastolic blood pressure, but the experimental group had a significantly greater reduction.[26]

Such groups as the patient-operated one mentioned above, self-help groups, and the groups at our diabetic-teaching luncheons also offer a second benefit: they encourage sharing among patients of coping techniques and useful hints. We believe, for example, that it is difficult for health professionals who have never had to struggle with an ileostomy or asthma to understand or be aware of the many problems of daily existence involved with those problems. The sharing and social support that occur in such groups can be augmented by technical assistance from health professionals, as long as they do not attempt to co-opt the group.

Another reason to use group teaching formats is to save the costs in time and money of using health professionals. If it takes 12 hours, as estimated by some dietitians, to teach a diabetic the fundamentals of diet, then obviously a group teaching session is going to save manpower and money.[27] Hassell and Medved found that when they used simple overhead transparencies in conjunction with instructor-led group sessions on diet, this experimental group performed significantly better on post-test scores than did patients in a control group, who were instructed in the traditional fashion with bedside training.[27]

Another benefit of group teaching that accrues to family members is the support they gain from health professionals and other patients and their families. Even if the group teaching session includes only the patients' family members, insight, knowledge, and support can be gained from the group teaching session. The fact that families gain support from one another is especially evident in pediatric settings and is one of the reasons for the success of the Ronald McDonald Houses for parents of critically ill children. This mechanism seems to transfer to more structured settings, such as group teaching classes, so that we see one spouse of a heart-disease patient sharing recipes with another. The feeling that "we're all in this together" is especially gratifying to family members, who are frequently more overwhelmed than the patient with the magnitude of the problem.

All of the data are not yet in on the advantages and disadvantages of group vs individual teaching and we would like to see more evaluation research conducted in this area. Whether to employ one or the other or a combination of the two is at the discretion of the health professional, who must constantly remember the individual needs of her patients.

Appendix A: Staff Workshop on Patient Education

The purpose of this program is to teach the RN and LPN/LVN the theoretical bases of adult education and to help each participant develop a teaching unit.

Learning Objectives

At the end of the learning activites the participant will be able to do the following:
1. Demonstrate her knowledge of adult-education practices by submitting the following in writing:
    a. An assessment of the patient's educational level and learning ability
    b. An assessment of the patient's current knowledge of the subject
    c. A summation of information that is to be taught to the patient with appropriate learning activities
2. Demonstrate her understanding of teaching methods and appropriate materials by developing a simple program, related to a particular prenatal teaching situation, with another staff person
3. Describe the evaluation model and monitoring system used for a particular type of patient

Course Outline

I. Principles of education
   A. The adult learner
      1. Characteristics
      2. Needs
      3. Assessment of the adult learner
   B. Instructional planning and design
      1. Instructional design model
      2. Education setting
      3. Instructional media

    C. Conditions of learning
       1. Motivation/attention
       2. Perception of goals
       3. Prerequisites of learning
       4. Presentation of material/learning
       5. Evaluation
       6. Feedback

II. Practical aspects of instructional presentations
    A. Application of instructional principles and design
       1. Instructional planning and design
       2. Conditions of learning
          a. Specific situations as examples
          b. Efficient communication
          c. Suggested materials to use
       3. Writing behavioral/learning objectives
    B. Methodology for teaching patients with special consideration given to the prenatal learner
       1. Experience
       2. Readiness
       3. Time perspective

III. Evaluation and documentation
    A. Feedback/return demonstrations
    B. Records and charts

Related Teaching/Learning Activities

A lecture and discussion format will be used. Students will be expected to participate with examples of experimental data. Patient-education materials developed by various institutions will be displayed. Simple arts and crafts supplies useful for developing programs will be available for participants.

Time Allotment

Three hours will be spent in class and a teaching unit that will be prepared during a break will require at least an hour of preparation time.

References

1. Simonds S: National Task Force on Training Family Physicians in Patient Education: A Handbook for Teachers, p 3. Kansas City, The Society of Teachers of Family Medicine, 1979
2. Neutra R: The frequency and determinants of compliance. First International Congress on Patient Counselling: Abstracts Volume. ICS (Amsterdam) 393, 1976
3. White C, Lemon D, Albanese M: Efficacy of health education efforts in hospitalized patients with serious cardiovascular illness: Can teaching succeed? Patient Couns Health Educ 2, No. 4:189–196, 1980
4. Sackett DL, Haynes RB, Gibson ES et al: Randomized clinical trials of strategies for improving medication compliance in primary hypertension. Lancet 1:1205, 1975
5. Knowles MS: The modern practice of adult education: andragogy versus pedagogy, New York, Association Press, 1970

6. Cousins N: Anatomy of an illness. New York, WW Norton, 1979
7. Illich I: Medical Nemesis: The Expropriation of Health. New York, Pantheon, 1976
8. Siegler M, Osmond HC: Patienthood: The Art of Being a Responsible Patient. New York, MacMillan, 1979
9. Piaget J, Garcia M: Understanding causality. Miles D, Miles M (trans): New York, WW Norton, 1974
10. Bille DA (ed): Practical Approaches to Patient Teaching, pp 276–277. Boston, Little, Brown, 1981
11. Abraham W: The early years: Prologue to tomorrow. Except Child 42:330–335, 1976
12. White BL: The First Three Years of Life. Englewood Cliffs, NJ, Prentice-Hall, 1975
13. Erikson EH: Childhood and Society, 2nd ed, pp 261–263. New York, WW Norton, 1963
14. Joint Commission on the Accreditation of Hospitals: Accreditation Manual for Hospitals. Chicago, American Hospital Association, 1982
15. Herskovitz A: What really makes a difference in learning from media. J Biocommun 6, No. 2:19–21, 1979
16. Cooper WJ, Fewings MJ, Snashall MG: Audiotape health messages through telephones in a general practice waiting room. Med Biol Illus 27, No. 2:87–90, 1977
17. Sackett DL, Haynes RB, Gibson ES et al: Randomized clinical trials of strategies for improving medication compliance in primary hypertension. Lancet 1:1205–1207, 1975
18. Knowlton C: How our audiovisual system upgrades and simplifies communication with patients. Pharm Times 45, No. 2:60–62, 1979
19. Chaisson GM: Patient education: Whose responsibility is it and who should be doing it? Nurs Adm Q 4:1–11, 1980
20. Benfer B: Defining the role and function of the psychiatric nurse as a member of the team. Perspect Psychiatr Care 18:166–177, 1980
21. Lancaster J: Community treatment for mental health's forgotten population. J Psychiatr Nurs 17:20–27, 1979
22. Feier CD, Leight G: A communication–cognition program for elderly nursing home residents. Gerontologist 21, No. 4:408–416, 1981
23. Burnside IM, Ebersole E, Monea HE: Psychosocial Caring Throughout the Age Span, p 478. New York, McGraw-Hill, 1979
24. Leininger M: Transcultural Nursing: Concepts, Theories, and Practices. New York, John Wiley & Son, 1978
25. Spector R: Cultural Diversity in Health and Illness. New York, Appleton-Century-Crofts, 1979
26. Nessman DG, Carnahan JE, Nugent CA: Increasing compliance: Patient-operated hypertension groups. Arch Intern Med 140, No. 11:1427–1430, 1980
27. Hassell J, Medved E: Group/audiovisual instruction for patients with diabetes. J Am Diet Assoc 66:465–470, 1975

Bibliography

Books

American Society of Hospital Pharmacists: Medication Teaching Manual: A Guide for Patient Teaching. Washington, American Society of Hospital Pharmacists, 1980
Backer BA, Dubbert PM, Eisenman EJP: Psychiatric/Mental Health Nursing: Contemporary Readings. New York, Van Nostrand Reinhold, 1978
Bille DA (ed): Practical Approaches to Patient Teaching. Boston, Little, Brown, 1981
Brink PJ (ed): Transcultural Nursing: A Book of Readings, Englewood Cliffs, NJ, Prentice-Hall, 1976

Burnside IM: Nursing and the Aged. New York, McGraw-Hill, 1981

Davis RM, Schenk B: Media Handbook: A Guide to Selecting, Producing, and Using Media for Patient Education Programs. Chicago, American Hospital Association, 1978.

Diekelmann NL: Primary Health Care of the Well Adult. New York, McGraw-Hill, 1977

Freedman CR: Teaching Patients: A Practical Handbook for the Health Care Professionals. San Diego, Courseware, 1978

Haber J et al: Comprehensive Psychiatric Nursing. New York, McGraw-Hill, 1978

Madnick ME: Consumer Health Education: A Guide to Hospital Based Programs. Wakefield, MA, Nursing Resources, 1980

Martyn DE: Source List for Patient Education Materials. Milledgeville, GA, Health Sciences Communications, 1978

Petrillo M, Sanger S: Emotional Care of Hospitalized Children. Philadelphia, JB Lippincott, 1980

Rossman P: Hospice: Creating New Models for Care for the Terminally Ill. New York, Association Press, 1977

Zander KS et al: Practical Manual for Patient Teaching. St Louis, CV Mosby, 1978

Journals

Cooper EJ, Cento MH: Group and the Hispanic prenatal patient. Am J Orthopsychiatry 47, No. 4:689–700, 1977

Doak LG, Doak CC: Patient comprehension profiles: Recent findings and strategies, Patient Couns Health Educ 2, No. 3:101–106, 1980

Redman BK: Curriculum in patient education. Am J Nurs 78, No. 8:1363–1366, 1978

Rosenthal RH, Thomas NS, Vandiver CA: Triage, education, and group meetings: Efficient use of the interdisciplinary team with chronic psychiatric outpatients. J Psychiatr Nurs 17:114–119, 1979

Stein D: Selecting and evaluating media for patient education. J Biocommun, 6, No. 3:22–26, 1979

Ventura FP: Counselling the hearing-impaired geriatric patient. Patient Couns Health Educ, 1, No. 1:22–25, 1978

Glossary

Affective. Pertaining to attitude development and valuing

Assessment. Process of collecting data systematically to identify accurately the needs and problems of patients and their families

Assessment tool. A guide or set of criteria that directs the nurse in the areas to be assessed

Chatterton model. Model constructed to examine closely the continuous decision-making process that the patient experiences as a health-care consumer; based on the Health Belief Model

Change-agentry skills. Those skills the nurse employs to effect planned change in the realm of patient education; change-agentry skills enumerated in this volume include *coordinating, collaborating, consulting, bargaining, confronting, reframing,* and *coercing.*

Client. *See* Outpatient

Cognitive. Pertaining to learning of knowledge or information

Community organization. A methodology that enables communities to develop their own human and economic resources; community organization as applied to health education connotes enabling communities to act in their own best interests to obtain needed health-care education and services

Compliance. The patient's response in conforming to a prescribed medical regimen; *concurrence* and *cooperation* are preferred synonyms for compliance because both terms suggest mutuality of goals, choice, and a patient–provider relationship based on respect and trust

Consumer. The consumer is the patient/client who uses the product—patient education

Documentation. The process of recording on a patient or client's medical record the objective facts pertinent to the process of patient education

Educational diagnosis. Definition of learning deficits or needs; includes identification of factors that inhibit or enhance specific health behaviors

Ethical dilemma. A problem or question that arises about what is right or what ought to be done in situations involving moral decisions about patients

Evaluation. The process of determining the value of a specific activity or program; evaluation is a component of the process of patient education

Evaluation research. The examination of a specific program for the purpose of evaluation using the problem-solving method.

Facilitators. *See* Inhibitors to Patient Education

Feedback. Data provided to the health-care system that informs the system of its success or failure in relationship to the process of patient education; feedback provides data that are useful in evaluating the efficacy of patient-education programs

Goal. An aim or end toward which intervention is directed

Goal setting. Negotiation of learning goals between the nurse and the client

Health Belief Model. Model constructed to predict preventive health behaviors; considers the patient's perception of disease and his decision-making process in the consumption of health-care services

Health-care providers. Persons who provide health care to patients or clients; traditionally, health-care providers were considered to be physicians only, but a more progressive definition includes nurses and other health-care professionals providing direct care to patients

Health-care services. Work or actions provided by health-care professionals; includes patient education

Health-care team. The group of all persons who provide health-care services to the patient and his family, with the patient being the fulcrum of decision-making

Health education. Patient education promoting wellness behaviors and the prevention of disease; often focuses on groups or communities

Holistic concept of man. View of the human being as a total, nonfragmented person who is the sum of all his parts

Implementation. The act of fulfilling or accomplishing; as applied to patient education, implementation is the actual doing of the patient education, or the undertaking of patient-education programs

Informed consent. A legal term referring to a voluntary act by which one person agrees to allow someone else to do something to him, after he has first received information about the procedure

Inhibitors to patient education. Those psychological, physiological, and environmental aspects of health-care settings that hinder or inhibit the patient's openness to, and acquisition, of patient education; *facilitators of patient education* are the converse of inhibitors, that is, those factors that assist the acquisition of health-management information

Inpatient. In this book *inpatient* refers to the *inpatient setting* where a patient is hospitalized for purposes of acute- or chronic-illness care in a secondary, tertiary, or extended-care facility

Input. In systems theory, *input* refers to the information or energy that the system brings in; with reference to patient education, *input* consists of the resources on which the process of patient education depends; *see also* Ouput *and* Throughput

Instructional media. Tools used by the teacher to help the learner retain, compare, visualize, and reinforce knowledge, attitudes, and skills

Instructional methods. Teaching formats and learning activities designed to meet specific learning objectives

Issues. Those questions, ideas, or matters pertaining to patient education about which disagreement or conflict may ensue; *philosophical issues* concern one's approach to patients and one's basic beliefs about how patient education should be put into operation; *political and power issues* concern matters of control—who teaches what, to whom, and when; *legal issues* pertain to those issues that involve the law, nursing, and patient education; *ethical issues* pertain to the questions about what is right or what ought to be done in situations involving moral decisions relating to patients and patient education

Learning contract. A tool used to formalize the agreement between the teacher and the learner; implies commitment to learning activities

Macroethics. Ethical issues pertaining to aggregates or such target systems as the community, the nation, or the world

Medical model. A model oriented toward identification of diseases, and the process of diagnosis, management, and prognosis

Medical regimen. Therapeutic measures prescribed for patients by physicians and directed toward management or cure of illness or disease

Microethics. Ethical issues pertaining to the individual patient as target system in the patient-education arena

Model. A prototype or system of concepts used as the matrix for decision making in certain situations

Needs assessment. The process of assessing or determining the needs of persons, groups, organizations, or communities for the purpose of providing programs such as patient education

Nurse. Licensed, professional nursing personnel, including the registered nurse. The licensed-practical or vocational nurse is not considered a professional nurse.

Nurse clinician, clinical nurse specialist. A registered nurse with advanced expertise in a specialized area of patient care or with a special patient population; the clinical nurse specialist must be prepared on the master's level

Nurse practice act. The legal provision of nursing and nursing services as defined at various states; Nurse Practice Acts protect the public from incompetent practitioners and most contain a definition of nursing and provide the legal basis for the provision of health teaching

Nurse practitioner. A registered nurse, with additional academic and clinical training in a specialty area, whose practice includes physical assessment, diagnosis, and management of common health problems

Nursing diagnosis. A nursing judgment based on sound data that have been systematically collected and analyzed; includes definition of patient needs and problems

Nursing practice. The performance of acts in diagnosis and treatment of patient health needs and health problems, in cooperation with medical management

Nursing process. Problem-solving model used in nursing practice; includes assessment, nursing diagnosis, goal setting or planning, intervention, evaluation, and modification of patient care

Objectives, behavioral objectives. Statement of what the learner will do as a result of patient teaching; a behavioral objective has three components: performance, conditions, and criteria

Outcomes. The resulting benefits to the patient and, coincidentally, to health-care providers of participation in the process of patient education

Outpatient. The *outpatient setting* refers to the client living in a community and receiving care in a home, clinic, office, or other primary-care facility; in this book the term *patient* is usually applied to people in the inpatient setting, the term *client* to individuals in outpatient settings

Output. The product that the system creates from its inputs or, in patient education, the actual patient-education program; *see also* Input *and* Throughput

Paternalism. An unequal relationship between health-care provider and patient, in which the health-care provider assumes a fatherly, protective role and the patient a subservient, obedient position

Patient. *See Inpatient; Outpatient*

Patient education. The process of influencing behavior producing changes in knowledge, attitudes, and skills required to maintain or improve health*

Patient-education coordinator. Person responsible for facilitating and coordinating the design, implementation, monitoring, and evaluation of a system of patient education and its teaching programs

Patient teaching. A component of the patient-education process; the actual imparting of information to the patient

Physician-nurse collegiality. A desired relationship between nurse and physician in which both cooperate to achieve desired patient-education outcomes

Protocol. A plan designed to give direction to the teaching/learning process for a specified topic or issue; includes definition of content, process, and resources

Psychomotor. Pertaining to learning of skills and performance

Right to know. A contractual agreement between a patient and a health-care institution, entered into when the patient presents himself for diagnosis and treatment; the patient's agreement to willingly present himself for treatment guarantees him the right to know what is wrong with him, what the results of tests and treatments mean, and what the prognosis is

Scientific method. Problem-solving model used by many disciplines to develop and apply new knowledge; the nursing process is based on the scientific method; steps in the scientific method and their adaptation to the nursing-process model are discussed in Chapter 6

Self-care activities. Activities performed by persons to maintain or improve their health and well-being

Self-help groups. Voluntary associations of people who share common needs or problems and use the group as the vehicle to handle the problem.

Significant other. The person who the client names as being most important in his life; this person frequently is the client's source of rewards, punishment, approval, and disapproval and should be included when possible in patient-education efforts

Support system. The group to whom a person turns for solace, aid, and information to assist in coping with the vagaries of daily life; support systems are frequently composed of family or friends and may positively or negatively affect the outcome of patient teaching

Systems theory. Examines man and his environment from the perspective of the smallest part (cellular level) to that of the largest part (international level) with attention to the interacting and integrated properties of each system; encourages assessment of the total patient and total family within the context of the community and the environment

Teaching/learning theory. Assumptions about the process in which knowledge, attitudes, and skills are imparted to and integrated by the learner

Third-party payment. Reimbursement and funding for health-care services by a person or group other than the patient or the health-care provider

Throughput. The process by which input is transformed and becomes output; the throughput in patient education refers to the implementation process of planning and establishing patient-education programs; *see also* Input *and* Output

*Simonds S: National Task Force on Training Family Physicians in Patient Education: A Handbook for Teachers, p 3. Kansas City, The Society of Teachers of Family Medicine, 1979

Index

Page numbers followed by the letter *f* indicate figures; those followed by the letter *t* indicate tables; those in **bold type** indicate Glossary terms.